Walking Through Cancer

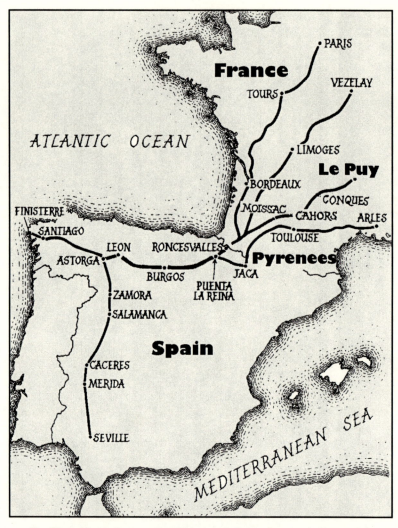

The Way of Saint James—Les Chemins de Saint-Jacques de Compostelle

Walking Through Cancer

A Pilgrimage of Gratitude on the Way of St. James

BY

Elyn Aviva

Buen Camino
on Life's Journey!
Blessings
Elyn Aviva

WALKING THROUGH CANCER
A Pilgrimage of Gratitude on the Way of St. James

by

Elyn Aviva

ISBN: 978-0-9790909-8-1

Library of Congress Control Number:

2009922140

Set in Adobe Caslon Pro 11 pt., with display in Handwriting - Dakota and Adobe Cason Pro in various sizes.

CONTENTS

ACKNOWLEDGEMENTS

I want to thank my beloved husband, Gary White, for his support and encouragement; my surgeon, Christine Hansen, for her competence and compassion; my copyeditors, Siobhan Houston, Karah Madrone of WordsmithEditing, and Rebekah Scott; Kathy Gower, Pat Farr, and John Galm for their cogent comments; Jake Eagle, Mary Jungerman, Rick Geertz, and Ali Galm for brainstorming sessions; Piedad Luna Tovar for her assistance; and Kate López, whose delightful watercolors adorn the cover and the text. All errors in the text are, of course, mine.

My deepest gratitude to Saint James, Sainte Foy, and the other companions who walked with us on the Way—and all the pilgrims, past and present, modern and medieval, ancestral and otherwise, whose footsteps we followed.

MAPS

ILLUSTRATIONS

Preface

Things happen. In my case, cancer happened. I don't know why. My struggle to deal with this radical challenge propelled me to walk a 460-mile-long pilgrimage road in France. *Walking Through Cancer* describes my three-stage journey on the Way of Saint James, a route that millions of pilgrims have followed, for a variety of motives, for more than a thousand years.

Humans are meaning-making creatures, making sense out of events by seeing them through filters accumulated during a lifetime of making sense out of things. Cancer offered me the opportunity to view my life through a fresh filter, a filter that colored my experiences with a new kind of significance. I chose to expand my meaning making to include the possibility of a compassionate universe filled with ongoing interaction with the Divine, however it manifested itself. Some might call this perspective grace; others might call it delusion.

Although I wrote up my travel notes after completing the first two stages of the pilgrimage, I put that rough manuscript in the bottom of a drawer. I wanted to forget all about having cancer. I wanted to look forward, not back.

Five years after surgery I statistically rejoined the general population pool. But statistics don't consider emotions, and I waited until the following year to look at the manuscript again. Eventually I expanded it into this book.

In reworking the manuscript, I have tried to respect how I was "doing myself" during the pilgrimage while incorporating how I have changed as I have brought new meaning to my experiences. I invite you to share my journey and to use it as an opportunity to explore your own ways of making meaning in the world.

Nota Bene:

(1) a "†" after a word the first time it occurs in the text indicates that the word is defined in the glossary (e.g., *auberge†*).

(2) An effort has been made to follow French punctuation rules when using French words or expressions; this usage may appear inconsistent because the rules are applied inconsistently in French.

(3) The scallop-shell motif in the book is a Photoshopped image of the fossilized scallop shells purchased in Conques.

Introduction

As soon as I heard the diagnosis—uterine cancer—and the treatment—complete hysterectomy as soon as possible, perhaps followed by radiation—I knew I had to go for a walk, a very long walk. Not just *any* walk, however, and not a walk that was "walking away" from my situation. I knew I had to go on a walk with a purpose: a pilgrimage on the 1000-year-old Way of Saint James.

If the surgery went well and the cancer was caught before it spread, I would make a pilgrimage of gratitude. If the surgery revealed that the cancer had spread, I would still make a pilgrimage of gratitude—gratitude for every moment that I was alive and still able to walk. My self-appointed task wasn't to find an explanation for what had happened but, instead, to create meaning out of it.

The idea of walking the Way of Saint James did not come out of nowhere. I had already walked the Camino de Santiago† (the Spanish part of the Way of Saint James) three times: once for my Ph.D. in cultural anthropology, once for my husband, and once to escape from marital discord. This fourth time would be radically different. It would be the first time I would make the pilgrimage with a spiritual motive.

In 1982 as part of my doctoral fieldwork, I walked the 500-mile-long Camino de Santiago for the first time. The Camino stretches from the Spanish Pyrenees across northern Spain to Santiago de Compostela, the supposed burial place of Saint James the Greater† (Santiago†), the first martyred apostle. In the Middle Ages this pilgrimage ranked in importance with pilgrimages to Rome and Jerusalem. Over the centuries it lost its cachet, but in the 1980s it started regaining popularity.

My motives for walking the Camino in 1982 were intellectual: I needed to experience the pilgrimage first-hand if I was going to write a dissertation about it. Spirituality? I wasn't even sure what "spirituality" meant. I had been raised as a humanist/agnostic Unitarian Universalist. Spirituality, like religion, was something other people had or did. During my first journey on the pilgrimage road, I was a tone-deaf person at a concert; I knew something was happening but I couldn't hear the melody.

In spite of my academic motivation, I was gradually transformed by my six-week journey on the Camino, a journey that stretched my physical and emotional limits. It taught me to be grateful for a place to rest at the end of a long day, for shelter from the blazing sun, for water to cleanse myself, for feet that could take me, however slowly and painfully, to my day's destination. Step by step I crossed Spain, following in the footsteps of the millions of pilgrims who had faithfully traveled that way for a millennium. [See my travel narrative, *Following the Milky Way: A Pilgrimage on the Camino de Santiago*, second edition.]

In 1997 I returned to the Camino. This time I made the pilgrimage with Gary, my husband of three years. He knew how important the Camino was for me and wanted to share in the experience. Our marriage was still fresh and new, and we still basked in the warmth of mutual admiration, deep affection, and sublime self-deception. We shared meditation and breathing exercises we had learned from the Sufi Order International, a non-denominational spiritual organization that honors all the world's religions. These practices gradually opened me to the possibility of a larger universe in which Spirit (or Divinity, or Ground of Being, or whatever one chose to call it) was more than just a word to analyze—it was something to experience.

We supported each other through debilitating heat, through exhaustion and illness, through loss of motivation and re-found enthusiasm. Unlike my first pilgrimage, which I hadn't wanted to end, Gary and I felt done with the Camino before we were finished. Only our determination and stubbornness (after all, we had said we were going to walk to Santiago!) kept us going.

Our shared pilgrimage brought us closer, but that intimacy did not last. By 2000 our seemingly idyllic marriage was in tatters, and mending its torn fabric seemed almost beyond hope. Struggling to gain a new perspective, I again heard the call of the Camino. This time I went without Gary, propelled by the need to get distance from our troubled marriage, to reclaim myself, to discover (or rediscover) who I really was—whatever that meant.

Afraid to travel alone (the Camino is safe, but I lacked both courage and endurance), I joined a small group of pilgrims traveling with a support vehicle. Together we walked the last 100 miles of the Camino. I had company when I wanted it and time to myself, which I claimed by walking alone.

"It is solved by walking," according to Saint Augustine, but it wasn't. Although some things became clearer during that ten-day pilgrimage, other things became murkier. Intensive and extensive counseling were needed before our broken relationship could be rebuilt in a healthier fashion. We persevered, just as we had on the Camino.

Our marriage counselor "held the faith" that we could transform our marriage and ourselves—though not, as we had erroneously thought, each other. Gradually I, too, began to develop a sense of faith. This was not the reassuring faith that things would turn out the way I wanted them to or thought they should. Instead, it was a faith that required letting go of all my expectations of what our marriage should look like. Paradoxically, it was this willingness to surrender, this acceptance that whatever happened would not only be all right but right, that enabled something wonderful to emerge in each of us and in our marriage.

As Gary and I let go of our expectations, our false images of ourselves and of each other, our old wounds and wounding projections, we began to create a relationship that was more supportive and more liberating than anything I had ever imagined. How limited my vision of relationship had been; how expansive were the possibilities.

Little did we know how important and relevant this work would be. Two years after our marital meltdown, I was diagnosed with uterine cancer. Although the cancer grew inside *me*, Gary made it quite clear that it was *our* cancer and we were on this journey together.

My newly developed faith in letting go and trusting was still tender and green, filled with lapses and fresh beginnings. It was a faith that required a leap as large as the abyss that separates people without cancer from those who have it. I felt gratitude for all that Gary and I had shared, for all the challenges we had overcome so that we could travel together through whatever trials awaited us.

We would make a pilgrimage through cancer together; we would make a pilgrimage of gratitude for all those experiences, like cancer or a strife-filled marriage, which we would never have chosen but that offered opportunities for living a fuller, more meaningful life.

Cancer had sneaked up on me when I wasn't looking. Suddenly cancer wasn't something that happened to someone else, with whom I could empathize from a safe distance, from the (presumably) cancer-free side of that great chasm. I was now forever on the other side of an unbridgeable divide. There was no going back. The diagnosis gave immediacy to magazine articles about preventing cancer, to press releases about new treatments, to Internet searches, to self-help books and support groups.

I didn't know why I had gotten cancer, but I tried to make meaning of it by considering numerous possibilities—including nutritional lapses, unresolved emotional issues and interpersonal conflicts, bad luck, and genetic predisposition. Some might say I was grasping at straws or engaging in the worst kind of New Age claptrap, but I found meaning in the idea that there is a relationship between mind and body, and that one's feelings impact one's health. At least that was something I could do something about.

Although my surgeon wanted to do a complete hysterectomy immediately, I refused; I wanted more information before I gave up all my reproductive organs. I was determined not to passively accept whatever the doctor recommended. With some hesitation, Dr. Williams agreed.

The first operation, on a Tuesday morning in June 2002, was exploratory. Since I wasn't permitted to drink for twelve hours before surgery, dehydration and my tiny, deep veins created a serious challenge for the nurses. First one nurse, then another attempted to insert the IV. They applied heat packs; they jabbed the side of my wrist but the needle perforated the vein; they tried a tiny needle on the back of my hand—the more they dug around, the more tense I became, constricting my veins even further. So much for letting go!

Finally I began doing a meditative breathing practice, and the nurse they called in from ER was able to finish the pre-op routine.

This operation was supposed to be simple, a D&C (scraping tissue from the uterine wall), during which the original diagnosis (first-stage uterine cancer) was indeed confirmed. The surgeon inadvertently punctured my uterus, however, so she did a laparoscopy as well, inserting a fiber-optic instrument through my navel in order to view the abdominal cavity and take samples for biopsies. I was unsettled by the prospect of microscopic cancer cells, freed from the confines of my uterus, swimming off to new venues, and I suddenly became eager to have the hysterectomy as soon as possible. It was scheduled for two days later.

On the way to the hospital that Thursday we stopped off at the Methodist church in downtown Boulder, Colorado, to walk the 35-foot-wide labyrinth painted on the basement floor. We had walked it many times before.

A labyrinth is an ancient symbol in which a single pathway leads in a twisting, spiraling fashion into the center of a circular design. Constructed using particular geometrical ratios, it is a wonderful tool for meditation. Since it is a single path, all one has to do is follow it. No decisions are necessary. Something about the rhythmic, repetitive turns can help one to open up to inner wisdom and to experience a state of inner tranquility.

There are different labyrinth designs. The one in the Methodist church was modeled after the twelfth-century labyrinth in the nave† of Chartres Cathedral†, just outside of Paris. Composed of eleven interconnected circles or circuits, the center is a six-petaled pattern thought to symbolize the Virgin Mary. According to esoteric lore, the pattern also represents the six levels of creation: mineral, vegetal, animal, human, angelic, and transcendent.

We parked the car and walked up to the church. Two rather oddly dressed women entered just ahead of us; with some misgivings we followed them down the stairs to the labyrinth. One was obviously having a "bad hair day"; inch-long white roots provided a startling contrast to her frizzy orange hair. She wore a black knit dress over beige pants. Her friend wore an oversized baseball cap and a dressy nylon blouse tucked into ripped, faded jeans. They sat down on two folding chairs, dropped plastic shopping bags and torn backpacks on the floor, and took off their shoes. All the while, the orange-haired lady was loudly whispering a great deal of misinformation about the labyrinth to her friend.

I wanted to walk the labyrinth to calm down before surgery, but instead I had to contend with these disruptive strangers intruding on *my* ritual! All thoughts of "letting go" disappeared out the window. Determined not to be a victim, I took immediate action. I slipped off my shoes, said a quick opening prayer, and stepped onto the labyrinth before they had the opportunity. Then, heart racing, I strode down the convoluted path.

My strategy failed. The ladies started right after me, and they walked faster than I did. Soon I stepped aside to let them pass by.

They hurried along the path as if it were a racetrack, reached the center, and then walked across the labyrinth to their chairs rather than retracing the path in reverse, which is the usual completion. As they put on their shoes I heard the orange-haired lady ask, *sotto voce*, "Well, did you feel anything?" Her friend shook her head. "Maybe next time," she commiserated. They picked up their assorted bags and went rustling out the door.

Suddenly I "got" it. I had definite ideas about what my marriage, my health, and even *my* labyrinth walk should look like, ideas that were both limited and irrelevant. Rather than struggling to make things turn out the way I thought they should, I needed to let go of expectations and be present to whatever happened. It had taken these delightful ladies to remind me.

I started to laugh, and soon I was crying tears of gratitude as, once again, I opened myself up to the surprising, amusing, bewildering theatrical production that we call life. Gary began to chuckle. We stood together in the center of the labyrinth, holding each other in a close embrace.

Gary whispered in my ear, "I think those bag-ladies were angels sent by central casting. They were just unusual enough to get us to pay attention. I wouldn't be a bit surprised if they disappeared once they got out the door."

"Angels? I didn't think you believed in angels."

"I do now."

Relaxed and in good humor, we went to the hospital. The receptionist remembered having seen me two days earlier.

"Back so soon?"

"Yup. I just can't stay away."

"No accounting for taste!"

This time the nurse had no trouble inserting the IV. Gary told me later that I had a smile on my face as they sedated me.

The operation went well. The cancer appeared to have been contained in my uterus, which was removed along with several other organs I would have preferred to keep. Letting go of expectations, letting go of what I thought was going to happen—even letting go of my ovaries.

Several friends came to give me Healing Touch and Reiki, forms of hands-on energy healing. I don't know whether it was the energy work, the prayers, or the relief my body felt at no longer having a diseased organ to contend with—whatever it was, I felt better than I had felt in months. A friend suggested I stay in the hospital as long as possible to recover, but my surgeon declared, "A hospital is *not* a healthy place to be."

I was released from the hospital less than forty-eight hours after my hysterectomy, as soon as the gurgles in my now more-spacious abdomen indicated that my digestive system was functioning again. A large vertical incision, held together by staples, lay hidden under discolored dressings taped to my belly. This sutured slit ran from my pubic bone to just below my navel. A horizontal bikini-line incision might have looked nicer but appearance was not high on the agenda.

With enormous gratitude, I returned home and settled into my own bed, surrounded by flowers, get-well cards, and love. I had only been in the hospital for two nights, but it seemed like a lifetime—and it was. My cancer-free life was over; my after-cancer life had just begun.

My dear son, Jesse, surprised me by flying out to be with me right after my operation. His father had died in 1997 from metastasized melanoma, and the news of my cancer (what an odd expression "my" cancer is, a mixture of possessiveness and ownership) had hit him hard. His loving presence helped speed my recovery.

While my body healed, Gary and I made our pilgrimage plans. Neither of us identified ourselves as Christian but we agreed that wouldn't keep us from walking an ostensibly Christian pilgrimage road; after all, we'd done it before. We decided to walk the Via Podiensis†, one of the four Chemins de Saint-Jacques† (Roads to Saint James) that spread out across France like the fingers of a hand; they cross the Pyrenees and become the Camino de Santiago in Spain. The Via Podiensis was unknown territory for both of us—just like our journey through cancer.

The Via Podiensis begins in Le Puy-en-Velay, in the middle of south-central France, in the Massif Central†. It stretches 460 miles on a southwesterly diagonal until it reaches Saint-Jean-Pied-de-Port, a Basque town at the foot of the Pyrenees in southwestern France. This route is the most picturesque—as well as the most strenuous—of the four medieval French Chemins, and it coincides with a popular long-distance hiking trail, the Grande Randonnée 65† (GR 65). The GR 65 guidebooks provide topographic maps and descriptions of local culture, architecture, and history. Because of its popularity with hikers, numerous hostels and B&Bs are located along the route.

We intended to walk to Conques, a tiny village 200 kilometers (130 miles) from Le Puy, but we agreed that we might not reach our destination. We would walk as far as we could each day, whether that meant one mile or two or ten, and we would walk for one day, a week, or more, depending on how we felt. We planned to stay in France for one month but we would take each day as it came. After all, what else could we do? What else can we ever do, despite our illusions to the contrary?

Our plane reservations were for early October, a little over three months after my operation. Dr. Williams, my eminently skilled surgeon, advised me that three months was the minimum recovery time before I could do anything strenuous. I healed rapidly, aided by my determination to get in shape in time to walk the Chemin. Going on pilgrimage was an inspiring goal—besides, I knew the preparation was good for my health.

Less than a week after surgery I started getting up early each morning to walk the flagstone labyrinth we had installed in our backyard. We had planted the earth between the stones with wooly thyme and sprinkled wildflower seeds around the periphery. The hot, dry Colorado summer proved ideal for weeds as well as flowers, so I spent part of each morning bending over and pulling up the intrusive seedlings. I had to be careful at first not to tear my stitches, but I knew that the exercise was helping me to heal.

Soon Gary and I began taking short daily strolls, then longer walks. Eventually we were hiking five miles every other day on flat land. We were quite pleased, even though we knew we would probably be walking further each day, on very hilly terrain, once we were on the pilgrimage. The foothills of the Rocky Mountains were only fifteen minutes from our home, but we were not quite ready to have a reality check.

In addition to hiking much more rugged terrain on the Chemin, we would also be carrying additional weight: Gary planned to carry a backpack and I would wear a large fanny pack. We intended to carry enough supplies with us for several days. A taxi or baggage-transfer service would transport our luggage, which was loaded with energy bars, vitamin supplements, changes of shoes and clothes, and so on. We were also taking an international cell phone. I had promised my eighty-eight-year-old father that he would always be able to contact us. Gary had programmed our cell-phone number into the memory function in Dad's phone, so all he had to do was punch a button to call us, whether we were in the US or France.

Pilgrims on the Camino argue passionately about whether it's a real pilgrimage if one doesn't carry everything on one's back—as well as whether it's a real pilgrimage if one doesn't walk every step of the way. Even though we planned to have someone else carry our luggage, I knew we were making a real pilgrimage and I really didn't care what anyone else might think. I had more important things on my mind.

As our departure approached, I read whatever I could about the route from Le Puy, including a charming autobiography, *The Little Saint*, by Hannah Green. In it, she describes her life in Conques and her journey on the Via Podiensis in the 1970s. She gives a vivid account of the annual festival of Sainte Foy (Saint Faith), the fourth-century martyr whose relics are preserved in Conques in a golden, jewel-encrusted statue seated on a gilded throne.

Sainte Foy was an adolescent girl who was executed before she had really begun to live—although I think she lived her short life more fully than many of us live our longer ones. The way she met her death gave her a kind of immortality, different from what the Church preaches about "life after death" but certainly more verifiable.

Born into a wealthy pagan family in Agen, in southwestern France not far from Conques, Foy was raised by a Christian nurse who had her baptized secretly. According to the legend of "her passion" (a word that, oddly enough, is etymologically related to the Latin word for "suffer"), the twelve-year-old girl preached publicly and converted many to Christianity. Unfortunately, she lived during a period of renewed Roman persecution of Christians.

When Dacien, the Roman enforcer, arrived in Agen, probably in 303 CE† (Common Era), most Christians took refuge in a nearby city but Foy either did not or would not. Perhaps she could not leave her family or perhaps she felt inexorably called to her fate, mixing the passion of faith with the passion of suffering. She refused to sacrifice to pagan deities, declaring, "I am ready to undergo no matter what torments you would choose for me."

According to the legend, Dacien took her at her word. First he had her tied to a brass grid and set a fire beneath it. Miraculously a dove extinguished the flames. Her persecutors did not give up: they successfully beheaded her—but that was hardly the end of her.

Sainte Foy's earthly remains were buried at a monastery outside the walls of Agen, and there they rested undisturbed for 500 years, until 866 CE when a monk from Conques stole them. (This act is known as *furta sacra†* or holy theft). He had insinuated himself into the monastery and waited until the opportunity arose to filch the holy relics. According to medieval reasoning, if Sainte Foy (that is, what was left of her) hadn't wanted to go with him to Conques, she wouldn't have.

Soon word of miracles wrought by her relics began to spread throughout Christendom. Theologically, it wasn't the relics per se that caused the miracles but rather Sainte Foy's continued presence in them. Her presence bridged the gap between the longings of this world and the longed-for response from heaven. Prisoners and the blind especially venerated her relics—and their faith was often rewarded, according to the *Book of Miracles of Sainte Foy*, compiled in the early eleventh century.

The presence of the miraculous relics in Conques attracted numerous pilgrims to the remote village, filling the abbey's coffers and enriching its treasury of valuable religious artifacts. Soon Conques' abbey church was a "must-see" stop for pilgrims en route to Santiago. Conques is the only site on the Via Podiensis mentioned in Book Five of the *Codex Calixtinus*, the twelfth-century French guidebook to the Way of Saint James. According to the author (thought to be Aimery Picaud),

> Then, the Burgundians and Teutons [French and Germans] who go to Santiago by the route of Le Puy should visit the most holy body of Saint Faith, virgin and martyr, whose most holy soul, after her body was

decapitated by the executioners on the mountain at the city of Agen, choirs of angels bore off to heaven in the likeness of a dove, and they adorned her with the laurel of immortality. ... Finally the most precious body of the blessed Faith, virgin and martyr, was buried with honor by the Christians in a valley commonly called Conques, above which a beautiful basilica† was built by the Christians in which, to the glory of the Lord, the rule of the blessed Benedict is observed even today with the greatest care; to the sound and to the infirm many favors are granted; in front of its portals is an excellent spring whose virtues are more marvelous than can be told. (Shave-Crandell and Paula Gerson, p. 78)

Sainte Foy's feast day is always October 6, but it is celebrated on the closest Sunday (on or after the 6th). October 6, 2002, was a Sunday, the day after my birthday. Since the fête actually begins the evening before, it would be taking place during my birthday.

Surprisingly attracted to this young girl who was willing to die for her faith, I wanted to be in Conques for both occasions. May I have that strong a faith, I thought, that much certainty when confronted with a life-threatening choice. After all, if my cancer metastasized I would have to make decisions about what treatment to pursue—and I might live or die by the outcome.

Medieval pilgrims took part in a blessing ritual that included donning special garb (a sturdy cloak, a wide-brimmed hat, and a small purse or pouch) and taking up a walking staff. This ritual usually took place at a church in their home town. It was a ceremony of leave-taking that invested pilgrims with special rights, privileges, and responsibilities. The ritual announced to the world that this was a pilgrim, someone who had made the socially sanctioned shift from secular citizen to sacred person.

On previous pilgrimages I had had no interest in getting a pilgrim's blessing. I had felt no need. This time, however, I longed for blessings from every source—Saint James, the Virgin Mary, Sainte Foy—whether I believed in them or not. Now I knew that every day I was alive was a blessing.

I decided that participating in Sainte Foy's feast day could serve as my blessing ceremony. I hoped to experience a change of state that would mark my separation from mundane life into sacred space—a stepping over the boundary of everyday existence into liminality†, a sort of time and space "in between," where all kinds of transformations are possible.

Thanks to modern transportation, we could begin our pilgrimage wherever we liked, even at such an unlikely place as where we planned to stop walking. We'd begin where we hoped to end, creating a Mobius-strip pilgrimage route instead of a linear one. Gary was more than willing to go along with my desire. We were both aware of how fragile life is and how uncertain each day.

We planned to arrive in Paris on October 4th and take the train from Charles de Gaulle Airport to Rodez, where we would spend the night. The next morning, my fifty-sixth birthday, we would drive a rental car to Conques, where we would stay for a few days, celebrate Sainte Foy's feast day, and get over jetlag. Then we would drive to Le Puy, leave the car with Hertz, and begin walking 130 miles back to Conques.

My limited French proved adequate for making hotel reservations in Rodez and Conques. Making arrangements was so effortless that it felt as if this plan was meant to be. Of course, *everything* is meant to be, including my cancer. I used to think that expression sounded both passive and fatalistic, but now I realized it was liberating: I was learning to accept what is, without attachment to outcome.

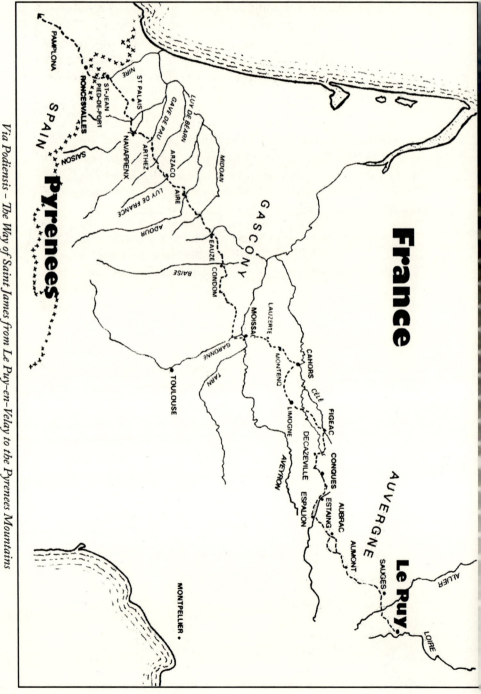

Via Podiensis – The Way of Saint James from Le Puy-en-Velay to the Pyrenees Mountains

October 2002 Pilgrimage

Friday, Oct. 4, 2002. Paris to Rodez.
Approximately 600 kilometers (375 miles) if we
had driven directly there; much further by train.

Planes, trains, taxis, and thirty hours took us from Denver to
Rodez. We arrived just before midnight. Danielle, a friendly, English-speaking taxi driver, drove us through the dark streets to the
Hôtel de la Tour Maje, an impressive stone building with a fourteenth-century tower lit up with golden light that dissipated into
the velvet-black sky.

Exhausted yet energized, we picked up our luggage and staggered to the reception desk. Christine gave us our key and pointed
us toward the elevator.

Saturday, October 5, 2002. Rodez to
Conques. 40 kilometers (25 miles) by car.

We slept through the night and woke at 8:00 a.m., our bodies
already adjusted to the eight-hour time difference. I rolled up the
light-blocking metal blinds and squinted out at a sunlit cobblestone
square lined with late-blooming flowers. Poking above the nearby
rooftops were the pink, fortress-like walls of the thirteenth-century
Cathédrale Notre-Dame.

Breakfast was an ample assortment of *fromaget*, cold cuts, hard-boiled eggs, croissants, *pain de chocolat* (a croissant pastry wrapped
around a chunk of bittersweet chocolate), baguettes, sweet breads,
cereals, yogurts, fruit juice, bananas, pears, and our choice of hot
chocolate (hot milk and a package of powdered Nestlé's), tea, or
coffee. The delicious array reminded me that I had to exercise willpower. At home my breakfast usually consisted of almond butter on
a sliced apple. I tried to avoid caffeine, sugar, and wheat in an effort
to minimize the swelling in my ankles, not that it seemed to do
much good.

For several years, my health-care providers had looked at my puffy ankles with concern, worried that this was an indication of either a compromised lymphatic system or a challenged immune system. Given my recent medical history, I shared their concern. So far nothing—neither lymphatic drainage treatments nor acupuncture nor elevating my feet—had made any difference. The latest suggestion was that the swelling might be related to food allergies. The most obvious culprits were caffeine and wheat; in addition, I was supposed to stay away from sugar on general principles.

Eating breakfast in France was not going to be easy—or rather, it would be too easy. I salivated at the sight of the flaky croissants and the *pain de chocolat*. The fragrance of fresh-brewed espresso filled the air, reminding me of how much I enjoyed savoring its bitter flavor.

Gary had no such dietary restrictions. He ate a bowl of granola, a croissant stuffed with sliced ham, and a container of sweetened yogurt while I discontented myself with cheese, cold cuts, an egg, and an unripe pear. I felt both deprived and self-righteous. At least I had used self-control. I remembered reading that willpower is like a muscle that must be exercised or it goes flabby. Clearly I would have lots of opportunity to build resolve on the Chemin.

We headed for the cathedral whose spires we had seen from our hotel room. Surrounded on three sides by massive grey stone buildings, it was squeezed into a space that seemed too small, like an overweight dowager billowing out of her overly tight corset.

Gary and I found our way in through a side door. Huge stone pillars soared upward to the distant vaulted ceiling. Chapels lined the walls, and an ornately carved seventeenth-century organ case, topped by wooden angels, dominated the north transept†.

We were on a mission, however, and it wasn't to admire the architecture. Like most French churches, the Cathédrale Notre-Dame provided an assortment of candles near the main entrance. Long and short white tapers, large and small votives encased in white or red translucent plastic, with a picture of the Virgin on one side, were arranged on shelves. We selected the candles we wanted and dropped the appropriate number of coins through a slot into the lockbox bolted to a stone pillar.

Then we walked around the cathedral, looking for a painting or a statue that attracted us and that had a nearby candle-rack. Virgins with various names and attributes, saints of all kinds, images of Jesus—at last we found one we were drawn to. We wedged our candles between the prongs on the circular, black metal stand and lit them, saying prayers of gratitude for our safe arrival, for whatever life brings. Then we sat quietly on a hard, wooden pew, enjoying the silence.

I took a deep inhalation and slowly exhaled. My dream had become a reality: we were in France, near Conques. In just a few days we would begin walking the pilgrimage road. Although that journey was filled with uncertainties, one thing was certain: It was much more pleasurable to be in France thinking about the Chemin than it was to be in Boulder thinking about cancer.

I turned to Gary. "What are you thinking about?"

He squeezed my hand. "Just thinking...."

After leaving the church we wandered through the extensive pedestrian zone, admiring the well-preserved medieval buildings. Some of them bore plaques describing events that had happened centuries ago when the town was an important ecclesiastic and secular center for the region.

We did some shopping, preparing our own version of the pilgrim's travel kit. Since my favorite Opinel knife had been confiscated at the airport security checkpoint, I bought a replacement: a folding knife with an olivewood handle and a tiny metal bee on the shank. The clerk informed me that my knife was a Laguiole, produced in a nearby town famous for its cutlery and its four-Michelin-star restaurant. We had thought we were in an isolated part of France, but appearances were deceptive.

We picked up our rental car and soon we were following road signs that pointed the way toward Conques, a UNESCO heritage site, designated in 1998 as part of the "World Heritage Sites of the

Routes of Santiago de Compostela in France."The Via Lacteat (The Milky Way, another name for the Chemin) was clearly an up-and-coming tourism attraction. We drove slowly down twisting country roads through scenic villages, around steep hills covered with chestnut trees, and alongside schist and granite outcroppings and deep gorges. I began to worry about whether we would to be able to walk up and down and back up those hills, day after day. Faith, I told myself, faith.

Our road grew narrower, the turns tighter, as we drove alongside the swift-flowing Dourdou river. We meandered past small towns and smaller hamlets, castles and manor houses before reaching the turn-off to Conques. A steep, winding road led up to a cluster of picturesque medieval half-timbered and stone houses clinging to the side of a nearly perpendicular hill. Vestiges of the old city walls, originally built in Roman times, remained.

The narrow one-way street into Conques was restricted to cars owned by the 362 residents, but we drove in anyway, looking for our hotel. The Hostellerie de l'Abbaye was not hard to find. Not surprisingly, it was located next to the medieval abbey church. We unloaded our suitcases, fanny pack, and backpack near the front door. While I guarded our luggage, Gary drove through the village to a large park-

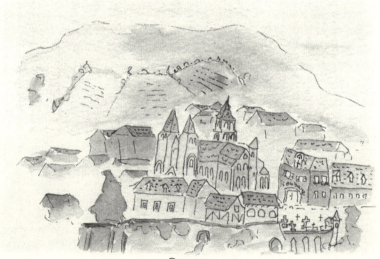

Conques

ing area reserved for tour buses and tourists' cars. Then he walked back, a bit winded from the exercise.

The innkeeper was not available, but his sturdy, elderly mother led us up a succession of creaking staircases to our room. I looked out the window. We were on the edge of a precipitous hillside, overlooking the gorge formed by the Dourdou. The river was so far below I couldn't see it, even when I leaned out the window. Suddenly the enormity of our undertaking hit home.

Gary and I rarely exercised, and even though we had been walking regularly for the last few months, we were hardly in good physical shape. Besides, I was still recovering from cancer surgery. One step at a time, I told myself, one step at a time. That's really all I have to do to walk the Chemin—and to journey through cancer. Don't look ahead too far; just look at what's right in front of me.

Pilgrims have walked this route for a millennium; we could do it too. Besides, we had much better gear than medieval pilgrims. We had state-of-the-art Gore-Tex hiking boots and Smartwool socks, high-tech Marmot rainwear, Polartec pile and Supplex nylon travel clothes, silk underwear, and spring-loaded Leiki hiking staffs.

The terrain outside our window was intimidating but the scenery was stunning. The colors of autumn were sprinkled like confetti over the hillsides, the trees changing from green to gold and orange, burgundy and rusty red. Blood-red vines spread like a stain.

After unpacking a few items, we went out to explore the village. A wedding was being celebrated in the abbey church, and a flower-bedecked antique automobile was parked on the cobblestone plaza that separated the church from a slightly bowed row of half-timbered houses.

Since we didn't want to intrude on the wedding we visited the pilgrim reception office in the Accueil Abbaye Sainte-Foy, located directly behind the church. The abbey's canons† and volunteers run the hostelry, which provides room and board for pilgrims. We explained to Canon Joel that we would start our pilgrimage in Le Puy but we had come to Conques for Sainte Foy's fête. Although he was surprised by our plans, he smiled at our devotion to the Little Saint.

We filled out a brief questionnaire and Canon Joel reached into a drawer and took out two pilgrimage credentials†. We would get these printed booklets stamped at each stop along the way, validating that we were pilgrims on the Way. He inscribed the credentials with our names and address, and noted that we would be departing from Le Puy on October 8, three days away.

Then he handed us our credentials. We were to write our signatures below a statement that, roughly translated, meant we promised to respect the spirit of the pilgrimage, the church, the pilgrims, our hosts, and nature. We were also to provide the name of our parish and the diocese to which we belonged.

Gary and I signed our names without hesitation, but we had difficulty with the rest since we didn't go to church. It would be problematic to explain our spirituality to Canon Joel, so I didn't try. We thanked him, mumbled something, picked up our credentials, and left. Once outside the reception office, we sat on the worn stone steps at the back of the church and debated what to write.

Our marital counselor, Jennifer, often said, "It's none of your business what anybody thinks of you." But at that moment it really did seem to matter what Canon Joel thought. After all, he was the custodian of the credentials. Torn between the complexities of self-disclosure and the discomfort of not speaking our truth, we decided not to do anything. We could always complete the credentials later.

We walked across the cobblestones to the nearby Treasury of Sainte Foy, located in what remains of the original abbey cloisters†. Sainte Foy's popularity brought not only fame but also exquisite religious art to this isolated village. The Treasury contains one the most important collections of medieval and Renaissance religious gold work in Western Europe.

In 1794, during the French Revolution, the National Convention ordered the confiscation of all precious metal objects—including religious—so they could be melted down. The people of Conques, fierce in their devotion to the Little Saint, ignored the decree. They did more than just disregard the decree; they hid the contents of the Treasury in their homes, gardens, and chestnut-drying sheds. After the Revolution all of the treasure was returned, including the golden reliquary statue of Sainte Foy.

We bought tickets and entered the narrow hall, its walls lined with glass cases displaying artistic masterpieces. At the far end of the room was the nearly three-foot-high, gold-and-gem-covered reliquary statue of Sainte Foy. During the tenth century, artisans had placed the oversized, head-shaped reliquary that contained her skull onto a seated statue, thus creating "Sainte Foy in Majesty," so-called because the figure is sitting on a throne. The emphasis on her skull has resonances with the ancient Celtic veneration of the head.

Legends abound about the martyred saint's playfulness and pleasure in fine things. In the Middle Ages she would appear in dreams, demanding gifts to adorn her statue, golden doves to sit on her throne, golden sleeves to complete her costume. She would offer something in exchange—perhaps the conception of a longed-for child or the curing of a chronic illness or disability—or maybe a less tangible sign that the gift of faith was rewarded.

I felt Sainte Foy staring at me, the black pupils in her white, wide-open eyes compelling my attention. She was a glittering, jewel-bedecked figure sitting on an elaborately decorated golden throne, her arms raised parallel to her knees, as if momentarily frozen in the middle of a gesture. She waited expectantly in the velvet-draped, stone-lined alcove, looking out into space, her serene, golden head (probably a Celtic or Roman face mask) too large for her body. Pointed, elongated, gem-encrusted shoes poked out from under her robe and rested on a red velvet footrest; a jeweled diadem crowned her oversized head.

From the ninth to the nineteenth centuries, grateful pilgrims had offered engraved crystals, gold, cabochons, enamels, and other precious stones, including emeralds, sapphires, rubies, topazes, carnelian, onyx, jade, amethysts, opals, bloodstones, garnets, and agates to embellish Sainte Foy's reliquary. Three cameos, thirty-one antique intaglios (carved gemstones)—one Roman, one Byzantine, and one Carolingian—and a ninth-century rock-crystal carving of the crucifixion adorned the sumptuous figure.

Her throne rested atop a sapphire blue, three-foot-high pedestal. Both the statue and the pedestal were enclosed in Plexiglas.

I marveled at the devotion that had crystallized into this jewel-festooned form, each gem a gift of hope, of gratitude, of faith. At first the idea of revering relics had seemed peculiar to me, but then I remembered that sports fans collect memorabilia of their favorite players; the signatures of long-dead presidents sell for hundreds of thousands of dollars; and people vie at auction for a strand of Elvis Presley's hair or Madonna's bustier.

What did Sainte Foy mean to me, I wondered, circumambulating slowly around her Plexiglas-encased throne. I felt she had a vital message for me, a message I longed to hear, a message I had traveled thousands of miles to receive. I stared patiently into her unblinking eyes. At last the answer came.

Faith, commitment, conviction, and trust were the words I heard echoing inside—words that stood for concepts I was beginning, by fits and starts, to bring into my life on a daily basis. This young girl—only twelve years old—was martyred in 303 CE because she lived her faith, and by so doing, died. She was a naive young girl, taking literally the Bible stories her nurse whispered in her ear. I longed for—I *craved*—that belief and determination, not in Christianity or martyrdom but in myself and in the choices I was making. For me, as it had been for her, these choices could be a matter of life and death.

At last I tore myself away from Sainte Foy to admire some of the other exceptional treasures. Safely locked inside large glass display cabinets were a large gilded letter "A" given to the abbey, it is said, by Charlemagne; two twelfth-century portable altars in silver, alabaster, and porphyry; the reliquary of Pope Pascal, complete with filigree work and diadems, also from the early twelfth century and said to contain pieces of the Holy Cross (how many of these pieces were real, I wondered, since there were enough scattered around the world to reconstruct a tree, if not a forest); the reliquary of Pepin (ninth to eleventh centuries), covered with embossed gold leaf, precious stones, and antique intaglios, including one of Persian origin; and an impressive processional cross.

But it was Sainte Foy's image that beckoned me. I made a silent promise to visit her again.

We walked across the cobblestones to the abbey church, one of the most important surviving Romanesque pilgrimage churches. It was begun in the eleventh century to replace a tenth-century basilica and designed so that it could accommodate the numerous pilgrims visiting Conques on their way to Santiago. It is constructed of reddish sandstone and warm, yellow limestone, filled in with local grey schist.

Twin towers with twin arched windows soar above the western doorway with its carved tympanum† of the Final Judgment. Faint hints of blue, red, and yellow paint still color the 124 characters that graphically portray the medieval vision of Paradise and Hell. Heaven is celestially peaceful, the serene Virgin Mary leading a procession of chosen people, including Charlemagne, the founder of the church, and an abbot, into Paradise. Hell is much more animated, filled with bizarre beasts and engrossing action.

In the center, Christ as judge holds court, surrounded by angels and seated on a throne in the middle of a mandorla, also known as a *vesica piscis*, which translates as "fish bladder." This almond-shaped geometrical figure is constructed by drawing the circumference of one identical circle through the center of the other. The central overlap creates an almond or bladder shape. The mandorla is said to represent the perfect balance of intuition and intellect, or the sacred marriage of spirit and matter, or Heaven and Earth combining into a new relationship.

We entered and sat down on a bench near the altar. The thousand-year-old church seemed silent, but I knew it was filled with the echoes of millions of prayers whispered by worshippers, murmured by pilgrims, recited by parishioners over the centuries. I could hear them faintly, filling the soaring interior space with the vibration of faith. Tears filled my eyes and I wept.

Eventually I stood up and walked around the church, admiring the carved capitals† on the columns and the sculpted Annunciation perched high on the back wall of the northern transept. Framed by a delicately carved archway, Mary seems in shock at the unexpected visit of the Archangel Gabriel. She hands her distaff to a young servant girl standing behind her, who holds a ball of wool on a spindle. The life-sized figures of the Annunciation look small because they are twenty-four feet above the floor.

The stained-glass windows are modern, designed by Pierre Soulages, a well-known French abstract painter born in nearby Rodez. He developed a new kind of glass for the project: grains of white glass are interspersed heterogeneously into a glass matrix, creating subtle variances in the color of light that shows through. Set into arched openings in the thick stone walls, the windows are stark and austere: thin, curving strips of variegated and streaked, off-white glass, with thin lead bands connecting the strips, each batch of translucent strips curving together in a horizontal, vertical, or diagonal direction—or sometimes in all three directions in the same window. To provide additional support, the opalescent glass is sandwiched between narrow horizontal metal bars.

Installed in 1994, the windows were designed to fit the austerity of the Romanesque architecture as it exists for us today, without the original wall hangings, frescoes, and paint. To me the windows seemed cold and jarring, like a blustery winter day. I didn't know what they had replaced, but I preferred the jewel-toned stained-glass windows I had seen in the cathedrals in Chartres and León, illuminating the interiors with rainbow light.

We lit candles in front of a contemporary wooden statue of Saint James wearing a gracefully draped cloak and a broad-brimmed hat adorned with the scallop-shell symbol of the pilgrimage. He would be our companion on this journey.

With each candle I said a prayer of thanksgiving for our safe journey, my successful surgery, my dear son, my beloved Gary—for whatever life offers. The fragrance of roses wafted through the air. Was it the candles, I wondered, or was it something else? The sudden scent of roses is said to indicate the presence of Spirit. Could it be a visitation from Sainte Foy or Saint James? I said another prayer of gratitude for the mysteries that surrounded me.

Before Sainte Foy's evening fête began, we celebrated my birthday at the four-star Hôtel-Restaurant Sainte Foy across from the church. Everything in Conques seems to be located across from the church, indicative of how small the village is. We hadn't thought we needed reservations, but Japanese tourists filled the restaurant. Nonetheless, the amiable hostess found a table for us in a relatively smoke-free part of the dining room; that, in itself, was a miracle.

We chose the most expensive *table d'hôte menu†* (the all-inclusive, fixed-priced, multi-course meal) instead of selecting à la carte. After all, we were celebrating my birthday, an occasion for which we were exceedingly grateful. We settled in for a leisurely feast. Dinner began with pumpkin soup adorned with slices of roasted veal tongue, followed by a fragrant rack of lamb accompanied by garlic flan and delicately steamed baby vegetables. Next came cheeses served with light walnut-oil dressing on a bed of greens. The tangy local goat cheeses melted in our mouths.

For dessert we had selected a walnut cake with chocolate mousse, but we ran out of time. It was already 8:35 p.m. and the procession was scheduled to begin at 8:30. The waiter promised our dessert would be waiting when we returned. As we ran out the door we realized we hadn't paid; the waiter waved us on, telling us to settle the bill later. Another miracle.

Just as daylight faded we gathered with forty or fifty other tourists, townspeople, and pilgrims (identifiable by their well-worn boots) in front of the abbey church. One canon played the guitar; another led us in songs; a young woman accompanied us on a flute.

Although Gary and I had thought we would only observe the proceedings, someone handed us tapers, which we lit from a neighbor's candle flame. Caught up in the spirit of the moment, we joined the procession through the narrow streets of Conques, singing songs of praise to Sainte Foy.

"Prie pour nous Sainte Foy," we sang. Pray for us, Sainte Foy. Yes, please, I whispered, pray for us, for each of us, as you have prayed for your devoted followers for centuries, for a millennium. Free us from our respective prisons, heal our unwillingness to see.

An English representative of a parish dedicated to Sainte Foy gingerly carried a small twelfth-century coffer containing some body part or other of the martyred saint.

> Reçois nos priers,
> Nos chants, notre joie
> Martyre douce et fière,
> O Sainte Foy
> Si jeune et si belle,
> Si proche de nous;
> Sois notre modèle,
> Protège-nous.

We sang in French, which I barely understood, and in Latin, which I understood less, and I wept as we stumbled up the worn cobblestone streets, our way lit by flickering candlelight. Surely pilgrims had walked in processions like this for a thousand years, pouring out their faith in song, holding candles aloft against the encroaching darkness.

My heart was overflowing. It was my birthday. I was fifty-six years old and thankful to be alive, to be in France, and to be going on pilgrimage with my beloved Gary. I wouldn't have been here if I hadn't had cancer.

We reached the top of the hill and the Centre Européen d'Art et de Civilisation Medievale, where a theatrical spectacle was about to begin, a combination Passion play and slide show. We had done enough, so we headed back to the restaurant to finish dessert and pay our bill. Or rather, we tried to. We got lost in the maze of alleys and stair-stepped passageways twisting up and down the side of the hill.

As we paused beneath a crumbling stone archway at a confusing crossroads a man with dark skin, long dark hair, and a very large nose suddenly appeared out of nowhere. He said something in French that seemed to indicate we were following the right way down.

I replied, "Ojalá!" which is Spanish for "God willing." The phrase is a corruption of the Arabic "in Sha'a Allah," enduring evidence of the lengthy Moorish occupation of Spain. I had no idea what prompted me to say "Ojalá"; the expression wasn't part of my normal vocabulary and besides, I was in France, not Spain.

The man looked startled, then started speaking to me in Spanish.

"Where do you come from?" he asked. And then, "Do you come from Kansas?"

Startled in turn, I asked, "Why do you ask about Kansas?"

"Just to say something..." he replied.

Although we now lived in Colorado, Gary had been raised in Kansas, and I had lived there for a number of years.

"Where are you from?" I asked.

He muttered evasively. He was a pilgrim, and he had walked from Fatima in Portugal to Rome, and from Le Puy to Compostela. At least that's what I think he said; his Spanish was difficult for me to understand.

We reached the abbey church and with a parting wave, he disappeared around the corner. Maybe he was Saint James in disguise, I suggested to Gary, half in jest, or maybe an angel. Miracles occurred in Conques, and not just in the Middle Ages.

Sunday, October 6, 2002. Conques.

The price of our room included breakfast, so we started the morning in the dining room. Someone had left a basket of sliced baguettes and a tray of homemade jams and marmalades at a table for two. There was nothing there I should eat. I had brought a large supply of energy bars, so I made do with one of them. It wasn't fair. Nor did I like the idea that I was paying for a breakfast I couldn't eat. How quickly I had stepped out of an attitude of gratitude, as easily as taking off a coat.

While I complained about the injustice of it all, the owner's mother came in and asked if we wanted coffee, tea, or hot chocolate. We asked for an *infusion†* (herbal tea) instead.

Sainte Foy's feast day is celebrated with a procession of the Little Saint and a high mass. I didn't want to miss any of it. After all, we'd traveled all the way from Boulder, Colorado, to be here for this occasion. I also wanted to be sure we got good seats in the church, so we arrived at 10:00 a.m., a half-hour before the mass was scheduled to start. The church was nearly empty, which seemed odd. Didn't other people want to get good seats? Several women busily arranged bouquets of flowers around the raised altar and on various columns.

A bright red banner on a post was propped up against the large stone column on the right side of the dais. Elaborate gold lettering spelled out "Saint Foi de Conques" and "Prie pour nous." In the middle, surrounded by gilt fleur-de-lys† and framed in a gold circle, was a romantic image of a very pale Sainte Foy, hands pressed together in prayer, a blue ribbon tying back her curling auburn hair, her head surrounded by a halo. In front of the banner stood a red-draped table with a vase of white lilies.

During the next half-hour several people came in and sat next to us. I felt a growing sense of expectancy. It was as if we were "behind the scenes," watching the preparations for a play—for that's in part what a religious ceremony is, complete with memorized lines, acts, scenes, and the build-up to the grand finale. But where were the rest of the audience and the performers? Where were all the people who were going to go to the Treasury to take Sainte Foy out on her annual excursion?

We waited. A canon appeared and scurried around the church, locking the doors. Over the public address system, I heard Canon Joel leading singing outside the church. Dismayed, I realized I had misinterpreted the printed schedule. I had thought the translation of Sainte Foy from the Treasury to the church would take place after the mass, not before.

The huge church doors were flung open and the procession entered, led by a middle-aged man in a gray suit carrying the heavy, gem-encrusted processional cross that was taller than he was. Behind him, four men carried Sainte Foy, encased in her Plexiglas container, on a palanquin. They set her down gently on the red-draped table. Suddenly the church overflowed with people—elderly women leaning heavily on canes, young couples whispering eagerly to each other, matrons holding babes in arms. We had missed the procession, but at least we had good seats for the rest of the ceremony.

The bishop of Le Puy officiated, wearing elegant white and red robes, along with several other priests. He called on the children to sit on the dais next to Sainte Foy. With a lot of giggling and shuffling, they came forward.

A christening followed and what seemed like a lengthy mass. Yesterday a wedding, today a christening. I supposed it was auspicious to celebrate these events near or on the feast day of the Little Saint; her blessing, like her reliquary, was presumably more accessible.

As I watched the ritual unfold I was struck by the juxtapositions of life and death. Christenings, weddings, martyrdom... . Behind them all was the promise of eternal life in Christ, exemplified in a concrete fashion by Sainte Foy's unfaltering popularity.

Inscrutable, she sat inside her Plexiglas shield, protected from touch and theft. Quite irrationally I felt sorry for her. She who was famous for helping to free prisoners was herself a prisoner of her own popularity, a popularity that had resulted in both her gold-and-gem-studded magnificence and her theft-resistant enclosure.

As the bishop droned on, my mind drifted off. Occasionally a familiar word floated through my consciousness: *pèlerinage* (pilgrimage), Saint-Jacques de Compostelle—words indicating the ongoing relationship between Conques and the pilgrimage to Santiago. At last the mass ended and everyone poured out of the church to receive an offering of sweet bread rolls.

We ambled around the village, treading carefully down the rue Charlemagne, one of the two medieval pilgrimage roads that passed through town. Houses lined either side of the lane. The narrow street is so steep that often a house has a front door for each of its stories. The pavement is composed of pieces of schist placed vertically at the edges and horizontally in the middle to channel water down the center of the road.

Window-shopping, we examined reproductions of nineteenth-century engravings of the village, contemporary stone sculptures of pilgrims and Sainte Foy, jewelry both quality and schlock, tourist souvenirs, postcards, and candies. At the Librairie (bookstore) Saint-Norbert, the enthusiastic young clerk proudly showed me Hannah Green's book, *The Little Saint*.

The clerk and I attempted to have a conversation but her English was worse than my French, and we were caught in a shifting mélange of only partly comprehended phrases. I understood her to say that she had known Hannah and that Hannah was always smiling. She also said that many people came to Conques because they had read Hannah's book. Of course, she added, a great deal had changed in the village in the thirty years since it had been written.

Sitting in silence next to the door was Father André, the canon whom Hannah had not mentioned kindly. He looked as if he were settling into senility. I wondered how the book had affected people in the village, since not all of Hannah's descriptions were favorable. Perhaps Father André's withdrawal was one response. I tried to ask the clerk, but the attempt was futile, greeted by an uncomprehending smile.

I wanted a tiny medal of Sainte Foy, a memento to wear on a chain or to fasten on my bag, but all the medallions in the display case showed a long-haired girl holding a miniature grill in one hand and a palm frond in the other. I was attracted to the gold-bedecked statue but not to her twin symbols of martyrdom.

We stopped at a rock and mineral shop located in one of the half-timbered buildings across from the church. It was so old that its walls had begun to bow outward. As I wandered through the store admiring the huge crystals, bead necklaces, and exotic stones, I noticed a large white block of fossilized scallop shells. It was approximately one foot high and one foot wide at its widest point; four large scallop shells fanned out across the face of it. According to the label, the fossils were from the Mesozoic or Tertiary period (from 245 million to 1.6 million years ago, a surprisingly large range of uncertainty).

The scallop shell (*pecten maximus* or *pecten jacobeus*, also known as *coquille St Jacques*) is the symbol of the pilgrimage to Santiago. It is also the symbol of Venus (commemorated in Botticelli's charming painting of Venus rising from the sea, her feet firmly planted inside an oversized scallop shell, her hands partially covering her breasts, her long golden hair coyly covering her genitals)—and, of course, of Shell Oil Company.

The "Veneranda dies" sermon, found in Book One of the *Codex Calixtinus*, asserts that the scallop shell stands for the good works pilgrims are expected to perform, the ridges along its back representing the fingers of the pilgrim's hand. The scallop shell is also associated with baptism and with the poverty of the pilgrim who, with open, outstretched hands, relies on the generosity of others.

Medieval pilgrims proudly wore the scallop-shell emblem—either a real scallop shell, gathered from the Atlantic shores, or a lead or jet replica—on a hat or cloak as proof of completion of their pilgrimage. But times have changed. Modern pilgrims adorn their backpacks with the scallop shell at the beginning of their journey rather than on their return to indicate that they are pilgrims, not excursionists.

One popular legend purports to explain the connection between the scallop shell and the pilgrimage. A bridegroom was riding his horse along the *rías* (salt-water inlets on the Atlantic coast near Santiago de Compostela) and his horse stumbled. He called on Saint James to save him from drowning. His prayers were answered and he rose from the sea, covered in scallop shells.

I was not convinced by the story or the sermon. The scallop shell is a symbol of the feminine, so what was it doing representing the Christian pilgrimage dedicated to Saint James the Greater, the first martyred apostle, patron saint of Spain? I thought it much more likely that it was a still-resonating echo of the cult of Venus, which had been brought to Iberia by the Romans, if not by even earlier conquerors.

Far from the sea, in landlocked Conques, I stared in fascination at the triangular block of chalk-white stone. The fossilized shells connected the sea with the land, the goddess with the saint, the far-distant past with the immediate present of our pilgrimage.

"I want it," I said to Gary.

He nodded, not surprised.

"If we make it all the way back to Conques, we'll buy it when we return," I declared, making a kind of "if-then" vow.

"Do you realize how heavy it is?" he asked, shaking his head. "Besides, how will we carry it home?"

"We'll empty one of the suitcases. By then I will have eaten most of the energy bars, so there'll be lots of room. Honey, just look at those scallop shells! They are the *original* scallop shells. And they look just like the modern ones."

Gary looked admiringly at the block of shells. "Okay, we'll do it."

The elegant shopkeeper had discreetly followed our discussion. Now she came forward with a smile. We explained our intention in a mixture of English and French. She nodded. Language is rarely a barrier where financial transactions are concerned. She gave us her card, explaining that if the store was closed for the season by the time we returned, we should call her at home. I worried for a moment whether the fossil would be there when we got back, but I decided that if we were meant to have it, it would be. Besides, there was a similar block on a nearby shelf. It was easy to shift from fatalism to serene acceptance—especially when there was a back-up plan.

Shops were closing for lunch, so we strolled back to our hotel for a festive fête-day meal (the words "festive" and "fête" are closely related: in French, the "s" drops out from "fest" and becoming a tiny inverted "v" over the vowel preceding it). Although all the tables were set in the dining room, we ate alone.

Later that afternoon we returned to the church and I sat on a bench in front of Sainte Foy, mulling over my attraction to a golden statue filled with the bones of a long-dead martyr. The medieval cult of relics depended on the idea that bits of bone or wood or cloth—physical objects that had once been associated with a saint or Mary or Jesus—retained the energetic imprint of that person. This concept is present in many traditions. Buddhists revere the Buddha's tooth; some Muslims visit the burial sites of departed saints; Hindus go on pilgrimage to locations associated with various deities; Hasidic Jews pray at the tombs of honored rebbes.

Artists have shown this energy radiating out of golden halos in medieval religious paintings, shooting out like arrows from the Bleeding Hearts of Jesus and Mary, rising up like flames from the head of the Buddha. These are symbolic representations of a sensed experience, an experience that is nearly impossible to measure scientifically and was discounted in the West during the Renaissance and the so-called Age of Reason.

Some processes, such as Kirlian photography, purport to capture images of etheric energy fields. Medical imaging technologies, such as MRI and NMR, rely on microscopic shifts in the human magnetic field—which suggests to me there is a scientifically verifiable basis for the symbolic representations.

I had a hunch that the cult of relics wasn't about superstition (although it may have decayed into that) but rather about sensory impressions that were once more widely experienced. I was willing to believe that the energy of saintly beings remained embedded in their physical remains, held on this earthly plane by their love and compassion. But whether it was efficacious to pray to these relics was another question entirely.

As I pondered Sainte Foy's reliquary I remembered a visit Gary and I had made to San Juan de Ortega, an isolated monastery on the Camino de Santiago. The priest's sister had taken us on a tour of the church, showing us the elaborately carved marble tomb of the twelfth-century saint. When I had asked to see another chapel—I was confused by a guidebook entry—she looked surprised, then led us across the courtyard, pulled open a rusting wrought-iron gate, and unlocked a small door. We entered an empty, dilapidated room, its blue plaster walls cracked and crumbling, an iron rod tying one wall to the opposite one to keep them from falling down.

As soon as I walked in, the hair on my arms stood up: I felt the presence of something I had never before experienced. I was surrounded by all-pervasive, unconditional love, love that enveloped me like a mother cradling her beloved infant. I started to weep. I paced around the room holding my hands over my heart and whispering softly, "Oh my, oh my."

The hair on Gary's arms also stood on end and, bewildered, he also began to weep tears of joy. Our guide watched us with a smile.

When I had recovered enough to speak, I asked her, "What *is* this place?"

"San Juan's tomb rested here for centuries. We moved him to the church twenty-five years ago because this room was no longer safe."

"He belongs here, in this room," I said.

She nodded. "Of course he does. We hope to bring him back soon."

Fascinated, puzzled, and bewildered, for months I tried to understand what had happened to me in that decrepit room. I talked with other pilgrims, some of whom said, "Oh yes, San Juan's a 'power place'"—whatever that meant; others, however, responded, "San Juan de Ortega? It was nothing special."

The closest I could come to explaining what had happened was that either we had experienced the etheric energy (for lack of a better term) left behind by the beloved saint or we had experienced the etheric energy (again, for lack of a better term) left behind by the thousands—perhaps millions—of worshippers who had come to that room and prayed before San Juan's tomb. I leaned toward the former explanation, since devotees would have been filled with longing, pain, hope, and suffering, as well as gratitude; what we had sensed was unmediated, undiluted love—the loving energy of San Juan, who had devoted his life to helping pilgrims on the Camino.

Why did we feel something at San Juan and other people feel nothing? I didn't know. I didn't feel energy radiating from Sainte Foy's reliquary, but I was willing to believe that others could. I had few answers and more questions. A few years earlier I would have scoffed at the concept of etheric energy or saintly energetic residues. Expanding my paradigm of reality was a pilgrimage of its own.

While I sat and contemplated the cult of relics, auras, halos, and energy fields, people came and went in front of Sainte Foy, standing in front of her, kneeling in front of her, reciting silent prayers, touching—or longing to touch—the Plexiglas cage that separated her from them. Eventually the priests returned and, after a brief ceremony, Sainte Foy was lifted back onto the palanquin and returned to the safety of her velvet-draped prison in the Treasury.

At 8:00 p.m. we and approximately twenty others returned to the church for Compline prayers and a pilgrims' blessing ceremony. We each received a printed program that including music and lyrics to various hymns; we sat in chairs arranged on the dais where the high mass had been celebrated.

Prayers were recited, Bible passages read in several languages, and once again we sang about what a flower Sainte Foy was and asked her to pray for us. Canon Joel asked how many of us were pilgrims and requested us to step forward to receive the blessing. The Spanish gypsy we had met the night before was present, but he did not come forward. Perhaps he'd had enough blessings.

A dozen of us stood up and formed a circle. We introduced ourselves by name, hometown, and travel plans. We were a mix of nationalities: Germans, French, Belgian, and two Americans. Some of us were beginning in Conques; others had started in Le Puy the previous year or this year. I wasn't the only one collecting blessings.

After speaking at length in French, Canon Joel led us in the "Song of Compostelan Pilgrims," the "Chant des pèlerins de Compostelle":

> Tous les matins nous prenons le Chemin,
> Tous les matins nous allons plus loin,
> Jour après jour la route nous appelle,
> C'est la voie de Compostelle.
> (Every morning we begin the Chemin,
> Every morning we go further,
> Day after day the route calls us,
> It's the Way of Compostelle.)

The rousing refrain was:

> Ultre-ïa! Ultre-ïa!
> Et sus eïa, Deus adjuva nos!
> (Go further, go higher, God, help us!)

The next verse didn't fit the melody quite as well, but the words were still inspiring:

> Chemin de terre et Chemin de foi,
> Voie millenaire de l'Europe,
> La voie lactée de Charlemagne,
> C'est le Chemin de tous les jacquets.
> (Road of earth and road of faith,

Thousand-year-old Way of Europe,
The Milky Way of Charlemagne,
This is the Road of all those going to Saint-Jacques.)

The refrain followed, and then the last verse:

Et tout là-bas au bout du continent,
Messire Jacques nous attend,
Depuis toujours son sourire fixes,
Le Soleil qui meurt au Finistère.
(And always at the end of the continent,
Saint Jacques waits for us
His fixed smile has been there forever,
The Sun that dies at Finisterre.)

"Ultreya. Ultreya. Suseya. Deus ayudanos." "Onward. Upward. God help us." These medieval words of encouragement still echo up and down the Chemin.

God help us indeed, I thought, my eyes filling with tears. I had thought that Sainte Foy's fête would be our substitute for a pilgrims' blessing; instead, we were getting the real thing. Although I wasn't Christian I found myself deeply moved—and blessed.

Canon Joel gave each of us a miniature gospel. Gary and I received the Gospel of Mark in English. Then he passed around a basket of stale rolls, hard as rocks. At first I was a disappointed by the stale gift, but then I realized that a time might come when I would be thankful for the sustenance. How quickly I had forgotten to be grateful. It had happened between one breath and another.

Then Canon Joel led us over to the beautiful carving of the Annunciation placed high on the north wall of the transept. Standing close together in front of it, staring up at Mary and Gabriel, we sang "Salve Maria" in Latin. Again, tears flowed down my cheeks. It was as if the well of my heart had been tapped, releasing emotions I didn't even know I had. Salty tears surged up from deep inside, uniting me with the ocean and the scallop shell.

Monday, October 7, 2002. Conques to Le Puy-en-Velay. 200 kilometers (124 miles).

I felt nervous as we prepared to begin our grand adventure, our pilgrimage of gratitude. Gary was preoccupied with packing. I wanted support, contact, interaction, but he seemed unavailable. Not a good sign.

We had a tentative plan for how far we would walk each day and where we would stay, based on the information in the *Topo-Guide† GR 65*; Alison Raju's guidebook, *The Way of Saint James*; and *Miam Miam Dodo*, the pilgrim's equivalent to a red *Guide Michelin* for the Via Podiensis.

The French Long-Distance Hiking Federation, the FFRP†, publishes the three-volume *Topo-Guide GR 65, Sentier de Saint-Jacques-de-Compostelle*. The guides include detailed topographic (topo) maps, cultural and gastronomical information, and descriptions of the route—all in French, of course, which limited their usefulness for us. At least we could read the maps and I could decipher some of the directions.

The Way of Saint James, by Alison Raju, is an English-language guide for pilgrims; it gives distances between towns, briefly lists notable art and architecture, and describes the pilgrimage route in graphic detail (gravel road, farm trail, stiff climb, etc.). The GR 65 is waymarked for hikers, so although it follows the historic Chemin de Saint-Jacques, it also includes scenic detours. Sometimes the GR leads the hiker up a ridge to a spectacular view, leaving the Chemin in the valley far below. Raju's guidebook, on the other hand, is intended for pilgrims en route to Compostelle who don't mind occasionally walking on a country road.

Miam Miam Dodo (French baby talk for "YumYum" and "Beddie-bye") is the accommodations bible for the Chemin. Updated annually, it includes a schematic map and detailed information about lodging along the route, including communal and private *gites†* (hostels), inexpensive hotels, *chambres d'hôtes†* (B&Bs), equestrian resources, campgrounds, and pilgrims' refuges. The guide lists the number of stars or wheat heads awarded to the accommodations and gives a *petit fleur* (little flower) to those renown for an extra-friendly reception.

Miam Miam Dodo also includes bars, grocery stores, restaurants, and other services, such as post offices, banks, clinics, and train or bus connections. This information is vital since one doesn't want to end up in a small town where all the services are closed during a holiday or Sunday afternoon or Monday morning—not unless one has reserved *demi-pension†* (dinner and breakfast) with one's lodging.

After consulting our guidebooks, we decided to leave our luggage in Monistrol d'Allier at the Hôtel-Restaurant des Gorges. According to *Miam Miam Dodo*, the hotel offered a baggage-transport service for $1.00 per kilometer. I had tried to contact Transbagage and Factage, but both had closed for the season.

Since Monistrol d'Allier was 20 miles (27.5 kilometers) up hill and down gorges from Le Puy, we allowed ourselves three days to get there. We would carry enough in Gary's backpack and my fanny pack to meet our daily needs and leave everything else behind in our two suitcases.

A French-speaking friend had written down several sentences that expressed our need to transport our baggage. We hoped that we would find innkeepers who spoke English and we wouldn't need to use the crib sheet, but if not, we had a fall-back plan. Although I had managed to make reservations in France when we were in the US, now I felt hesitant to make the attempt by phone, so we planned to stop at Monistrol on our way to Le Puy and make arrangements in person.

We took out our pilgrimage credentials. The time had come to make a decision about how to fill them out since later that day we would get them stamped in Le Puy.

I suggested, "Why not write 'Church of Universal Worship' for the parish? After all, that's the name of the worship branch of the Sufi Order International."

"Isn't it called the 'Church of All'?" Gary responded.

"Maybe so. When Bonney married us, she said she was a 'minister in the Church of All.' I don't really know what the Church of All is, but I do know what the Universal Worship is—a worship service that honors the world's major religions equally. I'm willing to go on record with that."

"Church of Universal Worship it is. Besides, I seriously doubt that anyone will look closely at the credential."

"You're probably right," I replied, "but I worry about these things. You know me, I want to do it right."

Gary nodded. He did indeed.

We wrote "Church of Universal Worship" on the blank line for diocese and parish, placed our credentials in Ziploc bags that we discovered were just a little too small to seal, and put them in our leather equivalents to the medieval pilgrim's wallet.

We made one final visit to the abbey church to light another candle to Saint James. Then we drove out of town, heading in the wrong direction. Navigation is not easy in a strange land, especially with an overly detailed map (the topo-guide), a too-general map (the Michelin road map), and vague instructions, accompanied by indecipherable gestures, from the innkeeper's mother.

I soon realized that Madame's instructions did not match the route we were taking. But we were already on our way. The wrong way. I hesitantly suggested this to Gary.

"Just tell me what you want me to do!" he snarled.

"I don't *know!*"

"I'm driving, you're navigating. Just make a decision, Elyn. It doesn't have to be the *right* decision."

I was stunned. It didn't have to be the right decision? *Any* decision would do? What a bizarre concept. But then I realized, what a liberating one!

I consulted the maps and realized that the road we were on would eventually take us to where we wanted to go, just not in the way we had planned. That sounded remarkably like my recent experiences. I took a deep breath and let go of my need to make the right decision, as if there was one, or as if there was *only* one.

Gary was right. It really didn't matter how we got where we were going as long as we got there. It didn't have to be the way I had thought we should go; it didn't even have to be what looked like the best way. All he needed was directions that would eventually take us to Monistrol d'Allier and then to Le Puy-en-Velay.

I sat in silence while Gary continued to drive down a narrow, winding country road in the general direction of Le Puy. I was engrossed in the novel idea that I could make a decision without agonizing over it. I breathed a deep sigh. Perhaps Sainte Foy, using Gary as an intermediary, was freeing me from my prison bonds. After all, pilgrimage is a journey full of metaphor, a journey that is not only physical but also emotional, psychological, and spiritual. There are many ways to reach a goal, whether geographic or otherwise. Although I had thought we would begin our pilgrimage in Le Puy, it had already begun.

We had gotten a late start, so we stopped at the first open restaurant we saw, the Relais† de Bruyers near Aurillac. It was a small, unassuming restaurant frequented by locals. The first course was a homemade vegetable puree, followed by roasted chicken, then a cheese plate, culminating with a fragrant, flakey, warm apple tart.

In a much better mood, we drove on, our route both surprisingly scenic (marked with a green line on the Michelin map) and unexpectedly slow. Near Saint-Flour the road was blocked. A rockslide had occurred, and we waited for more than an hour before a one-way path was cleared. Rather than getting frustrated, I used this opportunity to practice patience. It's all part of the journey, I told myself.

As we drove across a desolate, boulder-studded plateau, the weather abruptly turned cold and rainy. The car's thermometer registered between 6° and 11° Celsius (43° - 52° Fahrenheit). Cold enough for hypothermia, I thought with a shiver. Two exhausted pilgrims appeared at a bend in the road where the GR 65 crossed the highway, the wind whipping their rain ponchos. Silently wishing them a safe passage, I watched them until they were out of sight.

"There but for the grace of God go I," I thought to myself. Then I realized that soon, *with* the grace of God, I would be going there.

Odd, how traditional religious language kept coming to me even though I didn't find the traditional, anthropomorphic image of God meaningful. Did it surge up from an unknown part of me that longed to interact with the Divine and used the only language it knew?

Coming around a bend in the road we reached Monistrol d'Allier and the Hôtel-Restaurant des Gorges. "Gorges" is indeed an accurate description. The hotel is squeezed between the highway passing directly in front of it and a steep, tree-covered river gorge directly behind. We pulled up to the main entrance and parked.

The front door was locked so we rang the doorbell and waited. Just when we were about to leave, we heard footsteps approaching from a distance. The door opened and a disgruntled woman stared at us. We explained we wanted to leave our luggage and return in three days to spend the night. She motioned for us to come in and walked away, her worn slippers slapping on the tile floor. We heard a murmur of voices in another room. Soon a pot-bellied man came down the hallway, wiping his chin with a napkin. He greeted us a bit more warmly.

"Parlez vous Anglais?" I asked hopefully.

"Un peu … a little…." He replied.

We repeated our request to him, and he nodded. The hotel was closed for the season but would be open for us. Trusting that our luggage would be there when we returned, we left our two suitcases in the hallway and drove on.

Near Le Puy we ran into another detour and headed off into the unknown, following road signs whose meaning was lost in translation. We were encountering a surprising number of roadblocks, detours, and wrong directions as we began our pilgrimage. What, I wondered, was the metaphoric message? Persevere? The route is not always straightforward? Learn patience? Go with the flow?

We arrived in Le Puy-en-Velay, situated in a deep basin in the midst of a rugged volcanic landscape. Despite false starts and numerous detours, we had only taken half a day to travel by car 200 kilometers (124 miles) from Conques to Le Puy. It would take us two weeks to travel this distance on foot—if we were able.

Le Puy is a substantial town of 29,000 people. "Puy" means volcanic mountain, and the city is surrounded by them. It is built on several plugs, all that remain of the solidified lava that filled the necks of a once-active volcano. Of unknown antiquity, Le Puy was at some point a Gallo-Roman village. It has been a major pilgrimage center at least since the Middle Ages because of its location on the Chemin, its famous Black Madonna, and its elevated chapel of Saint-Michel-d'Aiguilhe (Saint Michael of the Needle). I knew from a previous visit that Saint-Michel-d'Aiguilhe radiated energy, perhaps due to the magnetism associated with its volcanic origins.

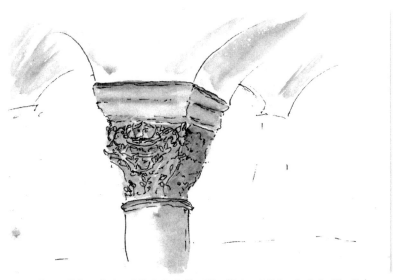

Green Man, Saint-Michel-d'Aiguilhe (Saint Michael of the Needle),
Le Puy-en-Velay

Sometime around 950 - 951 CE, Bishop Godescalc of Le Puy became the first pilgrim recorded to have traveled to Santiago de Compostela. Others had undoubtedly gone before, but his high ecclesiastic rank made his visit noteworthy. When he returned to Le Puy he built the chapel of Saint-Michel-d'Aiguilhe on top of a volcanic plug. He didn't start from scratch, however. He built on top of a Roman temple to Mercury, which was built on top of a Druid site, which was built on top of a megalithic dolmen†, whose massive slabs had been carved out of the top of the 275-foot-high volcanic plug on which it stood. A winding stone staircase with 268 steps leads to the chapel, the topmost tier of a religious layer cake.

An enormous rusty-red metal statue of Notre-Dame-de-France looms above the city, perched on top of another volcanic plug. She was cast from 213 melted Russian cannons. A statue of Saint Joseph holding the infant Jesus was erected on another plug. The two statues seem to be engaged in a lofty conversation, their immobilized gestures silhouetted against the sky.

We checked into our hotel, returned our car to the rental agency, and hurried over to the cathedral to get our credentials stamped. Our route took us into the still-intact medieval center of Le Puy. We walked quickly through the maze of twisting lanes, trying to keep the cathedral towers in sight. Then we turned a corner and saw the cathedral at the end of the rue des Tables, a steep narrow street lined with shops. Many of the store windows displayed examples of the famous local bobbin lacework, but this was no time for shopping. We had to reach the cathedral before the priest left.

The cathedral, too, was constructed on top of several volcanic plugs and giant basalt pillars. Initially built in the eleventh century to replace a fifth-century sanctuary—which had been built in turn over a Roman temple—the front of the cathedral cantilevers out into space, supported by an enormous staircase. It is an impressive sight.

The cathedral seems to overflow the space allotted to it, hemmed in on both sides by medieval buildings. Dark pink stone alternates with brown, creating a checkerboard and striped façade. Moorish arches and decorations abound, evidence of the extensive cultural exchange between southern France and Moorish-occupied Spain.

The cathedral looks like something magically transported from an exotic country and plopped down in the middle of a volcanic field in France—and in a way it was. In 1095 Pope Urban II named Adhémar de Monteil, then bishop of Le Puy, to lead the first crusade to the Holy Land. He was undoubtedly exposed to Middle Eastern architecture during his sojourn there.

Winded from climbing up the huge staircase, we hurried inside to get our credentials stamped. The first person we asked sent us to the sacristy, which was closed. Disappointed, we wondered what to do. I saw a nun and showed her my pilgrimage credential. I tried, using gestures, to ask her if she could help us find someone to stamp it.

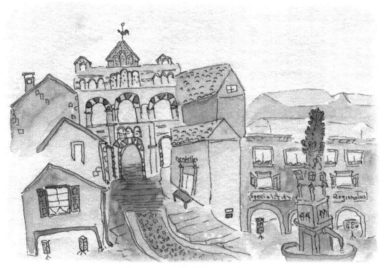

Cathédrale, Le Puy-en-Velay

"Of course," she replied in English, "I will do it."

As we followed Sister Marie-Geneviève down the hall, she suggested we attend mass at 7:00 a.m. the following morning and receive the pilgrim's blessing. I explained we had already been blessed in Conques since we'd been there for the fête of Sainte Foy. She nodded approval at our apparent devotion to the Little Saint.

Sister warned that it would be quite cold on the Chemin and that it would have been better if we had started in September. Pointing to my abdomen, I told her that we had had to wait for three months after my surgery before we could begin our pilgrimage. She commiserated and wanted to know if I was all right. Yes, I said, with a smile, hoping to reassure both of us.

Sister Marie-Geneviève unlocked the door to the gift shop and let us in. She took a large, low-relief rubber stamp out of a wooden drawer and, holding it by its wooden handle, rolled it back and forth on a red ink pad. Then she stamped our credentials with Our Lady of Le Puy. Our first stamp.

She signed and dated the credential below the stamp. "Our Lady will be with you while you walk," she assured us.

First a blessing from Sainte Foy, now the stamp of Our Lady given to us by a nun. We were making a real pilgrimage, even by Christian standards. We were held in God's hands—or perhaps the Goddess's.

I started to cry, and Sister Marie-Genevieve patted my shoulder. "Pray for us and we will pray for you," she said. Then she led us back down the hall to the main sanctuary.

Her words reminded me of the banner of Sainte Foy that read, "Prie pour nous." When I first walked the Spanish pilgrimage road, people asked me to pray to Saint James on their behalf. A pilgrim's prayers supposedly carried more weight—but I wondered if a nun's would carry even more.

Pray for us, I thought, and we will pray for you. I needed all the prayers I could get, but don't we all? Prayers of support, prayers of compassion, prayers of love and blessings. Prayers that mobilize the greatest good within both the person praying and the person prayed for. Modern scientific research indicates that prayer can indeed help in healing, especially if people know they are being prayed for. Besides, unlike some interventions, it couldn't hurt.

The Black Virgin of Le Puy stands in a place of glory above and behind the main altar. Her face and that of the infant Jesus, whose crowned head peeps out from the center of her robe, are black. She wears an elegant yellow satin robe embroidered with *puttis*, golden angel heads with wings. The tunic covers her body and that of the child. A delicate lace veil drapes gracefully from her golden crown down her shoulders and back. She looks like a mother kangaroo, complete with baby peeking out of her pouch.

Posted on a nearby railing was a plaque that read, "She is black because she labored in the fields in the sun (original figure burned 8 June 1794, Pentecost)." This Black Virgin of Le Puy was a nineteenth-century copy of the original, which, according to legend, had been brought back from the Crusades in the thirteenth century by Louis IX, also known as Saint Louis.

During the French Revolution the original Black Madonna was ignominiously removed from the church, placed in a trash cart, taken to the Place du Martouret in front of the Town Hall, and tossed onto a funeral pyre. *Her* funeral pyre. As she burned to a crisp, a tiny door on her back opened, and a small parchment roll fell out. Before anyone could save it, it too was reduced to ashes, leaving the truth of her origins forever a mystery.

Research indicates that the incinerated statue was probably an Egyptian effigy of Isis, whose cult was widespread in the first millennium. Isis and her child, Osiris, were often represented in the same seated position as the Black Madonnas found throughout Europe.

The Black Madonnas' darkness is a subject of much debate among scholars and clergy. Many (especially the clergy) claim the black comes from soot, or the color of the wood, or age, or is because artists thought Mary was sunburned during her sojourn in Egypt, or because she worked in the fields, or because Middle Eastern artists carved her with a dark complexion like theirs, or because Europeans carved her with a dark complexion like Middle Easterners, or.... All these explanations pointedly ignore that no other Christian European religious image is similarly black.

Regardless of the party line that attempts to rationalize away the significance of her blackness, her devotees know that Black Madonnas have a lot of miracle-making juju. Feminist scholars and Jungian psychologists hypothesize this is because the Black Madonna represents the chthonic forces of the Earth, the cave, the darkness of the soil from which seeds sprout, the recuperative powers of night or sleep, and the shadow.

Like other Madonnas, the Black Madonna of Le Puy incorporates two of the three aspects of the ancient triple goddess: the virgin and the mother. I think that her blackness embodies the third aspect: the crone. She is the wise old woman who approaches death. Virgin, mother, crone: youth, maturity, death—and rebirth. No wonder she is the object of veneration.

In a small alcove next to the altar is the *pierre des fièvres*, the Fever Stone, also known as the Stone of the Apparition. The black, flat, rectangular stone is all that remains of an ancient dolmen located where the cathedral now stands. In the early centuries of the Common Era, residents of Le Puy would spend the night sleeping on the stone, believing that it would cure their fevers. Gradually the stone was Christianized and brought into the church itself.

The practice so prevalent in Le Puy of confiscating and rededicating pagan sanctuaries and sites was neither accident nor aberration. It was official Church policy. Pope Gregory the Great (pope from 590 - 604 CE, the same pope who declared Mary Magdalene a prostitute, a misattribution that the Church eventually apologized for and rescinded officially in the 1960s) recognized that people are creatures of routine, especially in their religious practices. He wrote a papal epistle stating that pagan places of worship should not be destroyed. Instead, the idols were to be removed and the buildings purified with holy water. They were to be transformed into consecrated churches with the relics of Christian martyrs.

In other words, Christian priests were to co-opt pagan sacred sites, festivals, and deities by overlaying them with Christian chapels, holidays, and saints. That way, people could continue worshipping in the same place, at the same time, with just a slight shift of emphasis. Over the centuries, the original pagan devotions faded from memory, replaced by a new holy-day calendar and new personages.

This process of co-opting (some might call it assimilation) has been effective all over the world. For example, Our Lady of Guadalupe, Patroness of Mexico, is a not-very-thinly disguised transformation of Tonantzin, an indigenous Mexican goddess. Her shrine in Mexico City is located on the same site where Aztecs worshipped their mother goddess for centuries. And, of course, they still do—and some of them even acknowledge it.

Nor is co-opting limited to Christians. Several thousand years after Stonehenge was constructed, Druids used it as a ceremonial site. The Camino de Santiago—the Way of Saint James—may have been a pre-Christian pathway co-opted by one group after another. The association between the Camino and the star-strewn Milky Way (Via Lactea†) goes back for millennia. Some say the route was followed by migratory Neolithic hunters who relied on the stars to find their way home. Others suggest it was a Druid initiatic pathway that went from Paris to Finisterre, on the coast just west of Compostela. The Romans built roads over parts of this ancient route, which passed by many sacred sites. Medieval road builders used some of these roads for the Camino.

The church that expanded over the centuries to become the Cathédrale Notre-Dame-du-Puy was built on or near a sacred healing well and a ruined first-century CE Roman temple—which itself incorporated an ancient dolmen. According to one legend, in the third or fourth century a widow had a "malignant fever." She saw a vision of the Virgin Mary, who told her to go to Mount Anis, where stretching out on a particular stone (from the dolmen) would cure her. The bishop of the time heard of the miraculous cure and ran up to this pagan holy place just in time to see a stag leap out of a nearby wood. The stag traced the outline of the church with his hoofs in the snow—snow that had suddenly appeared, even though it was July.

According to another version, in the early fifth century the Virgin healed a sick woman near the dolmen on Mount Anis and urged Bishop Scutarius to build a church there. In a vision, the bishop saw the Virgin surrounded by angels, standing on top of the dolmen, the remnants of an earlier Gallo-Roman religious sanctuary. (Actually, a dolmen is a 4000 - 5000-year-old stone construction that pre-dates not only the Romans but also the Gauls. But never mind—we're in the land of legend, not archeology.)

The bishop built a sanctuary on the side of Mount Anis and included Roman masonry and funeral stones—and a slab from the dolmen, now called the Stone of the Apparition or the Fever Stone, as part of the sanctuary. Presumably the bishop got permission from Rome to put this erstwhile pagan object in the church.

Although no one in the religious hierarchy complained about locating the cathedral on top of a pagan site, subsequent Church authorities wanted the Fever Stone removed. Local clergy, however, believed that the stone had been exorcised at the time of the vision and was henceforth consecrated as the throne of Mary, hence its alternate name, the Stone of the Apparition. At some point a Latin inscription was carved into the slab, just in case anyone was still confused. "Those who lie on this stone and sleep are healed. Do you know why? The power belongs to the altar."

In the eleventh century the stone was reshaped and placed in the floor of the south aisle; it remained there for seven centuries and fever sufferers continued to fill the aisle. In the eighteenth century the clergy removed the stone from inside the cathedral. They were tired of sick people spending the night in the church—or perhaps they objected to the whiff of paganism that they smelled, however faintly, still clinging to the stone.

The stone was then placed at the top of the steps at the west front of the cathedral, where it remained until a few years ago. It was later installed next to the altar as a curiosity or historical artifact. Just to be certain there is no doubt about its Christianized nature—or no doubt about who is in charge—a large crucifix is suspended above it.

I sat down on the dark smooth stone, which felt unusually warm. I placed one hand on it, palm down. Much to my surprise, I felt a power surge go through me and out the top of my head. Gary sat down and put both hands on the stone and felt a circuit of energy running through his body.

We weren't the only ones to experience energy in the cathedral. In *The Little Saint*, Hannah Green described the telluric (earth) energy that she and her companions felt rising up through the cathedral, an energy that made them feel most uncomfortable. I wondered if what we experienced was related to the magnetic nature of the volcanic rock upon which, and out of which, Le Puy was built. The needle of a compass responds to such a pull, so why not the atoms in our bodies? After all, the human body has a measurable electromagnetic field; that's the basis for energy healing modalities and for high-tech medical imaging equipment.

We had had enough of feeling "buzzed," so we found a rack filled with candles. We purchased a number and lit them in gratitude for the pilgrims' blessing of yesterday and for Sister today, appearing just when we needed her. Gratitude for today and for tomorrow, whatever it brings. Gratitude for the whole messy catastrophe of life.

We lit another candle with prayers for a safe journey. Even though I didn't believe in the existence of intercessory saints, I asked for the help of Saint James. I prayed that he would travel beside us, guide us, push us if needed, and that the Virgin Mary in all her many forms would walk with us as well. It was odd to be praying to something I didn't think existed, but I was exploring how it felt to expand my paradigm of the world. Besides, it couldn't hurt to ask for help, whether that help came from beyond or within.

High on one wall I noticed the still-vivid remains of medieval frescoes. Christ was represented sitting inside the almond-shaped mandorla we had seen at Conques. The *vesica piscis* resembled a *yoni*, the sacred vulva of the Divine Feminine—a potent reminder that Mary gave birth to Jesus, the Divine Child of Light—and who was Mary, if not one aspect of the Eternal Mother? The same sacred symbol occurs throughout medieval church architecture—as well as in the twentieth-century chalice well cover in the Chalice Well Gardens in Glastonbury, England. The rust-red waters of the Red Spring that flow through the gardens are strongly linked with the Great Goddess.

It was getting late and we were very tired. Tomorrow would be a big day: we were going to start our pilgrimage walk. Thoughtfully, we returned to our hotel and an early dinner. The hotel restaurant highlighted the local gastronomy—walnut and duck salad, the green lentils of Le Puy, *confit†* (duck cooked and preserved in its own fat), and irresistible ice cream scented with local herbal Verveine liquor.

I lit a tiny votive candle and Gary and I spoke the words of our favorite prayer together: "Gratitude for today and gratitude for to-morrow, *whatever* it brings."

Tuesday, October 8, 2002. Le Puy-en-Velay to Montbonnet. 15 kilometers (9.3 miles).

We ate a large buffet breakfast at the hotel, feeling the need for plenty of sustenance for our journey. It was foggy and chilly outside, so I put on silk underwear, my Supplex travel shirt, black knit run-ning pants, a windblock vest, and a Polartec jacket. Gary, who didn't feel the cold as much, wore fewer layers.

We packed up our belongings and adjusted our gear, making sure the backpack and fanny pack fit as comfortably as possible. Ea-ger to begin, we set out to find the Place du Plot, the medieval start-ing point of the Chemin.

After getting lost again in the convoluted streets of Le Puy, we finally arrived at the square. A group of junior high girls and their teacher were taking photos of each other in front of three plaques on the wall of a large building. They saw us, giggled, and moved aside.

The first plaque is a commemorative inscription that states (translated), "Here is the beginning of the Via Podiensis, grand route of the Pilgrimage of Saint-Jacques de Compostelle." The second is a stylized equal-armed cross with a large scallop shell at the center. The third, the most elaborate, is a full-color map of Les Chemins de Saint-Jacques de Compostelle, highlighting in graphic relief the hills and vales along the Via Podiensis from Le Puy-en-Velay to Conques. The Amis de Saint-Jacques de Compostelle, one of many organizations dedicated to supporting the contemporary pilgrimage, placed the plaques there.

We asked the schoolteacher to take a picture of us standing in front of the plaques, poised to begin our pilgrimage. Then we waved goodbye to everyone. A few girls called out "Bon voyage" as we started to walk out of town on the Chemin.

We climbed out of the volcanic bowl of Le Puy and onto the flank of a long dead, eroded volcano. Alison Raju's guidebook is both accurate and explicit: "Climb steeply and steadily." Part of the road is signposted "the Route de Compostelle." Pausing frequently to catch our breath, we had plenty of opportunity to enjoy the expansive views and the enormous statues of Notre-Dame-de-France and Joseph, standing on their pinnacles below.

My legs began to feel like rubber. No, rubber legs would have felt springier. They felt like Jell-O, quivering with every step. At the top of the volcanic bowl we reached, ironically, a modern elastic bandage factory. Breathing hard, I hoped I would soon gain my stride.

After much too long, we reached a more level stretch of road and strolled along without a great deal of difficulty. In a nearby field we saw a man tossing a small, heavy ball. Pausing in his game of *boules*, he struck up a conversation with us. We were glad to stop walking and talk—or try to—in French.

Where we were going, he wanted to know. Where had we started? Where did we plan to stay? When we told him we hoped to reach Montbonnet, he suggested that we stay at the *gîte d'étape privé* l'Escole, a privately run hikers' hostel. We thanked him and, refreshed from our brief respite, continued on.

A large stone wayside cross peeked out of the bushes at the side of the road. Vines twined around its base and pebbles had been placed on top of the cross-arm.

An hour later and five chilly kilometers from Le Puy, we reached the hamlet of La Roche. On the right side of the road was a lichen-covered stone wall and a wooden sign decorated with a scallop shell and the words, "Via Podiensis, Santiago de Compostela, 1395 kilometers." 875 miles to Santiago. A covered box had been fastened to the top of the low wall. A note on the front requested pilgrims to write encouraging words in the *livre d'Or* (visitors' book).

We opened the lid and paged through the guestbook. "Ultreya!" Onwards! A Belgian pilgrim had written, followed by his name, hometown, and the date. A lengthy discussion in Flemish followed, along with phrases of support in French, German, and Japanese (I presumed it was support, though I couldn't translate the Japanese). I added words of encouragement in English: "Gratitude, gratitude, for whatever lies ahead."

Energized by our growing sense that we were part of a larger community of pilgrims supporting each other on the Way, we continued with more enthusiasm, enjoying the grassy track leading along a narrow ridge, thankful that the early morning fog had lifted. The ridge dropped off precipitously, and we would not have seen the danger if it had been hidden by fog.

The trees on the hillsides were turning color, some gold-tipped, some blazing bright orange and vermilion. Our path led us past isolated farmhouses, their walls, like the boundary walls in the fields, constructed out of black, brown, and sometimes pinkish volcanic rock. We walked beside fenced green meadows where black-and-white and golden-brown cows munched away. Tall thistles swayed in the gentle breeze, and bushes filled with ripe red berries lined the path.

Three kilometers further and we reached Saint-Christophe-sur-Dolaison. It was 1:00 p.m. and, despite the large breakfast we had eaten, we were hungry. Our guidebook said the bar across from the church would make sandwiches, but the guidebook was wrong. Besides, the bar reeked of cigarette smoke as dense as the early morning fog.

A pilgrim couple sitting at a table saw our uncertainty; they indicated we could buy bread and cheese in the village and bring it back to the bar, if we bought something to drink from the proprietor. But we would need to hurry: the shops were about to close. We thanked them and left. We looked around; there was no food shop in sight.

All at once we were tired, hungry, and concerned that we might not find lunch. Two petite middle-aged women wearing large backpacks were examining architectural features on the outside of the twelfth-century church. Hesitantly we went up to ask them for advice. Although they spoke French to each other, they directed us in perfect English to a nearby *boulangerie†* (bakery) and *épicerie†*, a small grocery that carries dairy products and cold meats.

Weary though we were, we trotted down the block and around the corner to the shops. We bought a crusty baguette, thin slices of dried ham (similar to Italian *prosciutto* or Spanish *jamón Serrano*), a round of local goat cheese, and two bananas. Then we found a bench in the shade near the church and prepared our picnic. The knife I had purchased in Rodez easily sliced through the crunchy bread crust. Fresh bread, tangy cheese, and salty ham. What a feast!

I was supposed to avoid eating bread, but cheese, ham, and a banana hardly seemed enough sustenance for a hard-working, long-distance-walking pilgrim. Beside, I had heard anecdotal evidence that French wheat was different from American wheat: less refined, fewer preservatives, a different genetic strain. I was willing to give it a try. How quickly I had convinced myself that my dietary choices were a matter of entitlement, rather than an opportunity to exercise willpower.

The same two Frenchwomen were taking photos of each other in front of the church. I offered to take a photo of them standing together, which delighted them. The woman with short, wavy auburn hair looked about sixty and spoke excellent British English; her slightly younger, dark-haired friend was much quieter but also spoke English. We soon learned that Collette (the former) and Danielle (the latter) had taught English to schoolchildren. Danielle hadn't spoken English for some time and was somewhat hesitant to engage in conversation, but Collette had no hesitancy at all. How pleasant it was to be understood without effort by someone other than Gary.

They said goodbye and started down the Chemin, heading the wrong way. They returned quickly and set off again in the right direction. We followed slowly behind them. The path was relatively easy—a country lane, a stony track, and then a grassy lane through a field—but Gary was tired. His feet didn't want to move.

It was sunny and warm. We shed layers and put on our sunglasses. What a glorious day. I recited the Navajo prayer: beauty before us, beauty behind us, beauty above us, beauty below us. Gratitude, gratitude, for whatever lies ahead.

One moment I was exuberant, the next, exhausted. Gary's feet felt like slabs of wood. My legs ached.

We caught up with Collette and Danielle, who took frequent breaks. Collette explained that, like us, she and Danielle had begun that morning in Le Puy. They had attended the pilgrims' mass, Collette commented, but hadn't seen us. She left the sentence dangling with an unspoken question. I explained that we had gone to the pilgrims' mass in Conques. She nodded in approval.

Collette said they planned to walk for one week, then catch a train back to Paris. They lived in Lille, a large city one hour north of Paris by high-speed train, where they sang in a local choir. They shared an interest in architectural history and, obviously, in pilgrimage.

As the kilometers slowly passed beneath our feet, we exchanged life stories—or rather, edited versions. I told Collette I had a Ph.D. in cultural anthropology and had written about the Camino. I also had published magazine articles about sacred sites, mystical places, labyrinth walking, and pilgrimage.

"Are you going to write about this pilgrimage, too?" Collette asked.

"I don't know. I'm not making the pilgrimage so I can write about it, but I am keeping a journal. I suppose that will become clear later."

After we had begun to establish a certain rapport, I asked, "Why are you walking the Chemin?"

Collette confided that she had had breast cancer a few years before. She was walking in recognition of her recovery, just as I was walking out of gratitude for my successful surgery. She hadn't made a vow per se, but she had known she wanted to make the pilgrimage for some time. Her friend, Danielle, had injured her knee in a skiing accident the past February and wasn't sure she could walk the Chemin, so this one week was a trial run.

I told Collette about my hysterectomy, and soon we were exchanging surgical experiences and medical opinions. She had gone to a Parisian oncologist, had chemo first and then surgery. Everything looked fine at her last checkup, she said, smiling. I smiled back. We were fellow pilgrims on the journey through cancer.

"You know," said Collette, "an experience like that makes you realize what's important. I no longer get so upset about small things."

I nodded in agreement.

"Surviving cancer," she continued, "makes life *so* sweet!"

Two objects stuck out of my fanny pack, objects that could have been the source of gentle amusement or scathing ridicule. Two small plush bunnies named Honey Bunny and Rustle Ears traveled with us. Collette saw them peeking out from the bag (usually they were hidden inside but I had forgotten) and asked about "the adorable creatures." She tweaked them on their chins and stroked their ears.

"Surely they have a story?" Collette asked, with a delicate tilt of her head.

And of course they did, a long, convoluted story. When I had first begun to have "female problems" (spotting, followed by abnormal cell growth) a year before my hysterectomy, I had had two D&C's. My nurse practitioner suggested that guided imagery was often helpful in correcting unhealthy uterine bleeding. Eager to do whatever I could, I set aside an hour each day for applying castor-oil packs and doing visualizations. To help me focus, I gave my uterus a name: Bunny. After all, what better name could there be for a womb than a name representing fertility and procreation? For months I diligently visualized washing my Bunny-womb clean of unhealthy tissue and saw it becoming pink and healthy once again. Over time the abnormal situation seemed to correct itself, and gradually I quit the practice and forgot all about Bunny.

The following May (a brief five months before this pilgrimage) we were vacationing in northwestern France, and I visited a toy store with a friend who was looking for gifts for her grandchildren. Hanging on the wall was a delightfully squeezable, cream-colored, floppy-eared bunny wearing a beige roll-neck sweater. The plush bunny seemed vaguely human; it could stand up (if held) or sit down. It was 13" tall when standing, 9" tall when sitting. I couldn't resist purchasing the rabbit, which I named Honey Bunny.

Back in the US a few weeks later in a bookstore, I purchased a Pat the Bunny (a popular children's book) plush bunny with stumpy arms and upright ears that rustled when touched. This bunny had a firm, springy torso and sat on its bottom, its stubby, almost non-existent legs stretched out in front. I named it Rustle Ears. Then, while waiting for a flight to visit my father in San Diego, I saw a collection of beanbag bunnies and bought several. Although I had had a collection of plush animals when I was a child—a collection that I lined up each night at the head of my bed—I thought it was peculiar that, as an adult, I was suddenly collecting plush bunnies.

Within two weeks of these purchases, I learned the test results from a routine Pap smear. I had uterine cancer. My subconscious, my inner guide, my higher self—my guardian angel?—had been trying to alert me that something was happening to my "bunny-womb," but I hadn't understood the message. Someone else might think the sudden appearance of all these bunnies was a meaningless coincidence, but I preferred to make meaning out of events, and to me the bunnies were an example of synchronicity. The universe had been trying to warn me.

Rustle Ears proved a great help while I lay in bed recovering from surgery. Whenever I had to cough as my lungs cleared out the remains of anesthesia, I would press Rustle Ears' firm torso against me to support my abdominal stitches. Honey Bunny's soft, squeezable body provided comfort of a different sort. Having them nearby felt good and I was grateful for their presence. Perhaps they reminded me of childhood, when life was simpler and reassurance could be found in the arms of a cuddly plush animal.

When we packed for our pilgrimage, we knew the bunnies had to come with us. Talismans, totems—I had no idea what they were or why they were important, but I knew they were part of my journey through cancer.

Sometimes they rode in my fanny pack, which Gary and I referred to as the "Bunny Bag." At other times they were stuffed inside my vest, heads peeking out. I usually hid them when we encountered anyone on the Chemin, but I had failed to do so before we caught up with Collette and Danielle. I could almost hear Honey Bunny saying, "What do you care what people think of you? You'll never see them again anyway!" But I did.

"Should I hide them before we reach a village?" I asked Collette. "I don't want people to think I'm weird."

"No, not at all!" She then quoted a French proverb that stated that those who keep their childlike imagination will go to Heaven. "And since it's in the Bible," she added firmly, "It must be true."

In the distance we saw Montbonnet, spreading up the side of a hill. I groaned. Suddenly I was too fatigued to go on. I was beginning to feel a slight chill, so I reached behind my back for the Polartec vest I had stuck through the stretch cords on my fanny pack. It was gone. With a weary sigh, I realized that I would have to retrace my steps. Frustrated and tired we said goodbye to our new acquiantances.

I dropped my fanny pack on the ground and left Gary sitting in the shade by the side of the road. It was surprisingly easier to walk without the Bunny Bag. I walked for ten minutes but my vest was not in sight. Since I didn't have the energy to go further, I turned around and headed back.

Gary had had a chance to rest and felt refreshed. We started again, going downhill before going up. We saw Collette and Danielle leaving the Chapelle Saint-Roch, an early thirteenth-century Romanesque chapel dedicated to a Frenchman (1295 - 1327) who became the patron saint of plague victims. The chapel had originally been dedicated to Saint James and later rededicated to a popular local saint. In the seventeenth century it was rededicated again, this time to Saint Roch, whose popularity was on the rise. Even saints pass in and out of fashion.

Collette and Danielle offered each of us a square of bittersweet chocolate, which we gladly accepted. Chocolate had been a mainstay

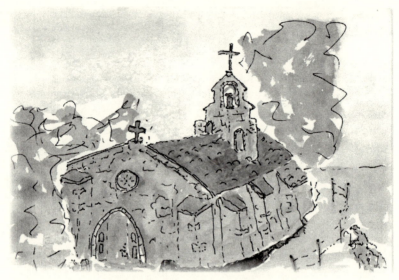

Chapelle Saint-Roch, Montbonnet

on our Spanish Camino, providing instant energy and a caffeine jolt. Throwing nutritional caution to the winds, I vowed to purchase several bars at the next opportunity.

Learning that I had not found my vest, Collette suggested, "Perhaps you can ask the innkeeper where you are staying to drive you back down the road to look for it."

I nodded. "Good idea. But we don't know where we'll stay tonight."

"Oh my," she replied, pursing her lips. "I booked the first night in advance. Since we are past the tourist season, many places are closed." She thought a moment. "Perhaps you would like to stay where we are staying? I made reservations at the *chambres et table d'hôtes†* of Monsieur Xavier de Grossouvre. I reserved dinner as well as a room."

Gary and I immediately agreed. It would be nice to spend more time with Collette and Danielle; besides, they would be able to translate for us if the innkeeper didn't speak English.

When we reached Montbonnet—or rather, the foot of Montbonnet, since the village extended upward toward the crest of the hill—Collette asked directions from a woman pushing a covered pram down the street. After a brief exchange, Collette headed up the street; we followed. How easy it is, I thought, when you speak the language.

But it soon became clear that Collette couldn't find the B&B. The directions were wrong or maybe they were incomplete. When Gary and I got lost in France, which happened regularly, we assumed it was because we had misunderstood the directions. Now I realized that wasn't necessarily the case. Collette was a native speaker and she, too, had been given poor instructions.

We were lost but soon we were found. Muttering something about how most *gites* have a sign posted on the side, Collette finally located the *gite*, a narrow, triangular stone building by the side of the road. Behind it were another stone building, presumably Monsieur Grossouvre's home, and a large open shed from which emanated a lot of noise. Monsieur Grossouvre was at work with some kind of power tool. Collette managed to get his attention at last, and he walked over to us.

A tall, distinguished-looking man with a graying beard and slightly graying hair pulled back into a ponytail, Monsieur did not look pleased. He and Collette had a heated exchange, something about how he had told her to send a deposit and she hadn't. She explained that was because she had only made the reservations a few days earlier and she didn't think the check would arrive in time. He declared he was not a *restaurateur* (a restaurant owner) and he was not prepared to make dinner after all. Collette tried to defend her perspective, but he did not seem interested.

Then Collette gestured toward us and indicated that we also hoped to stay at the *gite*. Monsieur looked us over and decided we were acceptable guests. Grumbling a bit, he agreed to make dinner after all.

The *gite* was an old storage building that he had recently converted into three guest rooms, one on each floor. Our room was on the second floor, reached by a curving wood staircase. The meter-thick stone walls of our room were covered with a thick coating of fresh white plaster; the furniture was new, the mattress firm, the toilet and shower modern. A radiator provided hot-water heat. We were grateful for the well-appointed accommodations.

Dinner would be at 8:00 p.m., Monsieur informed us, as he turned on the radiators. He would do what he could about dinner, he said haughtily, but given such late notice, we shouldn't expect too much. Then he left.

We discussed for far too long our host's bad temper. At last I changed the topic. "Tomorrow we have reservations at Monistrol-d'Allier at a large hotel. I am sure there will be room for you there, if you want to stay."

Collette smiled. "That will be fine."

We said goodbye and went to our respective rooms.

Wearily, Gary and I stretched out on the cold bed in our un-heated room. Nothing retains the cold like stone walls, so it would take a while for the room to warm up.

How quickly we had raised our level of expectation. Half an hour earlier we didn't know where we would stay or where we would eat dinner. Now we were complaining about the cold. So much for living in a state of gratitude.

We soon made several disturbing discoveries. First, although the radiators were on, they were providing no heat. Second, the toilet didn't flush. Worse than that, there was no water in the sink faucet. We had drained our bottles of drinking water while walking the Chemin, expecting to be able to refill them. Thirst suddenly became overwhelming.

I reconciled myself to not eating until 8:00 p.m.; I reconciled myself to the cold; but I could not reconcile myself to being thirsty. Dragging myself downstairs, I knocked on Collette and Danielle's door and explained the problem. They also had no water. So I went outside and found Monsieur Grossouvre. After a moment's puzzle-ment, he remembered that, indeed, there was no water; they were repairing the water storage system for the town, and the water would be turned off until 7:00 p.m. We would simply have to wait until then, he said dismissively.

Not willing to wait that long for something to drink, Gary and I walked up into the village. *Miam Miam Dodo* listed a café and a bar in Montbonnet. They were both closed, however, presumably because there was no water.

Trying to take my mind off my thirst, I decided to ask Monsieur Grossouvre if he would help me find my vest. This required some advance planning since I had to dredge my memory for a few French phrases that would explain my need. Hesitantly, I went up to the work shed and knocked. He stopped what he was doing and listened to my plea. Nodding affably, he said he would drive me back to find the vest, but his car was in the repair shop until 5:00 p.m. When it was ready, he would let me know.

I was filled with gratitude—not only that he was so agreeable but also that I had been able to make myself understood. I felt hopeful that we would be able to get our needs met on this journey, despite our limited French. Walking in faith, living in faith. Always another opportunity.

At 5:00 p.m. Monsieur Grossouvre fetched Gary and me and we drove back over country lanes, but there was no sign of my vest. I was ready to give up when I saw it, carefully placed on a fence railing by some pilgrim or hiker, waiting for me to reclaim it. Monsieur Crossouvre drove us back to the *gîte* while I thanked him profusely.

Soon Gary was snoring on the bed next to me. I was too cold to sleep, although the room was warming up. And finally there was water. How sweet it tasted.

Now that my thirst was assuaged, my hunger took precedence, but there was nothing to do but wait. Through the window, I watched the sky turn black. A cold drizzle descended.

At the appointed time the four of us braved the chill night air and hurried over to Monsieur Grossouvre's house. I had dressed for dinner by putting on my pile vest; Collette, on the other hand, had knotted a silk scarf around her neck. How very French.

The door to Monsieur Grossouvre's house was open a crack; bright yellow light spilled out into the dark, rain-flecked night. Our host, who had changed into a white shirt and black pants for dinner, greeted us at the door. A fire blazed in the fireplace.

The huge stone-lined hearth took up almost an entire wall of the large room; an embroidered cloth hung down a foot or so from the mantle to prevent smoke from drifting back into the room. Inside the fireplace—which was almost large enough to walk into—a large covered pot hung suspended on a rod over the flames. Lace curtains adorned the windows of the room; old wooden chairs were arranged around a rough table in front of the hearth. A worn Oriental rug lay underfoot.

Monsieur Grossouvre began by offering us a refreshing mixture of wine and cassis while we nibbled on chunks of sliced bacon. We warmed ourselves in front of the fire and had a convivial conversation—or rather, Danielle, Collette, and Xavier did. (We were now on a first-name basis.) Although at first everyone tried to speak English, it was difficult for Xavier, and the conversation soon shifted to French. I understood some of it, enough to know that when he bought the house it had been empty for fifty years; he had had to rebuild the interior from floor to ceiling; his daughter was an art student; and he actively supported local craftspeople, including makers of artisan farm products.

Periodically Xavier checked the contents of the pottery casserole, which was called a *diable* or "devil" and was filled with potatoes. Satisfied with the potatoes' progress, he invited us to sit down at the dinner table, a large, old wooden table in the other half of the living room. He, Collette, and Danielle discussed the wine selection at length. Then he served us a large salad of fresh, slivered carrots and plump raisins, dressed with vinegar and olive oil. We passed large chunks of bread around in a basket. The dark, chewy bread was one-quarter rye, according to our epicurean host.

While we devoured the sweet and tangy carrot salad, lamb chops sizzled on the grill. Xavier got up frequently to check them and the potatoes. Then he brought them both to the table and served us. The potatoes were fragrant, moist, and earthy, a perfect compliment to the meat. Scented with herbs, grilled over the open fire, the lamb chops were delectable. Xavier stated with pride that the lamb came from Bains' black sheep—a declaration that meant nothing to me but much to him. He opened another bottle of local wine and re-filled our glasses.

And then, with a flourish, the final course: cheese. And what cheeses! St Nectaire, soft and flowing, smelling of meadows, and a large wheel of blue cow's-milk cheese from nearby Mont Mezenc, called *la bouche du Mezenc*. It was creamy, smooth, and elegant, melting like butter in the mouth but with a delicious salty tang. Xavier instructed Danielle on the proper way to cut the wheel—horizontally, like Stilton, so that it would keep well—but either she didn't understand or she didn't pay attention. She cut it in wedges, slicing halfway down into the wheel. When he saw what she had done, his gracious demeanor disappeared for a moment, but he quickly recovered himself.

Several hours passed in convivial conversation and gastronomical delight. What an unexpected pleasure to spend the evening of the first day of our pilgrimage in a 300-year-old house discussing art, fine wine, and politics, and eating excellently prepared, thoughtfully selected food. Gradually the conversation, like the fire, died down, and it was time to go to bed. Well fed and happy, we waved goodbye and braved the chilly, damp night air to toddle across the yard to our now-toasty rooms.

Wednesday, October 9, 2002. Montbonnet to Monistrol-d'Allier. 12 1/2 kilometers (~7.7 miles). Every kilometer counts.

Xavier provided the standard French breakfast fare: coffee, tea, *infusion*, or hot chocolate; bread or toast; and *confitures†* (jams and fruit preserves). Emboldened, I asked for cheese. After a moment's hesitation, he took the cheese tray out of the pantry and set it before us. We demolished half of the delectable *bouche du Mezenc*—an indulgence that we paid for, since he added an extra charge to our bill.

As soon as we started walking, it began to drizzle. A stiff, cold wind drove the rain against us like tiny pellets. Immediately we ran for cover under a tree and quickly unpacked our raingear. Danielle and Collette donned hooded nylon ponchos that almost reached the ground and covered their backpacks, giving them a hunchbacked appearance. Gary and I struggled into our high-tech rain gear. The rain pants had full-length zippers, which meant we didn't have to take our boots off to put them on, but it took some practice to figure out what zipped to what.

Meanwhile the wind whipped our companions' ponchos, which they tried unsuccessfully to hold down. I remembered the wind-swept couple we had seen a few days earlier as we drove up to Le Puy. There but for the grace of God, I had thought. And here, by the grace of God, we were.

We walked steadily up a walled lane through a plateau with fields on either side. Eventually the rain stopped and the wind died down. The trail climbed steeply into the woods. At last it leveled out and became a forest path that meandered through semi-shaded conifer woods. Grey-green lichen hung down from the trees. Scallop shells painted on tree trunks reminded us of the overlap between the GR 65 and the Chemin de Saint-Jacques.

The red-and-white blazons of the GR showed the way; a large red and white "X" indicated the turns we were not supposed to take. Because the GR 65 is a hiking trail, it is clearly waymarked both coming and going. In contrast, the Spanish Camino is marked with yellow arrows painted on walls, sidewalks, and trees, which point in only one direction. Although historically pilgrims walked to San-tiago and then retraced their steps home (they had no other option), modern pilgrims usually walk only one way.

Collette and Danielle often walked ahead of us. Several times they went the wrong way at a crossing of trails, not noticing the red-and-white blazon on a tree trunk or road sign. We would whistle loudly and point them in the right direction. We showed them how to spot the blazons, but our instructions didn't help. Collette peered closely at the GR topo-map instead of the waymarked trees, and Danielle looked down at the path in front of her feet.

The forest was carpeted with mushrooms. Although we found the damp, chilly weather uncomfortable, mushrooms thrived in it. Some were large bugles, 6" across, resembling a kind of misshapen lily. Others were spotted bright red or yellow or brown. Collette warned us that, as a rule, the most beautiful ones were the most poisonous.

Every so often the forest would open up, revealing stunning vistas of distant hills burning with orange and crimson from the turning leaves. Our footpath descended into the hamlet of Le Chier, marked by a tall wayside cross. We continued to descend steadily, our path a narrow walled lane. At the bottom of the valley we crossed a slippery wooden bridge constructed of two parallel tree trunks stretched over a stream. Then we climbed back up to the country road and followed it into Saint-Privat-d'Allier, a village spread out along the side of a tree-covered hill. We had managed to walk seven kilometers (four and one-half miles) in time for lunch.

Although *Miam Miam Dodo* listed several shops, bars, and a *boulangerie* in the town, it was past the tourist season and they were closed. The Vielle Auberge, however, was willing to make sandwiches. Slabs of St Nectaire cheese arrived, wedged between thick slices of chewy country bread.

After lunch we visited the twelfth-century church and took photos. The walls were dark volcanic stone; modern stained-glass windows brightened the interior of the church. Collette and Danielle knew a great deal about church architecture; they told me more than I wanted to know.

Then it was time to go back on the road. Periodically the GR departed from the zigzagging country road and went steeply uphill on stony footpaths instead. I knew we were saving distance, but we were not saving energy. Were we following a more "authentic" route across country? I doubted it.

I asked Collette why Danielle was making the Chemin, and she said something mysterious about "She's going through an important life change."

Traveling companions on the Chemin are a bit like strangers on a plane, veiling and unveiling, revealing and disguising, as they share deep truths and shallow opinions with people they might never see again. Was it safer to share with people you didn't know, people who presumably have no judgment about you? Or did the Chemin bring out the desire to share the past along with sharing the present?

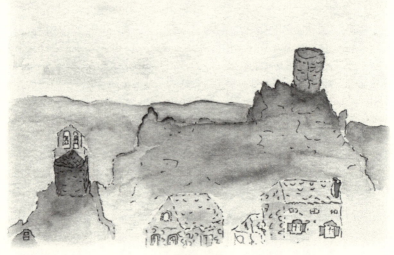

Rochegude

In the distance a large, crumbling tower thrust into the sky from a rocky belvedere above a group of brown stone houses with red tile roofs. The broken tower was all that remained of a once-impressive château. Next to it and slightly below was an open bell tower on top of the tiny chapel of Rochegude.

Bypassing the village, we continued up a rocky track to the chapel, walking carefully because the ground was slick with rain and the wind had returned in full force. The chapel, dedicated to Saint James, soared like an eagle but held on tight to the rock. Fighting each step of the way against the wind, we were grateful that the heavy wooden door was unlocked.

As soon as I walked in, I felt a huge rush of energy—from the bedrock that formed the floor? From the centuries of worship? Shaken, I sat down on a small bench. There was power in a place that for nearly 1,000 years had provided shelter for pilgrims, protecting them from raging tempests, from the wind that battered against the solid stone walls. For centuries the chapel had clung to the rock, a haven in times of storm—meteorological or otherwise.

Fresh flowers adorned the altar, and a small statue of Saint James stood on a stone ledge protruding from the wall. He was indeed with us on our journey. We rested for a little while. Then, after a prayer of thanksgiving, we started off again.

Our precipitous path went downhill. The views were awesome but our trail was treacherous. It was also exceedingly slippery when wet. Jagged rocks, slick stones, steps carved into the hillside—Gary and I appreciated having spring-loaded hiking staffs. They were adjustable in height for going up and down hill and cushioned the shock to our shoulders.

At the bottom of the gorge the GR 65 became a walled lane, then a grassy trail, then a footpath, which once again wound its way steeply down to the road, then up and down hills as it criss-crossed the highway. At one point we ignored the strenuous GR and opted for the gentler country lane. Then we forked off the road and followed another vertiginous stone footpath that led to Monistrol-d'Allier. We found our way down to the highway and walked along the narrow sidewalk until we reached the Hôtel-Restaurant des Gorges, where we had left our luggage two days before. It had taken us two and one-half hours to walk 5.5 kilometers (3.4 miles) from Saint-Privat to Monistrol.

This time the hotel had an "Open" sign propped against the front window. Again we rang the doorbell and waited. Again the disgruntled woman eventually answered the door. She was surprised to see four of us, not two.

Collette, the spokesperson for their pair, explained that they would like to stay there also. The woman said they were closed for the season, but she would see what she could do. She asked if we wanted dinner, and Collette asked what she would serve. Soup, turkey cutlet, vegetables, French fries, fruit, and cheese.

"How much?" Asked Collette.

"$15.00 each."

Collette whispered something to Danielle, then said, "We'll let you know."

"Let me know by 4:00 p.m. so I can buy groceries," the woman snapped.

"Of course," Collette replied.

As the woman led us to our rooms, Collette whispered that she thought $15.00 was a great deal to pay for such a boring meal. She was sure we could do better in the village. We didn't argue; after all, this was her country and surely she knew what was reasonable.

Our room was small but clean, and the luggage we had left a few days earlier was waiting inside. We had managed to be reunited.

Relieved to have a change of clothes, we washed the mud out of our pants. Our laundry supplies included travel soap, high-tech microfiber camp towels, and a rubber clothesline. We stretched the clothesline from the shower rod to the bathroom door hinge, forming a hazardous obstacle at throat height.

Then Collette, Danielle, Gary, and I followed the GR 65 into town, crossing a metal suspension bridge over the river Allier, which rushed wildly below our feet. The houses of Monistrol spread out on the other side of the steep gorge we had just struggled down.

As we walked into town we talked about our plans. Collette and Danielle intended to walk to Aumont-Aubrac and then catch a train back to Lille on Sunday, five days from now.

"Would you be agreeable to walking with us until then?" I asked, a bit shyly.

"Of course!"

"If so, would you make reservations for us where you are staying?"

Collette smiled and lowered her eyes coyly. "I would be delighted!"

We crossed the bridge over the river Allier and walked up the main street. Much to our dismay, all the shops and restaurants were closed, except for the ubiquitous smoky bar.

When Collette asked the bartender if he served dinner, he replied, "No." When she asked if he could make us sandwiches, he said, "No." When she asked if there was anywhere to purchase food, he said, "No." We got the idea.

Collette was downcast. "I was sure we would find somewhere better to eat!"

"What should we do?" I asked.

"We'll have to call Madame at the hotel and ask her to make us dinner."

"But it's already 5:00 p.m.. She said to tell her by 4:00 p.m.," I pointed out.

"I'll have to plead."

We wandered around town until we found a public phone booth. Collette closeted herself inside and carried on an impassioned conversation. She hung up the phone, looking relieved.

"Will she make dinner?"

"Yes. She was upset, but I told her we had been visiting the town and simply forgot to call."

Collette showed us several marked-up pages from *Miam Miam Dodo*. Did we have any preferences for the next nights' lodgings? We shook our heads. Where we stayed was up to her, but we would like a *gran lit* (large bed) and a private bathroom. She nodded and peered at the pages, holding them close to her eyes. Then she returned to the phone booth. After numerous calls, we had reservations for room, dinner, and breakfast for the next few days.

Sobered by our near-miss for dinner, we lost interest in sightseeing. We trudged up the road to the hotel and rested until 8:00 p.m.

Dinner was a pleasant surprise: carrot salad (apparently a typical regional menu item), juicy turkey cutlets, mixed vegetables, and a platter of delectable local cheeses. After complaining about our late notice, our hostess became quite affable.

Partway through dinner, Gary had difficulty swallowing. Whatever he was eating literally "stuck in his craw," and he was unable to swallow it or anything else, including liquid and his own saliva. This had happened before. Sometimes the spasm would release quickly; other times it took more than an hour; occasionally it required a visit to a hospital emergency room.

I knew what was going on because he gestured toward his throat. I also knew that trying to be helpful was not appreciated. He abruptly stood up and excused himself. As the minutes passed and he didn't return, Collette began to worry.

"Is he all right?" she asked me.

"He's having indigestion," I explained. "It happens sometimes." I didn't feel like explaining that he was having a throat spasm. That was his story to tell, not mine.

"Shouldn't we do something?"

"There's not much we can do."

"Will he want the rest of his dinner?"

"I doubt it."

I tried not to worry. As a friend of mine once said, "It's better to pray than to worry." So I prayed silently.

Making conversation, Collette asked what my religion was and I said, a bit disingenuously, "Unitarian Universalism." They understood about our plush bunny companions, but I wasn't sure they would understand about our Sufi practices.

Collette looked puzzled. "What's Unitarian Universalism?"

"It's a very liberal denomination.

"Is it Christian?"

"Well, sort of, but *very* liberal. It honors all religious traditions."

"So you believe in God?"

Again I hesitated, thinking that many UUs didn't. But I wasn't speaking for them, I was speaking for myself. "Well, yes, but not in a personified god that wears a white robe and sits in a throne in heaven. I believe in a universal presence, of which we are all a part, that is the perfection of love, harmony, and beauty."

Many UUs would have agreed with this statement, even though they might have difficulty with the phrase, "the perfection of love, harmony, and beauty," which was part of the Sufi Order's invocation.

Collette looked a bit puzzled. "So you believe that 'God is love'?"

"That's one way of putting it," I replied.

"Well, so do I!" she said enthusiastically, perhaps relieved to learn that although we weren't Catholic, we shared a basic theological understanding.

While I finished nibbling on some cheese, I pondered my prevarications. I preferred to be honest but I was worried about what our new friends would think if I said we weren't Christian. Why did I care? What was I afraid of? Why did I feel the need to hide who I really was? After all, the worst that could happen was that we would stop walking together. Maybe I wasn't really lying, I was just avoiding controversy—or so I told myself, rationalizing even further.

Madame suggested, "Would your husband like some hot tea?"

"That's a good idea," I said, eager to change the topic. I knew, however, that when Gary's throat was in spasm, he couldn't swallow anything, including tea.

Madame brought a cup of tea and I dutifully took it to our room, along with Gary's dinner. Eventually, as it usually did, the spasm released and Gary was able to sip the warm, flavored water.

"Any idea why it happened?" I asked, beginning a post mortem of the situation.

"I don't know. I never have liked turkey. Maybe my system was in revolt. Or maybe I wasn't paying enough conscious attention to eating."

"Are you hungry?"

"Not at all."

"You need to eat something."

"I'm not going to eat anything right now," he replied, a bit testily. "I don't want to eat just before going to bed. You know that always gives me indigestion."

"Right."

Exhausted by the events of the day, we were soon sound asleep.

Thursday, October 10, 2002. Monistrol to Saugues. 12 kilometers (7.5 miles).

After breakfast of bread and jam (I had given up trying to get protein), we lugged our suitcases down to the front desk. Our hosts had agreed to transport them to our next stop, the farmhouse "Chez Martins." I knew we would be repeating this scenario every day, and I wondered whether our luggage would always arrive where it was supposed to. Gary and I discussed whether we should lock the bags. If we did, it might look like there was something worth stealing. If we didn't, it might seem like an invitation. We decided to have faith that everything would work out the way it was supposed to—*and* the way we wanted it to.

The morning fog began to thin by the time we crossed over the bridge into Monistrol. We had to hike out of the river gorge, passing by the Chapelle de la Madeleine perched halfway up the hillside. The chapel, still shrouded in mist, looked Lilliputian. Huge rock outcroppings poked out from the trees that covered the precipitous walls of the gorge.

We crossed over the river Ance and began ascending a country road that zigzagged uphill. At a metal wayside cross we turned left up the stony track that led to the chapel. The rain splattered down. The track was treacherous, but eventually we reached the small chapel, nestling under an overhang of stratified rock, held like a delicate morsel within a gaping stone mouth. Shallow niches had been hollowed out of the cliff face to the side of the chapel, spaces large enough for someone to lie down in.

I had seen similar alcoves carved into the side of the volcanic plug of Saint-Michel-d'Aiguilhe in Le Puy. I was sure they had been used for dream incubation, an ancient practice where one slept near or in a holy place and asked for healing or guidance to come in one's dreams. Although the Chapel of the Magdalene had been built in the seventeenth century, the grotto was probably an ancient holy site co-opted by Christianity.

The chapel door was locked. A sign posted on a wall urged people not to use the place as a toilet. Apparently not everyone respected the sacredness of the place.

Our path became a series of steps with a hand railing on one side; without that, we might have slid back down the rain-slick trail. At the top of the gorge was the hamlet of Escluzels. Most of its houses were closed for the season. We walked on, continuing hard uphill on a wide forest path. At last we reached Montaure, another boarded-up village.

A sign advertised pilgrims' staffs. Curious, we strolled over to a nearby farmhouse. Alfred Cubizolles, farmer and craftsman, maker of staffs, proudly showed us his collection of hand-carved paraphernalia. Collette was looking for a hiking staff, but none of these was quite what she had in mind. I took Monsieur's photo and offered to send it to him, but he wasn't interested: he had lots of photos, he said.

"Are you going to mention him in your book?" Collette asked.

I smiled. "I really don't know. I'll have to see."

Collette didn't realize that being mentioned in a book is not always a pleasant experience.

We had climbed to the top of a high plateau where herds of sheep grazed peacefully in green pastures. A shepherd standing under an open umbrella nodded to us as we walked by in the rain. A sign advertised a *hôtel-restaurant/gîte d'etape†* twenty-nine kilometers beyond Saugues, proudly announcing they had been awarded the *petite fleur* of hospitality by *Miam Miam Dodo*. In medieval times, hostel-owners sent "front men" ahead to lure pilgrims to their establishments; modern-day innkeepers use wooden signs.

Hungry and wet, we found shelter from the rain inside a barn redolent with the fragrance of now-absent animals. I wasn't sure what might be hiding in the hay, so I propped myself against an iron-rimmed cartwheel to eat a meager snack of energy bars and an apple. The grocery stores in Monistrol had all been closed, and Madame at the hotel had not had any extra bread or cheese to make us sandwiches. I remembered with longing of the stale roll I had been given at the pilgrims' blessing in Conques. I had imagined there might come a time when I wished I had that roll; I hadn't expected the time to arrive so soon.

Collette plied us with questions about the Spanish Camino. Was it safe? Where would one stay? Could it be done if you didn't speak Spanish? I explained that, as far as I knew, it was safe; that there were numerous inexpensive pilgrims' hospices called *refugios†* along the Camino; and that she would generally be able to find someone who spoke French or English, although it would be wise to learn simple phrases in Spanish. Collette sounded alternately doubtful and encouraged.

The drizzle stopped while we continued hiking through semi-shaded woods, up and down forest trails and country lanes with fields on either side. At one point Collette and Danielle walked ahead and took another wrong turn. Although Collette had the GR topo-guide and looked at it frequently, her vision was so poor that she couldn't relate that information to the real world. The map was not the territory. I whistled loudly and waved my arms. They stopped and turned around, waiting for us to catch up.

"You're going the wrong way," I explained, a bit out of breath.

Collette was adamant. "No, this is correct." She held the guidebook map up to her thick glasses.

Gary explained, "You missed the blazon on the tree back there."

"Really?"

We nodded, walked back to the intersection, and pointed at the mark.

"Well, I guess you're right," she said.

I had often gotten lost on the Spanish Camino in 1982. Though the route was marked with yellow arrows, they were often lacking at crucial intersections. At the time it had been an opportunity to contemplate what it meant to lose one's way and how one found it again. I had thought the well-marked GR 65 would remove that metaphoric possibility, but instead it offered other opportunities.

As we walked together, Collette explained that she had bad cataracts but the doctors wanted to wait until they were worse before they did surgery. In the meantime she had difficulty seeing anything in the distance—and that distance, we realized, included anything further than arms-length away. Danielle, on the other hand, had no trouble seeing, but she seemed oblivious to her surroundings.

Collette whispered to me that Danielle's husband was initiating divorce proceedings, which she found excruciatingly painful. I wondered whether that explained her passivity or was the result of it.

When I walked beside Gary, I told him about Collette's limited vision. "I wonder what they would do without us to guide them," I mused.

"They would get lost a lot. Interesting, isn't it, how we help each other out? They speak French and help us make reservations, but they have trouble following the Chemin. We have difficulty making reservations but we have no trouble finding the way."

I nodded. "We each have something to offer each other. How fortunate that we found each other the first day on the Chemin."

"What do you think? Is it synchronicity or serendipity? A meaningful event or just plain good luck?"

"Synchronicity, of course." But after a moment's thought, I added, "Maybe it *is* just luck, but it feels more meaningful than that.

I feel like we're connected to something much greater than ourselves—and we're being given lots of reminders."

Gary nodded.

I continued, "And it doesn't just happen to us. It's something a
number of pilgrims comment on. How help shows up when they
need it; how they round a corner and find just what they were looking for.... When things like that happen, it's an opportunity to af-
firm the interconnectedness of everything—the *meaningfulness* of
what happens in our lives. At least that's how I make meaning out
of it."

We walked on in silence.

The route into the next village was flooded, so we hopped onto
tall stones that lined the path; gently holding onto the barbed wire
that was strung along the top of the stone wall, we managed to get
past the worst of it without falling into calf-deep mud. Eventually
the Chemin started descending again. In the distance were the red
tile roofs of Saugues, population 2000.

Our path passed by several large wooden sculptures. Dark and
abstract, they were constructed to commemorate the *Año Santo*†
1993. When Saint James's feast day (July 25) falls on a Sunday, that
year is a Holy Year during which pilgrims can earn a plenary indul-
gence† for their sins by going to Santiago de Compostela on foot
or bicycle, or by car, train, or airplane. The method of travel doesn't
matter, according to the Church, only the arrival and participation
in certain rites.

I wondered whether the Church didn't prefer the Catholic pilgrims who arrived in Compostela by bus or train, or on organized
excursions. They were a known quantity, unlike the hodge-podge
array of Christian and non-Christian people on a spiritual quest,
or having an adventure, or enjoying a hike, or seeking an esoteric
awakening, who walked the Camino. For this latter group the journey was what mattered, even if they looked forward to their arrival
in Santiago—or not. After all, we were making a pilgrimage on the
Chemin de Saint-Jacques that wasn't going to end anywhere near
Compostela—and yet I had no doubt it was a pilgrimage.

We made our way into Saugues. Carved, cast, and ceramic mushrooms of various sizes and shapes filled the shop windows, along with decorative wooden clogs (sabots) and posters showing "La Bête du Gévaudan," a large black animal somewhere between a mangy wolf and a monster. Obviously, the town catered to tourists.

We visited the information office to pick up brochures and get directions to the Accueil à la Ferme Chez Martins, a highly recommended (three wheat heads and a *petite fleur*) *gîte à la ferme†*, located at their farm. Chez Martins was on the outskirts of the other side of town. Drenched and tired, we arrived at last at a modern stone and stucco building. A large wooden scallop shell adorned the porch.

Madame Martins, a short woman with black hair, a red face, and a loud voice, greeted us warmly. Collette, I noticed, made a particular effort to respond courteously. I wished my knowledge of French would enable me to behave with proper etiquette, but it didn't. I could usually make myself understood, but not graciously.

Tea and cookies were waiting for us on the large plank table in the dining room. While we warmed ourselves inside and out, a bedraggled young woman knocked on the door. After a brief conversation with Madame Brigitte, she joined us at the table. The Swiss pilgrim was staying at the communal *gîte*, which, she informed us, was a nasty, cold pit of a place. She was inquiring whether she could stay at Chez Martin the following night. Why not tonight, I queried? She had already settled in and it was too much effort to move, she explained. We commiserated with her. Looking somewhat revived, she left.

Our rooms were upstairs. And they were warm. The wood-burning stove in the kitchen vented heat to the guest rooms. After changing clothes, I called my father on my cell phone to hear his latest medical report. His kidneys were not doing well; the doctors had lowered his heart medicines and now they were cutting his diuretic. They were trying to strike a balance between treating his congestive heart failure and damaging his kidneys. I assured him we were doing fine. Jesse had been keeping in touch with him, so even though I was far away, he knew that help was nearby.

Gary and I strolled back into town to see the sights and find something to eat. We bought a small quiche Auvergnate (named for the Auvergne region through which we were walking) at a *char-cuterie†*, the French equivalent of a deli. Potatoes, *bleu d'Auvergne* cheese, and dried ham filled the quiche. The clerk heated it up in the microwave and we gobbled up the fragrant snack.

Fortified, we began our sightseeing tour at the Église de Saint-Médard, with its octagonal twelfth-century Romanesque bell tower, a style peculiar to the Auvergne. (Spanish octagonal churches are associated with the Knights Templar, who built round and octago-nal churches after returning from the Middle East, where they saw such architecture. But that didn't necessarily mean the Auvergne bell towers were related to the Templars, even though there were numer-ous Templar establishments in France.)

An exquisitely carved, thirteenth-century Virgin in Majesty (so-called because, like Sainte Foy, she was seated on a throne) was dis-played behind a locked metal grill inside the church. She appeared solemn, serene, and inscrutable, the red, green, and gold paint on her carved robe still visible though faded with time. A close-fitting blue hood rimmed in gold covered her head. The Christ child sat on her lap, one hand raised to bless the world, the other holding a Bible. He had an adult face but a child's body. Mary held the child affection-ately, one hand on his left thigh, the other on his chest.

A nearby plaque stated, "The Virgin is the *sedes sapientae*, the fit-test throne to carry the eternal wisdom, the Son of God." Sophia, the ancient "seat of Wisdom," had become the lap that Jesus sat upon.

Gary suggested we light candles of gratitude, and I jokingly wondered if he had converted. In fact, we both had converted to the practice of giving thanks for all that life brings—at least when we remembered. We bought several tapers and lit them in thanksgiving for our journey.

Then we left the church and strolled around town, admiring the varied marketing ploys. Mushrooms, real and sculpted; wooden shoes, miniature and large; and the legend of the Beast of Gévaudan ensured that something in the town would appeal to everyone.

Saugues called itself the "Door to Gévaudan." Located between the Margeride mountains and the Valley of the Allier, it had been the center of the terrible deeds of the Bête du Gévaudan. According to the story (a mix of fact and legend), from summer 1764 to June 1767 a horrific beast killed 100 women and children and ate some of them. Soldiers tried to hunt it down. The bishop of Mende declared it a "scourge of God" and ordered public prayers. The beast ignored the prayers and traveled widely, slaughtering as it went.

On January 12th, 1765, the monster attacked a group of seven children near Saugues. The eldest, a twelve-year-old boy, defended them bravely and was congratulated by government officials. According to the story, his valor enabled him to study to become an officer. The next month 20,000 troops, along with numerous local men and foreign bounty hunters, tried to locate the beast, hoping to win the huge reward offered by the King. It was not to be found. In August, a courageous woman defended herself with a bayonet and hurt the beast—or a beast. But the slaughters continued.

On September 20th, 1765, Francois Antoine killed an enormous 130-pound wolf, which he had stuffed and took to the king at Versailles. As a reward, he obtained the right to put the Beast of Gévaudan on his crest. The beast was dead and the matter finished, as far as the authorities were concerned.

But it wasn't. The killings continued and people were terrified. Was it really a wild animal causing such mayhem? One had to wonder, given its carefully selected victims. Finally, on June 19th, 1767, a large, woman-and-child-eating, wolf-like creature was killed by Jean Chastel and quickly but inadequately preserved. It was five feet long, two and one-half feet tall; its mouth opened seven inches, and its jaw was seven inches long.

Chastel took the beast to the king, hoping to gain a reward; after all, *this* was obviously the real monster, wasn't it, since people had continued to be killed until he slaughtered it? Unfortunately, by the time he arrived at the king's court, his trophy had become exceedingly gamy. The king ordered it buried without so much as looking at it. Chastel returned empty handed. Grateful locals included him in the legend, a legend that says as much about human avarice, self-promotion, and political expediency as it does about a marauding beast.

A twenty-foot-high wooden sculpture of a fearsome wolf-creature rears up on its hind legs on a nearby hillside, visible from the highway. Brochures provide detailed directions for driving excursions to nearby towns where statues and steles commemorate "the Beast" and various combats. Saugues has a Bête du Gévaudan museum, complete with diorama, and there is talk of constructing a wolf sanctuary. I hoped that the modern wolves would remain safe from people with over-active imaginations.

Dinner was at 8:00 p.m. We joined Jacky and Brigit Martins, their teenage children, and several other relatives at the large dining table. Brigit ladled steaming vegetable puree, made from home-grown vegetables, into large, shallow soup bowls. After finishing the first course, the family members cleaned their bowls with a piece of bread, so we did the same. We were learning French etiquette—or at any rate, farmhouse etiquette.

A salad of pickled beets, tomatoes, and corn followed, spooned into our now-empty bowls. It was deliciously fresh, grown in their garden and prepared in their kitchen. Following the family's example, I again cleaned my plate with bread. I tried to avoid eating bread, but what could I do?

Brigit then served an oh-so-politically-incorrect main course: stew made from veal fed only on its mother's milk. Jacky joked that we didn't need to worry about mad cow disease—he knew *exactly* what the baby calf had eaten, since they had raised it from birth. The cheese course followed, including a luscious *bouche du niege* (a log of blue and snow-white cow's milk) and a fresh homemade cheese. The latter was dry, crumbly, and sharp, tasting of earth and manure. And then the final course: fruit.

I had eaten in restaurants where every course brought new silverware and dishes; here we ate multiple courses from the same bowl. But our meal was as good as any I had eaten.

Friday, October 11, 2002. Saugues to Chanaleilles. 14 kilometers (8.7 miles).

I kept trying to figure out how to do my morning meditation practices, given that I was never alone. If I woke up before Gary, I could spread a towel out on the floor to form a sacred space and silently recite my prayers and do my breathing practices. Usually he woke up before me, however, and once he was awake it became difficult to focus. I *had* to find a workable routine; otherwise I would end up abandoning my practices, just as I was abandoning my dietary regime. So far my lack of willpower didn't appear to be causing me any health problems, but I was worried—though not enough to do anything about it.

We packed our suitcases, then went downstairs for homemade cheese, plopped out of small plastic containers; homemade jams, including rhubarb and apricot, and banana; toasted bread, left over from the day before; and hot milk, fresh from the cows and then boiled. Collette arranged for transport for our luggage to Chanaleilles.

I asked Brigitte how far it was to Chanaleilles and what the Chemin was like. "Twelve kilometers and flat," she asserted. She was wrong on both counts, but we didn't know that when we started out in the cool (50° F) morning mist, which turned to rain as we walked back into town.

Collette and Danielle had decided to begin the day by going to mass, and Collette was quite pleased when I said we'd go with them. mass was celebrated in a tiny chapel near the medieval Hospital of Saint James. Approximately twenty elderly people attended the service, singing with heartfelt and quite melodic passion. Afterwards the parish priest stamped our pilgrimage credentials with an imprint of the Virgin in Majesty we had seen in the church. The sacred feminine was honored on the Chemin, even if her attributes had been a bit altered over time.

It was market day in Saugues, which was convenient for us since we needed luncheon supplies. Saugues hosts the fourth largest sheep market in France, and open-sided butcher vans displayed various cuts of lamb. Numerous produce sellers had spread their wares on folding tables, protected from the drizzle by colorful, rectangular umbrellas. Banners touted *produits regionaux* (regional products) and *fromages fermiers* (farm cheeses). The fresh mushrooms, the gorgeous cheeses, the crusty breads tempted me, but Gary reminded me that he would have to carry on his back whatever I bought.

I couldn't resist an oversized, hand-felted white beret I found at a tiny shop called "Association d'Insertion au Pays de Saugues." The association helped people who had "had troubles" (e.g., been in prison or psychiatric hospitals) re-enter into community. While I was in the store buying my beret, Collette at last found the staff she wanted. It was wood and had a metal tip, a compass on top, and a strap.

Carrying and wearing our purchases, we hiked out of town and back into the forest. An amazing variety of mushrooms—velvety red ones, shiny brown ones, others that appeared to be covered with melted shredded cheese—poked out of clumps of grass and sprouted from tree stumps.

At one point we had a heated exchange with Collette, who was sure we should take a different route. Adamant, she pointed to the GR topo-guide. Equally adamant, I read aloud from Raju's guidebook, which states that the GR route is a variant that would take us far out of our way. Unwillingly, Collette gave in.

The two guidebooks often coincided but sometimes they didn't. The GR route is for hikers looking for an interesting walk; the Raju guide is for pilgrims willing to walk on pavement occasionally and not wanting to miss important monuments. Neither book consistently follows the original route (which may no longer exist), nor has there ever been just one authentic Chemin. Medieval pilgrims just walked, choosing one route or another depending on the season, the popularity of different shrines, and the availability of companions.

In Spain, the yellow arrows supposedly mark the authentic Camino, and some pilgrims and villagers critique a pilgrimage depending on whether one followed this putatively historic route. In reality, the traditional Camino is frequently buried under highway asphalt or is otherwise inaccessible because of urban development. A modern network of forest trails, country roads, and hiking trails has replaced it, designed to get pilgrims off the highway and into nature or at least less-populated areas. Nonetheless, the debates rage on, emphasizing not the inner quality of one's journey but an irrelevant criterion.

The rain continued. Our high-tech rain jackets didn't cover our packs, which I hoped were waterproof. Collette and Danielle resembled humpbacked, winged creatures, their grey and blue ponchos flapping in the wind. Our feet squished as we trampled on the packed damp leaves. Gary and I walked silently, heads slightly bowed to keep the rain from dripping off the tiny hood visors into our eyes.

As I plodded along, I thought about my interactions. Collette was *very* determined and liked things her way. What annoys us in others is often a reflection of ourselves, so I supposed she was providing me with an opportunity to see something about myself. But it was a distorted reflection, wasn't it? After all, I wasn't *that* opinionated—or was I? Many times when I made a suggestion about where to go or when to stop, she would immediately say "no!" But then if instead of pressing the issue I said, "okay, fine, whatever…." she would reconsider.

Danielle seemed passive in contrast. Collette wanted to walk further than Danielle did (Danielle was concerned, I presumed, about her injured knee), but each day Danielle would go along with Collette's decision. Once I said something about Danielle's injured knee and Collette replied, "Oh, her knee's okay!"

With a sigh, I realized this was an opportunity to examine my habitual patterns of judgment and control. We are all actors, creating our lines as we go—and projecting onto others the roles we want others to play, whether they (or we) realize it or not. It was time to take responsibility and realize that Collette wasn't annoying me; I was annoying myself.

Brigit had said the road was flat but it was not. Perhaps she thought it was level because we weren't descending river gorges—or perhaps because she had driven it but never walked it. We walked through forests carpeted with mushrooms, past trees emblazoned with grey-green lichens and fields speckled with dark green and yellow broom or with the chartreuse sprouts of winter wheat. Black and white cows grazed in meadows. Stone outcroppings lined the trail. Gary, who knows about such things, said the stone is a mixture of feldspar, granite, and schist. I looked more closely and saw a jumble of white, black, and orangey pink crystals.

We passed huge grey and brown stone houses with large attached barns, darker stone frames setting off the doors and windows. The bright-colored flowers in their courtyards softened the somber buildings.

Near La Clauze we found shelter in a woodshed stacked high with kindling. There was a just enough space for us to stand inside, protected from the rain by the overhanging roof-tarp. I took a picture of Gary, Collette, and Danielle leaning nonchalantly against the woodpile, thick slabs of bread and cheese raised to their mouths. Travel-worn Honey Bunny and Rustle Ears had popped out of my fanny pack, which was propped on a stack of firewood.

Suddenly my cell phone rang. Heart pounding, I wondered whether it was my father calling with a health emergency.

"Hello?" I said, breathlessly.

"Hallo," a heavily accented voice replied. It was Dr Penoel, a Provençal specialist in medical aromatherapy†. I had read several of his books, translated into English, and I hoped that his skills could help me avoid a recurrence of cancer. I had tried to arrange an appointment with him from the US but had been unable to reach him. Now, in the depths of *France profunde*—Collette's expression for this isolated countryside—we agreed to meet at his office at the end of October.

I had given up seeing Dr Penoel, yet he had called and the timing for the appointment was perfect. It always is perfect, even the disappointments, even the apparently missed opportunities—but given our limited vision, sometimes we are blind to the perfection. How could it be perfect sometimes and not all the time?

Here in "deepest France" I felt cared for, protected, and watched over. I felt held in God's hands. I surprised myself with this expression, since I didn't find meaning in the concept of an anthropomorphic masculine deity with hands. Yet "held in God's hands" was the feeling that kept coming to me as I opened myself up to embrace and be embraced by a compassionate universe.

We developed a walking routine with Collette and Danielle. If they walked ahead and came to an intersection, they waited for us. If we walked ahead, we made sure they could see us before we continued. That way, they didn't get lost and we didn't have to go find them.

After walking gentle and not-so-gentle uphill and downhill trails through forests, fields, and tiny hamlets, including Le Falzet, we took a kilometer detour off the GR to Chanaleilles. Collette had booked rooms in the local *gite*.

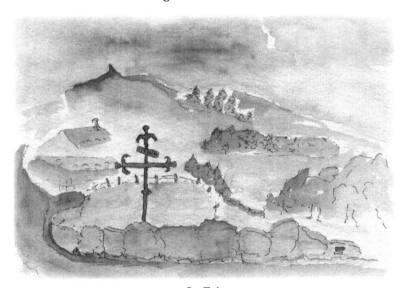

Le Falzet

The *gite* was a new two-story concrete building located at the edge of the village. The main level included a shared public room with a kitchen, fireplace, large table, various books, sofa, chairs, coffee pot, and other paraphernalia.Upstairs were three bedrooms, each with two sets of bunk beds, and a large dormitory that slept twelve. One bedroom was already occupied, so we chose between the other two.

Leaving Collette and Danielle behind, we walked into the village to find the Café du Post; its owners ran the *gîte*. The café was the equivalent to a rural Quick Shop, stocked with everything from candy bars to children's toys to soap to canned *cassoulet* (a thick bean, duck, sausage, and bacon stew) to a large selection of wine—after all, we were in France. We arranged to rent sheets and towels, reserved dinner for the four of us at the café, and made a few purchases, including chocolate, postcards, bread, and cheese.The proprietor made us sandwiches.

While we ate, we conversed in English with a young French pilgrim named Emmanuelle. He was walking thirty kilometers a day and had stopped in Chanaleilles for a mid-afternoon snack. I mentioned I had walked the Spanish Camino twenty years before, and he wanted to know what it was like now. I told him what I knew. Were the dogs really fierce? Not usually. Were there places to stay? Yes, there were inexpensive pilgrims' hospices, called *refugios* or *alberguest*, every day's walk or more frequently along the Camino. He thanked us and strode out the door, eager to reach Spain.

We strolled back to the *gîte* and settled into the communal area. Two Swiss women and a Frenchman were already staying at the *gîte*. One of the Swiss women was slim and attractive, with highlights in her carefully done blond hair. She wore bright red lipstick, lots of eye makeup, and gold jewelry. She looked as if she were on a stroll through downtown Zurich instead of on a pilgrimage. Definitely a fluff-head, I decided, wondering why she was subjecting herself to the discomfort of life on the Chemin.

Her stolid friend had dark, seriously pouffed hair and was intently reading the Bible. Although she indicated she did not like being disturbed, she soon joined in the conversation. She remarked that she walked in the Alps every weekend, but she found the Chemin tiring and had developed painful blisters on her feet. I supposed it was like the difference between a sprint and a marathon.

The Frenchman had met the two women on the Chemin. They were staying an extra day at the *gîte* because the weather was so bad. Tonight he would have to sleep with the ladies, he explained with a smile, since we had reserved the other two rooms in advance.

Collette suggested the Swiss ladies could sleep with her and Danielle, since there were four beds in their room, but Michel assured her they all got along "quite well." I made some comment about a *ménage a trois* and he laughed heartily. Collette whispered to me that my French was really *quite* good.

Gary and I climbed up the hill behind the village to the Romanesque church. The fourteenth-century bell tower had six bells, rung in medieval times to help pilgrims find their way through the fog.

We couldn't find the light switch inside the church, but gradually our eyes adjusted and we saw a statue locked behind a filigreed grate. This is the famous Black Virgin of Villeret. She is carved out of chestnut-colored wood; if she once was painted, all color is gone. Vertical cracks run through her head. Her hands are large, and her arms and torso are disproportionately long. Perhaps at some time the statue was chopped off somewhere below the knees, accentuating these odd proportions. Deeply carved folds in the Virgin's robe and the Christ-child's garment give the sculpture an unexpected gracefulness. She has a weary, pained expression on her face, as if she has a premonition of the suffering she and her child would experience.

It was cold in the church and we couldn't find any candles, so we didn't stay long. Outside, Gary and I wandered through the cemetery, puzzling over the peculiar symbols on some of the tombstones. One was decorated with a twisted rope carved into the stone. We didn't understand the code, but we attempted to make meaning out of it.

Looking out across the fields to the distant hills, I admired the autumnal colors of the hillsides and mused about the countryside we had walked through. I felt both a sense of accomplishment that we'd made it this far—and great humility for all the help we had received.

Sitting on a bench and holding hands, Gary and I discussed the rest of our journey. So far, making arrangements had been easy: Collette had made them. She spent a great deal of energy calling, leaving messages, and then calling again. It was a time-consuming, frustrating process even though she spoke French. The problem (or the challenge) wasn't the language, it was that many *gîtes* and hotels had closed at the end of September. The few that were open were often full or only had one room available, not two. The few lodgings that were open required reservations for room and for dinner; otherwise we would have nothing to eat.

Did we want to try our luck and "take it on faith" that we could find room and food at the inn without reservations? Not likely. Especially not off-season. There's an Arabic saying: "Trust in God but tie your camel to the post." We had brought more supplies (energy bars, supplements, clothes, etc.) than we could carry, so we had to arrange to transport our suitcases—which also meant we had to know in advance where we were stopping for the night.

Collette and Danielle would be going back to Lille in a few days. Would we be able to make the necessary arrangements without them? This was an opportunity to "let go" and practice trust, but I felt anxious, and I couldn't decide whether my concern was reasonable.

Our bodies were holding up surprisingly well. We were a bit stiff but that was to be expected, considering the terrain, the rain, and the chilly temperatures. I found that twelve kilometers (7.5 miles) was a comfortable distance to walk in one day. My legs got tired before that, but if we stopped for a while and rested, I could continue on a bit further.

At 7:30 p.m. we gathered for an early dinner at the Café du Post. Collette and Danielle, Gary and I, the two Swiss women (who had dressed for the occasion), and Michel sat down at a large table in one corner of the café. The woman I had talked with earlier served the meal, running to the kitchen and returning with heaping platters of food that her husband had prepared.

Dinner began with homemade pork-liver pâté and the local *charcuterie d'Auvergne*—regional pork-based products that were justly famous, according to Madame. When Gary and I lived in Spain, we had concluded that the Spanish included pork in every dish from scrambled eggs to mixed vegetables because they wanted to make sure no secret Jews or false *conversos*† had stayed behind after the 1492 expulsion. What better way to unmask them than to serve pork in every course except dessert? But such an explanation was unlikely for the ubiquity of pork in this meal. Maybe it was just inexpensive.

An ample platter of *boeuf bourguignonne* (beef braised in red wine, onions, mushrooms, and bacon) followed the *charcuterie*. Buttered noodles dotted with sautéed *cépes*†, meaty mushrooms picked that morning in the nearby forests, came next. For those of us who still had an appetite, fresh pears were served for dessert.

While we demolished the meal, we had a heated discussion. The Bible-reading Swiss woman proclaimed in excellent English, "I am very disappointed. The Chemin isn't spiritual enough. People are walking it as a *randonnée*†, a long-distance hike, with no sense of the true spirit of it."

I jumped right in. "Even if people begin as excursionists, the Chemin can impact them at a deep level. They can become pilgrims. They have the opportunity to walk in nature, which is where some people get close to God."

She looked at me with icy disapproval. "This is supposed to be a *spiritual* journey, but I see too many people having a good time, enjoying themselves. Like this meal, for example. It's not a proper pilgrimage when you indulge yourselves so much." Never mind, I thought, that she ate as much as any of us.

Michel began to rave about Neale Donald Walsch's book *Conversations with God.* "That book tells the truth. Everything is God," he said. "This tiny crumb of bread is a tiny bit of God! Life should be enjoyed."

Collette added, "Christ enjoyed life, and he had a body, after all, and went around with his disciples, eating grilled fish and drinking wine."

The dark-haired woman vehemently disagreed. "Pilgrimage is not about the body, it is about the soul. Laughing, having a good time—that's not a pilgrimage."

Soon the conversation switched to French, little of which I understood.

After a while, the blond-haired Swiss woman said in English, "All this talk gives me a headache. You're confusing religion and spirit." And she changed the subject. She told us she had a degree in economics (stock-market related) and used to teach but quit two years ago. She wrinkled her nose and said that she could "smell" that Gary was a professor. He grinned and acknowledged that he was a retired music professor.

After my initial, unappreciated foray, I had decided to listen to the conversation and not participate. I immediately noticed how often first impressions were deceptive. Evaluating the blond woman as a "fluff" because she wore makeup and gold jewelry on the pilgrimage, I had decided she wasn't a serious pilgrim. That was just the sort of judgment her friend was making about the rest of us: we were enjoying ourselves so we weren't real pilgrims. As further demonstration of how badly I had misjudged, the blond woman was witty and intelligent, while her dark-haired friend was ignorant and narrow-minded. Wryly, I realized my tendency to be judgmental was like an onion: I peeled off one layer only to discover another.

Saturday, October 12, 2002. Chandeilles to Saint-Alban-sur-Limagnole. 16 – 18 kilometers (10 – 11 miles), depending on whom you believe.

A dream filled with violence and death. Something about my mother... but she had died five years before... I woke shaky, uneasy.... I couldn't remember the details but was determined to shake it off.

We took turns washing up in the bathroom down the hall, packed up our meager possessions, and prepared to go downstairs for breakfast. The door across the hall was open, and I saw Michel sitting on a bed in tight blue briefs, pulling on his socks. He flashed me a big grin.

Breakfast was, as usual, a choice of hot drinks and dry bread with jams. I had given up asking for anything different. Besides, my ankles weren't swelling. Maybe all I really needed to do was get enough exercise. That was easier, and much more pleasurable, than exercising self discipline.

The morning was once again chilly and misty. Striding quickly to warm up and gossiping enthusiastically about the Swiss women and the Frenchman and what they might or might not have been doing the night before, we started out walking in the wrong direction. Gary realized we were going the wrong way but didn't say anything; he thought the road we were on would eventually join the Chemin.

Fortunately, before we had gone too far a car drove by and stopped beside us. The driver leaned out the window and informed us that we were on the wrong road. We thanked him and turned around.

Collette smiled and said, "Our four angels were talking about how to get us back on the Chemin, and they decided to send him."

"Angels?" I asked.

"Everyone has a guardian angel. Surely you know that?"

I hadn't. "An angel? I don't see any."

"Of course not. They're invisible. Besides, they need humans to do their work."

Gary and I had joked about the two women on the labyrinth in Boulder being angels sent from central casting. But we had been joking, hadn't we?

Even though we had angels watching out for us, at least according to Collette, I still felt sad because of my dreams. Quite illogically I whispered in Gary's ear, "There'll be nobody to call me Honey or Sweetie once you're gone—so call me Honey a *lot*—and often!"

He looked surprised but whispered back, "I love you, Honey."

There was no reason to think Gary would die before me. He was nine years older than I but, after all, I was the one who had had cancer.

We decided not to take a detour to the Domaine du Sauvage, a former Knights Templar's compound whose current residents were dedicated to producing organic produce and protecting the Aubrac breed of cattle. I would have liked to visit the Domaine, to experience what it felt like, even though it had been nearly 700 years since any Templars had inhabited it.

The Templars (the Order of the Knights Templar of Saint John of Jerusalem) were a highly controversial group of lay knights established in 1103. The order rapidly rose to great importance and became the first international banking organization (aside from the Jews) in medieval Europe. King Phillip IV of France abruptly disbanded the order on Friday, October 13, 1307, when he raided French Templar strongholds, took many of them prisoners, and arrested their leader, Jacques de Molay. Some say that's why Friday the thirteenth is considered unlucky.

Legends abound about their missing treasure, their secret, perhaps heretical rites, and their mysterious powers. Some alternative historians link them to the origins of the Freemasons; others associate them with the Holy Grail (interpreted as the holy bloodline of the progeny of Mary Magdalene and Jesus) and the Priory of Sion, another mysterious organization. The stories were fascinating, but now was not the time to visit their *domaine*. We had many miles to go that day.

After climbing up a small hill we stopped at the Chapelle Saint-Roch, also known as Chapelle de l'Hospitalet du Sauvage. Destroyed on several occasions, the chapel was last rebuilt in 1901. Originally the location was a hospital for pilgrims and travelers, founded in 1198 and dedicated to Saint James. At some point, Saint Roch had supplanted Saint James, as he had elsewhere on the Chemin. Why a dead French saint was deemed a more potent advocate than a dead apostle I didn't know—unless it was because Saint Roch was a fellow countryman.

The original chapel had been built next to a spring with healing waters. The spring had undoubtedly been there for thousands of years, long before the chapel. A small statue of Saint Roch with his dog was ensconced behind a metal grill in a grey, concrete edifice. Unfortunately, the monument covered up the holy waters.

Country lanes. Light rain. Narrow trails going up and down the hillsides. Attractive new signposts made of wood, waymarkers decorated with the EU's stylized yellow-gold scallop shell on a blue background. Yellow shell, blue background: sun and sky? Seashell and water? Another mystery.

Collette and Danielle walked ahead of us harmoniously singing French and English children's songs. We joined in when we could. I enjoyed hearing Gary sing. A retired music professor and composer, voice had been his chosen "instrument" in college, but it had been years since he had sung in public. I hoped that this pilgrimage would prove meaningful to him in unexpected ways.

Sometimes together, sometimes apart, we walked through conifer and birch forests, admiring the gorgeous mushrooms sprouting everywhere. Grey-green lichens covered the trunks and lower branches of the Scotch pines. Fire-burnished autumnal colors—dull gold, rusty reds and deep burgundies—mixed with dark and lighter greens cloaked the hills. Fallen leaves softened our path. Forest alternated with fields where light-brown cattle with horns and limpid brown eyes encircled by a dark brown ring grazed on the grass. A cardboard sign nailed to a lichen-covered tree proclaimed, "Love is the Way."

Later that morning on the GR we encountered an agronomist who educated us about Scotch pines, birch trees, lichens, and local cows. Lichen is used in the perfume trade to "catch" the essence of flowers. Economically important, it is illegal to gather lichen from private land—hence the frequent "Private Domain" signs posted on fences and nailed into trees. The cows, like the lichen, were also something quite special. They were purebred Aubrac cattle. According to the expert, the ancient Greeks complimented a beautiful woman by saying that her eyes looked like the eyes of a young female calf. This would seem to be unlikely praise, unless you had seen the eyes of the Aubrac cows.

The agronomist pointed out some unusual rocks with large, oblong, clear-colored inclusions. This is horsetooth granite, he explained; the inclusions are feldspar. His information expanded my experience beyond a simple judgment that something was beautiful or something else was not.

When his wife and another couple caught up with us, he quit expounding on the glories of nature. They were on a weekend hike on the GR. With a friendly nod, he strode off with his companions.

We came to a chubby, equal-armed, lichen-covered roadside cross on a stone pedestal, its horizontal arms and the pedestal covered with pebbles and small stones. Danielle explained that in France people put rocks on wayside crosses to symbolically "lighten their load."

There is a sacred place called the Cruz de Ferro on the Spanish Camino, west of León in the mountains of the Maragatería. It is a huge mound of rocks topped by an iron cross attached to a tall wooden pole. Originally sacred to the Celt-Iberian settlers of the region, later it became a "mound of Mercury" dedicated to the Roman god, and people brought stones to the crossroads as an offering. The pile of rocks was Christianized in the Middle Ages with the addition of the iron cross, but medieval pilgrims continued the practice of bringing a stone to place on the ever-growing pile. Modern Camino lore instructs pilgrims to bring a stone from their homeland, a stone that symbolizes a burden or a sin, which they then leave behind at the Cruz de Ferro. Curious, this practice of leaving pebbles on sacred spots, as if one could deposit a feeling in a stone. But then again, maybe one could.

Danielle was exhausted. We had almost reached Saint-Alban-sur-Limagnole, but she wasn't sure she could walk any further. She explained that she had injured her knee the previous winter, but the doctors refused to do reconstructive surgery because she was too old. With a shrug, she added that she was only in her late 50s.

We took a short rest stop, even though we were only a few kilometers from Saint-Alban. Then, when Danielle looked a little less wan, we started up again. The GR led us alongside a soccer field, between buildings of the regional psychiatric hospital, and down a steep flight of stairs. The town, built on the side of the hill we were descending, was further below. Danielle stumbled wearily behind.

At last we reached Saint-Alban-sur-Limagnole. We walked down another flight of stairs to another street, trying to find our inn for the night. In one hotel Collette had an animated conversation with the clerk, who could not find our reservations. It turned out we were in the wrong hotel.

Michel, the Frenchman from Chanaleilles, called out to us from the doorway of another hotel.

"Where are your Swiss friends?" I inquired.

"They decided to go home. Blisters, you know."

We waved goodbye and walked down a side street to the Hôtel-Restaurant Le Breuil, located near the church. Madame was sitting at a table, picking through a large bowl of orange mushrooms. She did not seem very friendly, but maybe she was just preoccupied and overworked.

Wiping her hands on a towel, she led us to our third-floor rooms, squeezing past a drying rack full of clothes on the top landing. We had a bed, bidet, and sink in our tiny room. The shower and toilet were next door in a large room that doubled as the laundry drying room. Sheets and towels dangled from clotheslines stretched wall to wall. The shower was a pipe with a showerhead, located over a drain in one corner of the room, without a curtain.

After looking at the accommodations, Collette whispered to me, "Madame doesn't seem very friendly. And the place isn't very nice. It's hard to tell from the guidebook, you know. The other places I tried were full. Now it's too late to change."

"Don't worry about it," I reassured her. "The room looks clean and that's what matters."

"Yes, well, I suppose you're right. The sheets are clean; the place is quiet. I suppose it's not so bad but it's not what I expected."

"How could you know what to expect?" I asked.

Collette started to reply, then stopped and smiled.

Collette made reservations for dinner at the hotel, and we agreed to meet later. Gary and I did some hand laundry, commandeering part of a clotheslines strung across the bathroom-laundry room.

Then we went out to buy fruit and cheese for the next few days. We asked directions to a grocery store and were told to go left. We did. We walked until we were nearly out of town, then gave up. If there was a grocery store in that direction, it was further than we could reach on foot. As we wearily walked back to the hotel, two people came towards us carrying heavily laden grocery bags.

"Oú est le marché?" I asked. They looked puzzled; apparently that wasn't the proper word for grocery store. I pointed to their bags and they pointed to the right—and then went with us to show us the way.

This seemed to be a day for angels. What would happen, I wondered, if I started noticing helpful encounters and gave the credit to angels? Would I have more such encounters? Would I simply be more aware of the divine interventions that occur on a daily basis? Or would I be giving supernatural credit to human kindness?

The small supermarket had everything we needed, including *saucisson* (dried duck sausage) and Pérail, a locally made raw-sheep's-milk cheese. It resembled a ripe Brie, soft in the middle and bowing out at the rim. We also bought apples and pears.

After we returned to the hotel, I asked Madame about the *menu* posted outside the front door. Did we want the *tête du veau* (veal head) she asked? Absolutely not, I indicated, with a slight shudder. What about *truffade* or *aligot*? I asked. Madame explained that *truffade* was a mixture of potatoes, cheese, and bacon, and that *aligot* was made from mashed potatoes and fresh local cheese. My food vocabulary was relatively large (indicative of where my interests were), so I understood most of what she said.

"Truffade, s'il vous plaît," I requested.

She shook her head. There wasn't enough time to prepare it. Instead, she would make the *aligot*.

When we first arrived, Madame had seemed surly and noncommunicative, but she became quite animated when asked about dinner specialties. Once again, first impressions had been misleading. After all, what did I know about her life? Perhaps she had had a fight with her husband. Or maybe she was tired of trying to understand demanding pilgrims who barely spoke French.

We went out again. A tall, thin Asian-looking man with round wire-rim glasses, thick black hair, and a mustache was standing outside a nearby hôtel-restaurant, looking at the posted *menu*. In heavily accented English, he asked us what we knew about the place. We told him we didn't know anything because we were staying somewhere else.

Akira was a Japanese pilgrim walking the Chemin. He traveled all over the world on pilgrimage. I was fascinated by pilgrimage so I invited him to have coffee with us.

"How do you find your way on the Chemin?" I asked.

He took a French guidebook out of a large bag.

"Ah, so you read French?" Gary said.

"Not really, so it is difficult. I follow the GR 65 signs and this map." He pulled out a large-scale map, lacking in detail.

Gary and I exchanged glances, amazed that he had been able to follow the route. I carried several maps and guidebooks at all times, and I still complained that the maps weren't accurate enough—even though I knew that the map is not the territory and finding one's way on a pilgrimage is not about having a compass. It's about following the roadmap of the soul.

I asked, "What do you know about the Shikoku circuit? I think it takes place on a small Japanese island with lots of mountains."

"I have done it four times. The Shikoku pilgrimage takes forty days minimum to travel on foot to the main eighty-eight shrines, although there are 210 shrines in all." He shook his head sadly. "Now it's not so pretty. Lots of concrete, lots of highway traffic. Cars, noise everywhere. Not like this! This journey is so beautiful. I am very surprised."

"Who goes on the Shikoku pilgrimage?" I asked.

"Mostly older people. They retire and think, what is my life about? What is its purpose? Its meaning? Pilgrimage to Shikoku is a time to get away from the incessant 'noise attack' of society."

Akira explained that he was a misfit in Japanese society. He refused to own a computer or cell phone. Sometimes he traveled with friends or acted as a guide because he was an expert on pilgrimage and Buddhism—Tantara (Tantric) Buddhism was his specialty, although he grew up practicing Zen. Shikoku, he said, is the center of Tantara Buddhism. His mother didn't understand his life, he added.

Always the anthropological fieldworker, I asked, "So why do you go on pilgrimage?"

"To compare the religious buildings and pilgrimages. There is a big distinction between Japan, a land of wooden buildings, and the French stone churches. I am interested in the energy that I feel—the energy meridians impacted by the architecture. The Romanesque, which I love, is very different from the Gothic, which really doesn't interest me very much."

"So why pilgrimage?" I queried.

"To move higher spiritually. To give meaning to my travels...."

Akira added that he taught Leiden University students who specialized in Japanese studies. One of their doctoral requirements was to complete the Shikoku pilgrimage. He instructed them on how to do it.

Akira explained the distinction between pilgrimage, which is linear and goes from one spot to another, and the *shugan*, a Japanese practice that involves going up and down mountains to reach sacred shrines on the summits. The mountains themselves are also important. We were back to stones, the energy of stones....

As well as spending a year on pilgrimage in India and a great deal of time in Thailand with the forest monks, he had also traveled to Bali, Greece, Jerusalem, Rome, Iran, Pakistan, Egypt, and the US, including a Zen center in northern New York. He knew about the Breton pilgrimages in northwestern France and Skellig Michael off the coast of Ireland. He suggested we visit the three sister churches of Senac, Sirracan, and Rutreney—three Romanesque abbeys in Provence.

Finished with our coffee, we walked together to the church near our hotel. He pointed to the plaque near the door and asked, "What does *église* mean? I have seen that word several times."

Surprised that he didn't know, given his architectural interests, I replied, "It means 'church.'"

His eyes widened.

It was getting close to dinnertime and we invited Akira to join us. Although he had been in France several times, he'd never been outside Paris before and he had never ventured inside a restaurant. He bought his food at grocery stores or carried it with him from Japan.

I mused: What faith it took—or was it self confidence?—to go on pilgrimage in a foreign land where you didn't speak the language, didn't feel comfortable eating the food, and didn't know the local customs. Would I walk the Shikoku pilgrimage without being able to speak Japanese, without knowing my way around? I doubted it. And what would it mean for me, a Westerner, to go on the Shikoku pilgrimage? What did it mean for Akira, a Japanese Buddhist, to go on the Chemin? It meant whatever meaning we gave it.

We went back to the hotel and I stretched out on the bed for a few minutes. Suddenly I began to feel chilled and shaky. Was it a reaction to walking so far or to the bread and chocolate I'd eaten that day? Or both? I self-medicated with vitamin C and several essential oils that we carried with us: peppermint, tea tree, and a blend called Resiste. I followed Dr Penoel's advice on using high-quality essential oils as medicine, not just aroma. After fifteen minutes, I began to feel better.

At 8:00 p.m. Akira joined us at the hotel. This gangly Buddhist pilgrim who was traveling a Christian pilgrimage road intrigued Collette and Danielle. Of course, we weren't Christian either, but I still hadn't made that clear.

Dinner, served by Madame and cooked by her husband, began with homemade leek soup, followed by *aligot*, the famous local specialty, made of mashed potatoes, garlic, and fresh *tomme de Cantal* (Cantal cheese curds), no more than three days old. The mixture was beaten extensively until the cheese and potatoes formed a kind of stretchy batter that could be pulled like taffy and cut with scissors. It was bland but tasty. Adding salt helped.

Next, Madame brought us pan-fried beefsteaks and sautéed chanterelle—lovely pale-orange wild mushrooms, probably picked that morning in the forests we had been walking through, followed by curly endive salad and cheeses. Dessert was warm and fragrant *pain perdu* ("lost bread"), a kind of bread pudding made from stale cubed bread, milk and eggs, sugar, prunes, vanilla, and raisins. The bread had been soaked in milk, the other ingredients added, the whole thing baked and cooled, and a custard sauce poured over it.

Collette cooed over the bread pudding and, throwing caution out the window, I ate too much of the delicious concoction. I had decided to have faith that nothing bad would happen if I ate whatever I chose. I was exploring the power of faith rather than the power of will.

Although a little hesitant at first, Akira soon ate everything on his plate. He enjoyed the wine that came with dinner, so Collette and Danielle ordered more. Akira informed us that he led tours of Saki manufacturers and offered to take us on a tour if we ever went to Japan.

By the time we finished eating and drinking it was after 10:00 p.m. Akira thanked us for giving him the opportunity to experience

French dining and said goodnight. I wondered if we would ever see him again.

Sunday, October 13, 2002. Saint-Alban-sur-Limagnole to Aumont-Aubrac. 14.5 kilometers (9 miles), depending on whom you believe.

Breakfast waited for us downstairs: bread, jam and butter, brewed coffee, and instant hot cocoa. I ate half of a sliced, slightly stale baguette and sipped at a cup of hot cocoa. Tea, coffee, and even *infusions*, I had discovered, resulted in the need for frequent toilet stops, which was quite awkward on the Chemin—so I was switching to hot chocolate, even though it was full of sugar. Besides, I knew we had a long walk ahead of us and I wanted to be sure I had enough energy. I was beginning to believe my own rationalizations.

So far, I didn't seem to have swollen ankles or blood-sugar problems from taking the path of least resistance and greater pleasure. Maybe all the exercise I was getting was improving my metabolism. Or maybe it was faith.

It was a gorgeous, sunny day in the mid 60°s F. On the way out of town, just off the main road, we passed a large display on the pilgrimage to Saint-Jacques de Compostelle. Posters protected under glass described the meaning of the scallop shell, showed various trails, and provided melodies and words to popular medieval pilgrimage songs. Some group in Saint-Alban obviously was eager to promote the pilgrimage. Aside from spiritual benefits, the economic importance of the pilgrimage was obvious.

Collette asked, "Are you going to include Akira in your book?"

"I don't know. Maybe," I replied, annoyed by her frequent inquiries into the content of a book I might or might not write. Besides, I felt that what she really wanted to know was whether *she* would be included in the book. She might be surprised.

"Maybe *you* should write a book," I replied with a forced smile.

"Oh no, I couldn't do that," she responded.

Just then a tall lanky pilgrim wearing a bright yellow jacket walked up the path: it was Akira, carrying an enormous canvas pack strapped to his back. We greeted him warmly and he walked with us for a while, but he had a faster stride and he soon said goodbye.

We hiked up hills and down, through conifer forests and across fields. In this part of the Auvergne there were fewer deciduous trees to turn flaming colors, so the countryside had a quieter, subtler beauty. Cows of various sorts chomped on meadow grasses.

A wooden hiking staff leaned against a fence. Gary noticed that it had a crudely carved scallop shell at the top. Sometimes when "nature" called, people would drop their packs and staffs as an indicator not to follow them into the woods. But there was no trail at that point; there was only a fence with a decorated staff leaning against it. Almost as an afterthought, Gary took the stick with him.

A Swiss woman soon caught up with us. She was going to meet her husband in Aumont-Aubrac; he was arriving by train. They would rent a car and drive home.

Suddenly I realized that this day was the last day we would be walking with Collette and Danielle; Monday they would take the train from Aumont-Aubrac back to Lille. The time had passed so quickly! I would miss their companionship, their bell-like voices lifted in song. Admittedly, there were moments when I longed for quiet and regretted that Gary and I weren't alone. Trade-offs. Silence vs. song; quiet companionship vs. the pleasure of new friends. Whichever I was experiencing, I knew I would feel nostalgia for the other—at least until I reached a higher level of spiritual development, at which time I would accept everything with gratitude, whatever it was, and feel longing for nothing except God. I sincerely doubted I would live that long.

I remembered the synchronicity of our encounter with Collette and Danielle. We had met them on the first day of our pilgrimage, two English-speaking French women, one of whom, like me, had had cancer and was walking the Chemin as a result. They had helped make our journey much easier as well as more entertaining. Were they angels on our journey? Perhaps so. Of course, we had kept them from getting lost numerous times, so perhaps we were angels as well—or rather the vehicles for angels. Perhaps we were all angels, offering succor and support to those in need.

There is a Hasidic story about a nearly defunct monastery in the forest. One of the monks consults a rabbi and asks him how to rejuvenate the dying order. The rabbi says, "Go back and tell your brothers that one of you is the Messiah." Puzzled, the monk goes back and tells the others what the rabbi has said. Gradually a transformation occurs in the community as each person treats the others—and himself—as the Messiah. Soon people begin to visit the monastery again, drawn by its revitalized spirit, by the aura of love and respect that now permeates the environment.

We stopped for lunch by the side of the road, perching ourselves on convenient rocks. I used my knife to cut through the hard crust of the sourdough rye bread, to slice the duck *saucisson* and the squishy, pungent disk of sheep cheese. We offered some to Danielle and Collette. Collette demurely accepted; Danielle politely declined; she had more than enough cheese of her own. She offered us part of an orange and we accepted it. Then I pulled out a bar of bittersweet chocolate and we shared that as well.

"I'm sad," I said to our companions, "that you will be leaving us tomorrow."

Collette had tears in her eyes. "We must meet again. We must plan to walk more of the Chemin together."

That brightened me up considerably. "Yes, let's do that!"

"Perhaps next spring?" Collette offered.

"That sounds great! We'll keep in touch. We'll make plans!"

A gentle breeze wafted the scent of chocolate and orange into the air. Sitting on the rock, basking in the sun, life was very good indeed. I didn't know what would happen tomorrow; I didn't know how Gary and I would make reservations and arrangements to transport our bags; but that was all right. That was tomorrow.

We packed up the remains of lunch and started up the trail. In the distance I saw a man collapsed by the side of the road. It was Akira, resting against his heavy pack.

"I'm not feeling well. No energy. This pack," he said, with a grimace, "is too heavy. I don't know why. I carried more around Shikoku."

"Do you know where you'll be staying tonight?" I asked, concerned.

He shook his head.

Collette pursed her lips with a worried look. "Oh my, that isn't good. It's difficult at this time of year. Why don't you come with us? We'll see if there is room for you."

Akira smiled gratefully. Then he stood up, heaved the rucksack onto his back, and began walking with us.

Gary handed him the staff he had found. "Maybe this will help you."

Akira took it, admired the carving, and nodded. Companions on the road helped ease the burden in more ways than one.

"What do you carry in that heavy pack?" I asked.

"Japanese food."

"Food?" Collette repeated, incredulously.

He nodded. "Rice, a cook stove, canned and dried foods. I want to be sure I have my regular diet."

I pondered his commitment to maintaining his nutritional regime, a commitment that included hauling supplies all the way from Japan. I, on the other hand, jettisoned my regime at the first opportunity and happily savored croissants, fresh crusty bread, hot cocoa, and bittersweet chocolate. Obviously I lacked discipline. I told myself that I was practicing having faith that everything would be all right no matter what I did; I had a sneaking suspicion, however, that this was a somewhat delusional approach.

Raju's guidebook indicated a very long slog uphill and it was, but talking and singing with our companions helped ease the difficulty. We shifted from children's songs to Beatles' songs. Collette particularly enjoyed "When I'm 64," since she had just celebrated hers.

We emerged into a small clearing at the top of the hill and then descended. I was beginning to dread walking downhill since it usually meant we would have to go up again. We reached a shady walled lane running parallel to the road and, after catching our breaths, walked another few kilometers to Aumont-Aubrac.

Our shelter for the night was the Gîte du Barry, located at the Ferme du Barry (the farm of Barry), 200 meters from the train station. Our suitcases had arrived before us and were leaning against a stone wall next to the road.

"I can't believe they left your suitcases like that! It's not safe," Collette exclaimed.

The risk had occurred to me before, but this time I wasn't bothered. "Well, they're here," I replied, "and I guess the innkeeper must know what's safe and what isn't. This isn't Paris, after all."

Gary walked into the compound. Soon he returned. "Nobody's here."

We found an open door leading into a large dining room, so we rolled our suitcases inside and waited. Soon other pilgrims arrived. We all waited, sitting around several large trestle tables.

Eventually a corpulent, red-faced man stomped into the room, smelling of cigarettes and—could it be?—alcohol. He was our host, Monsieur Robert. With a friendly smile, he assigned us rooms. Danielle and Collette had a room to themselves and so did we. Akira also got a private room, much to his relief. The other pilgrims were staying in the large dormitory across the courtyard.

We left Danielle and Collette huddled in conversation with Monsieur Robert and went to our room. It was clean and cold. Thick stone walls are hard to heat, and we were still on that cusp between natural warmth and the need for artificial heat. Although it felt very chilly to us, the heat wouldn't be turned on until November.

Gary needed to rest, so Collette, Danielle, and I strolled into town so they could confirm their reservations at the train station. Along the way we stopped in a bar and sampled the local specialty, a delicious aperitif called Gentiane-cassis, a mixture of bitter liqueur made from the roots of yellow-blossomed gentian flowers and sweet black-currant liqueur. I was grateful to be traveling with congenial people who knew what to order. Without them, I would have missed a great deal of the local cuisine and etiquette.

While we savored our drinks, Collette and Danielle informed me that instead of taking the morning train to Lille they would walk with us to the Ferme des Gentianes; then Monsieur Robert would pick them up and take them back to Aumont-Aubrac to catch the night train. Collette had also arranged for Monsieur Robert to take our luggage to Nasbinals, our stopping point the day after.

I felt like jumping with joy. They would be with us another day! Although we had only been walking together for six days, we had grown quite close. My fondness for them grew out of shared experiences on the Chemin: getting lost, getting found, struggling up and down treacherous trails in the rain, exchanging chocolate bars and orange sections, basking in the sun together, encouraging each other when all we wanted to do was drop from exhaustion, conversing with "the bunnies" over lunch, meeting each day with open hearts and gratitude. With hugs and kisses all around the table, we ordered another round of Gentiane-cassis.

"Don't forget to mention that in your book!" Collette reminded me.

This time I smiled. Then, despite their protests, I paid the bill.

Collette explained that we needed to bring food with us if we wanted to eat at the Ferme des Gentianes; the owners wouldn't be available to cook dinner. As we strolled down the streets, I stopped to buy *saucisson* and cheese at a regional specialty shop, and Collette pointed out Prouheze, a nationally acclaimed restaurant. Even in *France profunde* outstanding dining was available. I fantasized about eating there but, like many of the interesting souvenir shops we had passed, it was closed for the season.

When we returned to the *gîte*, Gary was sunning himself in the garden. I told him that Collette and Danielle would be with us for another day and he was delighted. More kisses and hugs.

At dinnertime we sat on benches on either side of a large trestle table. Our dinner companions included the Swiss woman we had walked with earlier; Akira, from Japan; a priest from Quebec; three Germans; two Frenchmen and a woman; two Americans (us); and two more Frenchwomen (Collette and Danielle). We were a jolly international group, even before the wine began to flow. Dinner was provided by a *traiteur†*, a caterer who delivered numerous large trays covered with foil. Monsieur Robert brought the courses to the table.

Our meal began with local *charcuterie*: sliced salami and processed ham wrapped around mixed vegetables and slathered with mayonnaise. Next came tomatoes doused with herbal vinaigrette. Then our host proudly presented the main course, the famous green lentils of Le Puy, dotted with bits of crisp bacon and layered with large grilled sausages. It was heavy, Germanic (to my way of thinking), and tasty.

Unfortunately, Gary's throat went into spasm during the main course and he abruptly left the table.

Collette whispered to me, "Don't you need to go help him?"

I shook my head. "We've been through this a number of times. He doesn't want my help. Besides, there's nothing I can do. He'll be okay."

Collette frowned in the direction of the hallway. Obviously, she felt I was remiss in my wifely duties.

More wine, more conversation in a mélange of languages, and then dessert. Monsieur Robert brought out several cheese trays, each laden with five kinds of cheese, including two blue and several St Nectaire. Then he sat down at the edge of the bench and joined us.

I asked Collette to ask him how many pilgrims he had seen this year. She translated.

"About 5,500 people have stayed in the *gîte* since April."

A communal gasp went around the table.

"That many?"

He nodded.

"From what countries?"

"Lots of French and Spanish, five Japanese pilgrims…"

Akira was startled. He had thought *he* was the first Japanese pilgrim on the Chemin.

"Australians, and many others."

I wondered how many were hikers and how many were pilgrims, but there was no way to tell.

For someone who had been hesitant to try French food, Akira no longer had any disinclination. He ate and drank heartily, turning from one side to another to catch a bit of one conversation or another. I noticed, however, that the fine points of Western dining etiquette were unfamiliar to him; he cut his bread into big pieces with his fork and knife, and then stuffed each piece into his mouth.

I remembered the summer of 1981 when I had first visited Spain in preparation for doing fieldwork for my Ph.D. I stayed at a Benedictine guesthouse in Sahagún, where I shared the table of an elderly Spanish couple. The solid, well-fed matron was horrified at my table manners and, convinced that her way was the only way, she quickly set about teaching me the proper way to eat: the right hand was always to remain in sight (to demonstrate that I wasn't hiding a sword under the table); fruit was to be peeled and eaten with a fork and knife; and nothing larger than one bite was to be put into one's mouth. She told me always to tear off a small piece of bread rather than nibbling from a large slice.

After listening to numerous stories and various innuendos exchanged by the three Germans (just who *was* sleeping with whom?), I brought Gary a plate of food and a cup of hot tea. This time he had recovered more quickly than before and he was, in fact, hungry. But not for sausage.

"What do you think is setting off the spasm?" I asked.

"I don't know. Maybe eating something I don't want, something that literally 'sticks in my throat,' like pork sausage. There was a lot of noisy conversation and I just wasn't paying attention to swallowing."

Never mind that normally he didn't have to pay attention to swallowing.

"I'm glad you're okay now."

"It's over, but my throat is a little sore from the spasm. Thanks for the tea."

"Maybe it would help if you drink warm tea while you eat?"

"Maybe so."

I pulled on my silk long underwear and hurried to bed. The room was cold (62° F) since the heat had not yet been turned on. We snuggled together and soon we were warm enough to fall asleep.

Monday, October 14, 2002. Aumont-Aubrac to the Ferme des Gentianes (near Finieyrols). 15.5 kilometers, plus a few. (9.5 miles plus a few).

Breakfast was day-old croissants, yesterday's cheese, and coffee, tea, or hot cocoa. Monsieur Robert explained apologetically it was Monday and hence the *boulangeries* were closed. One bakery was supposed to be open, but the owners were sick. Most of the pilgrims had already left by the time we got up—they were walking further than we were that day—but Akira, Danielle, Collette, Gary, and I enjoyed a leisurely, convivial breakfast.

It was another lovely day for walking. We set out together, a contemporary *Canterbury Tales* melange of pilgrims, singing and telling stories. Life was good.

We took a short break at Chez Regine Café, located near Les Quatre Chemins. I photographed Gary, Danielle, and Akira sitting at the plastic picnic table, sipping cocoa and coffee. Akira's large canvas pack leans against the whitewashed side of the café, and chickens scurry around.

This was our last day on the Chemin with Danielle and Collette. They sang songs in French or English; Collette was the alto, Danielle the soprano. Sometimes Gary's tenor would harmonize, and sometimes I would join in as well. I felt sad, I felt happy, a confusing mixture of emotions passing through me as rapidly as clouds speeding across the sky.

The day warmed up. It was cloudy but occasionally the sun would break through. The countryside shifted rapidly from thick evergreen forests to rolling, open fields filled with big boulders and occasional clusters of juniper or cedar. Cows and sheep grazed the land. The Chemin itself changed from a forest trail to a sometimes-boggy gravel path. Stone farmhouses dotted the countryside. We had traveled from the Lozère region into the desolate, wind-swept Aubrac plateau. Akira, who had read extensively about the history of the Chemin, said that many medieval pilgrims lost their lives here due to marauding wolves or the lack of shelter from violent storms that surged across the plateau.

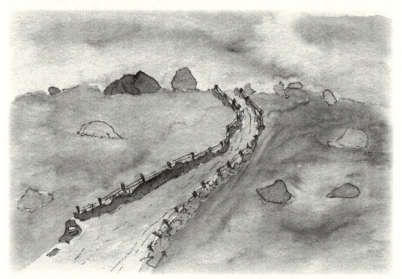

Aubrac

The style of roadside crosses changed as well. Tall, openwork metal crosses perched on three- to four-foot-high concrete platforms replaced the squat, lichen-covered stone crosses. The filigree design allowed sky and clouds to show through. These crosses also had rocks piled on them, but the only place to leave a pebble was on the base. The stone crosses evoked the Rock of Ages, the permanence of faith; the metal crosses reminded me of the impermanence and pieced-together nature of life. Of course, they only looked delicate. They had weathered many a storm.

Fortunately, we didn't have to worry about storms. We were in the middle of an Indian summer. The air was fresh, the temperatures pleasant. I felt rested and walking was a pleasure. I felt better than I had *ever* felt. Better than before I had had cancer surgery. Akira, however, was exhausted and had trouble carrying his pack. I wondered whether the French food and wine were disturbing his metabolism. He stopped to rest. Although we told him how to find the *gîte*, I had an intuition he would get lost.

When we reached the isolated Ferme des Gentianes a note taped to the front door of the farmhouse directed us to go to the *gîte*, a two-story building just behind the main house, and settle into our room. Settling in was not so simple. Two German pilgrims had already arrived and taken one room. We claimed another room, with three beds. The Germans looked at us with suspicion and inquired if we had a reservation. We replied that we did. Then a Swiss woman arrived who claimed she had a reservation for the dormitory, which was locked. What to do? We didn't want to sleep with her, nor she with us, so we moved the cot out of our room and put it in the anteroom next to the dorm. She was satisfied. Where would Akira sleep, I wondered: with the Germans?

And where was Akira? He should have shown up by then. Gary walked back down the road to find him but he was nowhere to be seen. Collette thought maybe he was meditating and simply hadn't arrived yet, but I was sure he had missed the turn and walked on.

The thought of Akira lost, alone, and exhausted disturbed me, so I set out to find him. Without my heavy fanny pack I felt almost buoyant. I walked a kilometer or so, plaintively calling out Akira's name like a mother who has lost her child. There was no reply.

Maybe he was waiting in the next village. That's what I would do. So I walked on to the next village, but still no Akira. I saw a group of people working on farm equipment in a field, and I asked if they had seen a tall pilgrim. They shook their heads. I continued through the village.

Suddenly I saw Akira in his bright yellow jacket walking toward me. Beside him was the Canadian priest we had met the night before. Relieved to see me, Akira explained that the priest had shown up right after we had left him. They had been deep in conversation and he had missed the sign to the *gite*. When they reached the village they had seen no signs for the GR or the *gite*, but since there was no one to ask, they had kept on going. At last they had turned back because they thought they had missed the route.

I told the priest he was, indeed, on the GR. Since he planned to reach Nasbinals that day, he said goodbye and started back up the lane alone.

"You came all this way to find *me*?" Akira asked with disbelief.

I nodded happily. After all, I had just had another encounter with angels. This time, the priest was the angel bringing Akira back to me, and I was the angel coming to find Akira. As we retraced our steps, he told me he was completely done in. He was very grateful that I had found him.

When we got back to the *gite*, our friends greeted him with hugs and kisses. We discovered another unlocked room, with several beds, and suggested that Akira claim it as his for the time being.

Just then Monsieur Robert drove up and honked his horn. It was time for Collette and Danielle to leave. We said goodbye, hugged, kissed on both cheeks and then once more for good measure. We were in tears, even though we planned to continue the pilgrimage together the following spring. As they drove away I remembered that Collette had asked Gary to sing "When I'm 64" one more time, but we all forgot.

I was sad to see them go, but it was all perfect. It had been wonderful to walk with them, and now it would be different. Not bad, just different. It would be quieter; we would be moving at our own pace, starting and stopping when we wanted. When I stayed in the moment I knew that everything was exactly the way it should be, and I was content.

Akira invited us to tea later in the afternoon and we eagerly accepted. In the meantime we were hungry, so we went into the kitchen and I prepared bread, cheese, and sausage for a midday snack. We shared the cramped space with the two taciturn German pilgrims. Our exchange consisted of one of them pointing toward the dish drainer and indicating that I should turn the water off in the sink while I washed dishes. I tried not to take their criticism personally; they were probably very tired.

Gary was fatigued and in pain. He had carried a heavy pack filled with our food supplies and something had happened to his left foot. The top of the instep was swollen. It was a hard, raised bump, almost as if the bone was bruised. We decided to take it easy the next few days. After all, we were not in any hurry and the two of us could decide to walk as much or little as we wanted to.

After resting for a while, we went to Akira's room. He had brewed toasted rice tea, one of the many precious food items he had carried from Japan. As we slowly sipped the fragrant tea, Akira talked at length about Buddhism and meditation. He told us the goal was to expand the present moment as long as possible.

That's what walking the Chemin was like, I realized. A walking meditation. Being present to the miracles that occur at every moment. The miracle of breath, of heartbeat, of sun, of tree, the miracle of friendship and love and interconnection. The miracle of simply being alive. Gratitude, gratitude.

When we stood up to leave, I noticed a copy of Alison Raju's guidebook on the small bedside table. To lighten my load, I had only brought the section from Le Puy to Conques, and I had wondered what I would use for a guide if we decided to walk farther. I was forming a plan to continue walking fifty-one kilometers farther to Figeac, but I had worried about how we would find our way without an English-language guidebook—the very guidebook that had now been serendipitously—or synchronistically—provided for us.

Just then the owner of the farm returned. An energetic, solid lady, she immediately began organizing who was sleeping where. We'd already pulled the cot out of our room for the Swiss lady, and she approved of that arrangement. Madame declared that the two Germans would share a room with Akira, and we would have a private room for ourselves.

I followed Madame to the *chambres d'hôtes* next door to buy postcards, and I asked if I could buy Raju's book. She thought that a pilgrim must have left it, so I could have it as a gift.

How likely was it that this particular book would show up on Akira's bedside table? Not likely at all. First of all, it wasn't available for purchase in France; second, it was in English; and third, whoever had brought it could hardly have intended to leave it behind. Our needs were being met in the most spectacular way. We were held in God's hands. I said a silent prayer of gratitude. It was, of course, easier to have faith when things turned out the way I wanted than when they didn't: my goal was to reach a point where I was grateful *whatever* happened. After all, I had had cancer.

Later that evening I went back into the kitchen and prepared dinner. Dry sausage, soft cheese, sardines, and fruit. Dessert was a special treat, "Marías," dry round cookies that I found in a cabinet in the kitchen, next to several boxes of tea.

The two Germans were sitting at the small kitchen table. One seemed slightly friendlier than the other, but that wasn't saying much. Don't take it personally, I reminded myself. They're probably just tired. They'd walked twenty-five kilometers that day, more than twice what we had managed.

That night we took our silk sleepsacks out of the pack and slipped them under the blankets. The radiator was set at 65°, but the room never got that warm.

Tuesday, October 15, 2002. Ferme des Gentianes to Nasbinals. 11 kilometers (7 miles).

I woke up sore and aching. The mattress was the worst I had slept on, on the Chemin: it was so hard that my legs hurt, my hips hurt, and even my breasts hurt from lying on my side. In addition,

I had had very strange dreams. According to Gary, I woke up in the middle of the night whimpering.

That morning we ate breakfast in the main farmhouse. I had my "Peace, not War" button pinned on my vest. When the two Germans saw it, they smiled and shook my hand. Suddenly they were eager to talk in English about everything from politics to pilgrimage. Their aloof behavior the day before had indeed not been personal: it had been directed at all Americans.

Heinrich became loquacious and was eager to hear about the American anti-war movement. We spoke passionately and at length while munching on fresh bread and homemade preserves. He told us that he had walked from Burgos to Santiago in 1999, an *Año Santo* (Holy Year), and that the Camino had been very crowded. In his view, people were taking to the French routes because they were less developed, an important consideration for younger people walking the Way.

Gary interjected, "First Spain, now France. Where next? Italy? Germany?"

Madame took Akira into another building so he could call Japan. When it came time to depart, we looked for him. He had already left, but without his hiking staff. Gary took it with us, hoping to catch up with him. Even though we walked quickly we couldn't catch up with Akira. I worried that he had gotten lost again, but a pilgrim we met later that morning assured us that he had seen Akira hiking strongly, far ahead.

Gary left the staff leaning against an openwork metal cross on the Pont de Marchastel. Rivers and streams were aesthetically important to Akira, so in memory of him and our brief time together I took a photograph of Gary and the staff on the bridge, the river Bès running below, the treeless fields of the Aubrac extending to the horizon.

Angels were everywhere, some more visible than others. Someone had left the staff behind. Gary had found it and given it to Akira to help him on a particularly difficult day. Now Akira had left it behind and Gary had left it for someone else in need. Perhaps the staff was an angel, or at least an angel's instrument.

We were crossing the Aubrac, land of an annual spring tran-shumance† festival during which golden-brown cattle, wearing fan-ciful, decorative head ornaments of pompoms and miniature trees, are transported on foot (or hoof) from one part of the region to another. It is a landscape of abandoned farmhouses, a windswept, nearly treeless plateau that reminded me of the Flint Hills of Kansas. But up close, which was one advantage to walking, we saw bushes bursting with rose hips, purple flowers springing up in green mead-ows, and trees heavy-laden with red berries.

Although the GR led us up and down over rolling terrain, we somehow managed for a short while to match strides with the two Germans, who were now quite eager to talk about themselves, Ger-many, and the United States. We soon parted company, however; they wanted to follow an ancient Roman route across the Aubrac. Since it was not waymarked, they would use their compasses and head out across country. Wishing them well, we said goodbye.

As we strode along, I felt that we were being held in God's hands. Much to my ongoing bemusement, these were the words that kept coming to mind; that was the feeling that enveloped me. We were in harmony, walking through beauty, surrounded by love.

It was easy to feel this when synchronicities abounded. At such moments how could I *not* believe we are held in God's hands? But to know that this is *always* true required that I be present, notice events, and not dismiss them as chance. It meant believing that there is order in the universe, that there is a reason for things happening—that events are meaningful, not random.

When things went according to my limited perception of what "going well" should look like, I relaxed into the sense of a compas-sionate universe. When they didn't—when I was diagnosed with cancer, or when a friend suffered a horrendous accident, or when my marriage was breaking apart—it was much harder. Yet that is when faith is most important.

The challenge was to have faith that even cancer is an opportunity for something transformative to happen. And indeed it had. My cancer diagnosis and subsequent operation had propelled me deeper on my spiritual journey and had literally set my feet on the Chemin. It had brought me new friends, new experiences, and a deepening sense of gratitude for all that life brings. I looked around me. Seasons come and go; life renews itself in a constant ebb and flow of giving and receiving, of creation, maturation, and transformation. How could it not be so? Everything is held in God's hands—in the interconnected web of Being, of which we are all a part.

We only walked a short distance that day, but Gary was already footsore. Fortunately, we soon reached Nasbinals and turned right, expecting to find our hotel in town. We were wrong. Our hotel was half a kilometer outside of town in the other direction. We had to trudge uphill to the Hôtel La Randonnée, a two-star establishment with twenty-one rooms. Our room was clean and quiet, with a private bathroom with a bathtub. What a treat!

We washed all our clothes except for what we were wearing. We wrung them out by rolling them inside our microfiber travel towels and stomping on them. Pants dangled from the clothesline we stretched across the bathroom, shirts dripped from the shower rod, and socks drooped from the top of the electric heater, which we cranked up to high.

For lunch, the clerk directed us to the Bastide restaurant at the Hôtel d'Argent, back in town. The same people who owned the Randonnée also owned the d'Argent. As we strolled into town, delighted not to be weighed down with our packs, I noticed a monument commemorating a local hero, Pierre Brioude. The large bronze bust rested on a cement pedestal adorned with a pair of cement crutches and the words, "Hommage a Pierrounet." Brioude was a nineteenth-century bonesetter and joint manipulator, said to have (successfully, I presumed) treated nearly 10,000 people a year.

Around the corner from a small Romanesque church was the restaurant, bustling with activity. When we explained La Randonnée had sent us, they seated us immediately. We chose a light salad and an omelet with freshly gathered *cépes*.

Given Gary's recent throat spasms, I suggested we needed an "intentional time" before eating. Although we always said a short grace before eating ("O Thou, Sustainer of our bodies, hearts, and souls, bless all that we receive in thankfulness"), it was easy to recite the grace by rote, without really paying attention. The difference when we slowed down and savored the words was immediate. I realized how speeded up we had become, busy walking, busy talking, busy figuring things out.

Many important local citizens were having lunch in the restaurant, judging by the frequent hand-shaking, back-patting, and occasional cheek-kissing taking place among formally dressed people. It was instructive to watch the customs of another culture.

Rejuvenated by our brief rest and delicious meal, we went sightseeing.

The shops and tourist office were closed for lunch, but the eleventh-century Église de l'Assumption was open. Simple and charming, the church has blind arches around the outside of the apse and an octagonal bell tower. Another octagonal tower. I wondered whether the eight-sided shape recalls the Christian association of eight with resurrection and rebirth (Christ rose from the grave eight days after entering into Jerusalem)—which is why many baptismal fonts (symbolic of spiritual rebirth) are eight sided.

Although most of the church is constructed of grey granite, a mixture of colorful volcanic stone alternates with granite on the portal on the south side. The upper archivolt† (curved carving on the arch over the doorway) on the southern portal is black basalt.

Inside, a wooden stand displayed a large, hard-bound guest book. After my eyes adjusted to the dim light, I paged through the *livre d'Or* and discovered an entry made that morning in Japanese.

"Akira was here!" I exclaimed.

Although neither Gary nor I could read Japanese, the date was in English and we were certain the short message was from Akira. I was glad to know he was not lost on the Chemin. He had been here about an hour and a half earlier, judging by what little we could decipher. I had decided to look for angels, and our angel of the day was news that Akira was on the right path.

Two brightly painted, naïf carvings of Saint Jacques and Saint Roch stand on wooden platforms jutting out from the wall at eye level. A bearded Saint Jacques wears a dark blue cloak, red robe, purple sash, and green money belt; a white shell adorns his broad-brimmed black hat. Two large, white-petaled flowers with bright yellow centers rise up out of the green grass that sprouts around his feet. Saint Roch isn't as colorful, but he is accompanied by a dog holding a loaf of bread in his mouth. Both Saint Jacques and Saint Roch lean on hiking staffs, much like the one we had left behind on the bridge.

Near the altar, a marble Madonna holds a pudgy Christ child. She stands on top of an ornate, four-tiered, white and gold platform that reminded me of a wedding cake.

Sitting quietly in the cool, tranquil church, I centered myself and tried to feel the energy that Akira said he perceived in the Romanesque churches. I sensed a gentle, pervading sweetness.

On our way back to the hotel we encountered a teenage girl standing next to a heavily laden donkey.

"Peregrino?" I asked, using the Spanish word for pilgrim. She looked blank. "Pèlerin?" I tried again, using the French word. She smiled and nodded. Eva-Marie explained she and three other family members had traveled from Switzerland with their donkey, Germaine. Although using a donkey to transport luggage was more picturesque than using taxis, it was much more complicated. They had to feed, shelter, and pasture the animal, and keep away from cities and paved roads.

Having exhausted the town's attractions, we strolled back to the hotel. Gary slept while I spent the rest of the afternoon writing postcards. Gary's right ankle hurt on the outside, and the large bump on the top of his left instep was painful. He had taped a small disk-shaped magnet over it, however, and that seemed to help.

That evening we ambled back into town to the restaurant. The *demi-pension menu* was soup (chicken stock filled with carrots, onions, celery, cabbage, and potatoes), followed by a *bouche de reine*, a puff pastry with creamed bacon inside. Next came two local specialties: *truffade* (similar to scalloped potatoes with bacon and melted Cantal cheese, with parsley sprinkled on top) and *andoulette*.

The couples at the neighboring tables were intrigued by our selections and did not hesitate to give their opinions. They particularly enjoyed my wrinkled nose and obvious distaste for the *andoulette*. It was a large grilled sausage made of pork tripe that had been lightly seasoned and rolled, forming alternating layers of light and dark grey innards. It was very piggy.

The restaurant patrons were eager to find out what we were doing in this small town. We explained that were walking the Chemin and they nodded; they knew the GR went through Nasbinals. A couple at the table next to ours spoke English—at least the husband did. He was "in oil" and from Montpellier, and he had spent time in Texas. They were enjoying the nearby thermal resort. Their vacation package including staying at the hotel, eating at the restaurant, and spending the day in the hot springs while getting a massage, enjoying the Jacuzzi, or taking advantage of other spa offerings.

Gary turned to me enthusiastically. "Sounds like a great idea, don't you think? Maybe after we've finished the Chemin, we can come back here and relax."

"Maybe so," I replied, contemplating a life of ease.

A couple from Belgium informed us they were hiking in the area. When we said we had walked eleven kilometers that day and would walk nine kilometers tomorrow to the village of Aubrac, the young woman laughed disparagingly. "It's cheating to walk such a short distance!"

Since when had the validity of one's pilgrimage been based on how far one walked in a day? I restrained my impulse to defend myself. I also restrained my urge to inform her that I was recovering from cancer surgery. It was easy to be judgmental, as I knew well.

The Swiss woman from the Ferme des Gentianes entered the dining room and looked around for a place to sit. We gestured for her to join us. We tried to talk, but our languages rarely intersected. I understood that she was walking for three days; the next day her husband would meet her and they would drive to Conques to spend some vacation days together.

After eating too much—the tripe and *truffade* had been followed by a cheese tray and bananas flambé—we said goodbye to our new friends. I browsed for a few minutes in the hotel gift shop, examining numerous books that touted the regional tourist attractions (wild flowers in spring, thermal baths, hiking trails) and admiring a two-foot-wide donut-shaped, sugar-coated sweet bread called *fou gasse, fouasse*, or *fouace*. The clerk offered me a taste of this Auvergne delicacy, but I was too full to be tempted.

Wednesday, October 16, 2002. Nasbinals to Aubrac. 9 kilometers (5.5 miles).

I awoke reverberating with the aftershocks of terrible dreams— with a struggle, I put the quickly fading images aside. They made no sense. I got up and started packing.

We went downstairs for breakfast, an ample buffet of cheeses, ham, sausage, yogurt, fruit croissants, bread, and tempting slices of *fouasse*. This time I sampled it; it resembled a brioche, yellow with eggs and sweet with sugar.

Several tables were already filled with hikers who were probably not pilgrims. This area of the Aubrac was quite popular for day excursions, and Josette, the desk clerk, had told us that a group of twelve had arranged to stay at the hotel for five days. Each day they walked a different trail with a local guide.

Josette agreed to bring our luggage, without charge, to the hotel in Aubrac as part of her daily errands. She was going that direction anyway and it was less than ten minutes away by car. Walking nine kilometers would take us most of the morning because we were still tired. Besides, we were not in any hurry. We might have been able to go further, but we had to make hotel reservations so Josette would know where to bring our bags. Maybe for our next stage on the Chemin we would only bring what we could carry.

As soon as we started walking I felt queasy. Perhaps it was the *andoulette,* maybe it was the *fouasse,* or possibly it was just eating completely off my normal regime. Gary's foot and ankle continued to bother him. He didn't complain, but I could tell by the slight frown on his face and his withdrawal.

Fortunately, it was another gorgeous day for a walk: sunny, fresh, and breezy. The Chemin led through town and uphill, soon turning into a stony forest path matted with golden leaves. We followed it up and over treeless hills, then through cow pastures and across an undulating plateau. After awhile, our route ran parallel to the woods. We lost sight of the GR markers so we followed Raju's guidebook instead.

Thickets of trees nestled in the folds of the hillsides; isolated stone farmhouses sat on top, commanding views of rolling, empty fields. The group of twelve hiked toward a distant building, perhaps one of the *burons†* (houses that sheltered shepherds and their flocks in summer) that dotted the landscape. We didn't have the energy to walk over and find out.

As we hiked up a wide path of beaten ground, partly hidden by grass, we encountered a well-dressed gentleman, his sport coat thrown casually over his shoulders, his tie loosened around his neck. "How far to Nasbinals?" he asked.

We wished we knew.

While we paused for breath, he informed us we were following the Grande Draille, the traditional transhumant trail across the Aubrac. He added that in the spring the fields are carpeted with wild flowers of all descriptions.

Up and down, through stiles and gates, along stone walls, through an empty cattle pen, past a statue of the Virgin, we eventually descended to a road. To one side was the Royal Aubrac Sports

Resort, which includes holiday lodging and various sporting opportunities, but it was closed between seasons. In *The Little Saint*, Hannah Green describes getting lost in this area and ending up at the top of a ski run. I was thankful we had found our way.

In the distance I saw several large buildings and two towers, all that remain of the church and monastery of Notre-Dame des Pauvres and the Tour des Anglais. The GR led down into the valley and then back up to the buildings, but we stayed on the country road that gently curved its way into the town of Aubrac. Why, except in the name of putative authenticity, would we go down and up when we could stay on level ground?

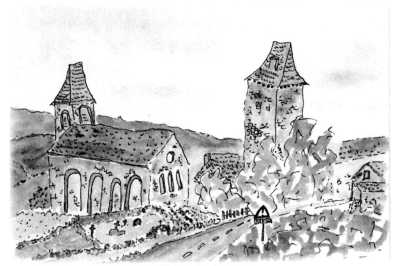

Dômerie, Aubrac

Aubrac was founded in 1120 as the Dômerie d'Aubrac by a Flemish viscount, Adelard de Flandres. He had been traveling to Santiago de Compostela when he was attacked at Aubrac by bandits. He survived and made it to Santiago, but on his way back he almost died in a snowstorm at Aubrac. Rather than focus on the near-disasters he had experienced, he chose instead to be grateful for his double deliverance. He founded a refuge for pilgrims at this desolate spot, 1360 meters above sea level, a site prone to bitter winters and glorious springs.

In its halcyon days, the Dômerie was a large fortress that included a washhouse, kitchen, infirmary, and separate dormitories for knights, pilgrims, and noble women. Twelve priests, twelve monks, twelve ladies, and twelve knights dedicated themselves to helping pilgrims. It became an exemplary model of how to serve those in need and, in recognition, received numerous special privileges, including the protection of a pope. According to the *The Pilgrim's Guide*, "The knights would defend them from bandits and wolves, the ladies would wash their feet, the monks would serve them" (page 123), and the priests would recite prayers and serve the poor.

Little remains of the town's former glory except a few three- and four-story stone buildings clustered around a central plaza. We walked down the street that ran through the tiny village, past a granite mansion called "Hermitage Himalaya," with a yurt in the front yard and a sign warning people to stay out. Next to that was the Hôtel-Restaurant de la Dômerie, another large grey granite building with a more welcoming sign on the door.

An elderly gentleman checked us in. He spoke no English but informed us that his daughter had lived in England and would be able to speak with us later. Could we eat lunch at the hotel, we asked? He shook his head. The restaurant was only open for dinner this late in the season. He wasn't sure where we could eat, he said, with an indifferent shrug.

After washing up we strolled over to the nearby plaza, surprised to find that the day had turned chilly. A sign in the window of Chez Germaine indicated it was open and cheese soup was available. We walked in and the waitress enthusiastically ushered us past a dessert-laden counter to a small table near a fire blazing in the huge stone fireplace.

The soup was hot, delicious, and filling, made with fresh Cantal cheese, a few minced greens and carrots, bread, and stock. I pulled gooey sheets of cheese-laden bread from the bowl, cutting it with my knife. The accompanying salads were enormous, a mixture of fresh greens, hot bacon, walnuts, and a delicate walnut-oil vinaigrette.

In between mouthfuls of scalding soup, we started talking with a Swiss woman at the table next to us.

Marie said, "You're from Colorado, aren't you? And you've walked the Camino five times."

Startled, I replied, "Yes, we're from Colorado, but I've only walked the Camino three times. How did you know?"

She smiled a Mona Lisa smile, then explained. "The pilgrims' telegraph." She had met the Belgian woman who had told me at dinner, "It's cheating if you only walk eleven kilometers." They had stayed together at the *gîte* in Nasbinals. News traveled faster than we did on the Chemin—and became distorted in the process.

Marie had started in Switzerland and hoped to get as far as Figeac this year. Ruefully, she pointed to her feet. "I developed bad blisters a few days ago. Fortunately, I was able to find a pair of hiking sandals in Le Puy so I've been able to keep walking."

"What if it rains? Won't your feet get wet?" I asked.

"That is a problem. But it's still better than the pain."

Marie wanted to know whether the Spanish Camino was boring and whether she could walk it without speaking Spanish. I was surprised that Marie, who spoke several languages, was worried. Was there something about Spain that made her—and Collette—uneasy? After all, we spoke little French but that hadn't stopped us from walking the Chemin. Then I remembered that we had felt some trepidation about our limited French and had been grateful for Collette's assistance that first day and every day afterwards.

I would have been hesitant to walk alone in Spain, even though I spoke the language and knew the Camino, just because I was hesitant to walk alone. And I never would have attempted to walk the Chemin by myself, given the language challenges. I appreciated Marie's courage.

After lunch we visited an odd little shop, the "Comptoir d'Aubrac of Catherine Painvin," located in a hulking, four-story building across the plaza from Chez Germaine. It had originally been built in 1862 as a hotel for pilgrims on the Chemin. The charming young clerk explained that Catherine Painvin, the founder of Tartaine et Chocolate, a French luxury brand of children's clothing and home furnishings, had converted the building into an outlet shop and fashionable B&B. Painvin had developed the *comptoir* (an antique word for trading post) during a very low period in her life—an anguished divorce that occurred at the same time as her cancer diagnosis.

The *comptoir* sold seconds and past-season merchandise. Clothing of various sizes and descriptions was piled on large tables or tossed into boxes. Luxurious silk bedcovers, wool blankets, pewter candlesticks, children's backpacks, toiletries, and other paraphernalia were displayed in open cabinets. I found several large scrapbooks filled with pictures of Catherine Painvin and news articles about her life and business. She owned over 140 boutiques worldwide and had been awarded the French Medal of Honor, as well as being selected Businesswoman of the Year. I wondered why she had chosen the isolated Aubrac as a retreat.

After trying on various hats and being reminded by Gary that we would have to carry whatever I bought, I purchased a small pewter scallop shell. The clerk helped me find a piece of cord so I could fasten it to my bag.

Then we returned to the hotel. I felt tired. I was so busy *doing* that I was not really *being*. I was always walking or writing postcards or doing laundry or talking to people in a mixture of languages or eating or trying to bring my journal up to date or doing something else that kept me occupied. I wasn't devoting much time to being inward, silent, and reflective.

Exhausted both physically and mentally, Gary and I took a late afternoon nap. I had a headache and the beginning of a sore throat, so I started Dr Penoel's "melaluca oil regime." By the end of the hour, my throat and stomach were markedly improved.

At 7:00 p.m. we went down to dinner but we were an hour early, so the elderly owner seated us in a large lounge area next to the fireplace. He brought us tea and a half-dozen photo albums filled with thirty years of his photographs of the flowers of the Aubrac. There are over 2000 varieties in the area, many of which he had managed to capture. Gary began to talk eagerly about returning to the Aubrac in May, the peak season for wildflowers.

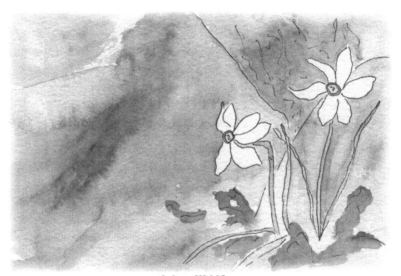

Aubrac Wildflowers

The innkeeper's daughter arrived and began speaking with us in rapid-fire English. She had studied and traveled in Australia and San Francisco. Now, however, she was living in this tiny village where there were almost no young people, because her family needed her help.

Eventually we were allowed to enter the dining room. Two middle-aged women and a man sat at one table.

One of the women asked, "Are you Mr. and Mrs. White?"

I decided not to quibble that my surname wasn't "White." "Yes," I replied, "but how do you know?"

"The Camino telegraph." They had met Akira in Saint-Chély, the next village down the Chemin, and he had told them to look for us. They were from England. He was a retired professor traveling with his wife and their mutual friend, Claire, a doctoral student. Her topic had something to do with secular and religious impacts on the Way of Saint James. At least that's what I think she said, but what I understood didn't make much sense, even though we were both speaking English. At least I thought we were.

Claire focused on collecting written documents (newspapers, magazines, books, etc.) rather than on interviewing people. But she wanted to have some first-hand familiarity with the Chemin, so they would drive somewhere and stay for several days while they walked selected parts of the Chemin, combining research with recreation. I doubted that walking a few days would give them a meaningful experience of the pilgrimage, but then I realized I was being judgmental. Or maybe I was just being realistic.

The professor regaled us with tales that demonstrated his erudition. One story was relevant to the pilgrimage, so I paid more attention. The previous year on the Spanish Camino they had met Tomás, a neo-Templar who has established a *refugio* at Manjarín in the isolated mountains of León. Although the Knights Templar had been disbanded in the early fourteenth century, various organizations claimed to continue some of their traditions.

Although Gary and I had stopped by the *refugio* in 1997 on our pilgrimage and I had also been there in 2000, I had never met Tomás. It was a peculiar place, unclean and unkempt, with geese, chickens, and a donkey wandering in the courtyard of a decrepit stone house that lacked running water and toilet facilities.

Our dinner companions said that Tomás had been wearing a white robe, similar to that worn by the medieval Templars. He also showed them a sword that he claimed was a Templar's sword. When pilgrims approached, the geese would start clacking and a microphone would activate a tape of Gregorian chants.

Dinner arrived, ending our conversation for the moment. It consisted of vegetable soup, grilled trout, boiled potatoes, and salad with Laguiole cheese. Although it sounded good, the meal was indifferently prepared—or maybe our standards had been raised by fresh farm fare. Our talkative neighbors were provided with a different *menu*.

Seeing my puzzled glance, the older woman said, "We insisted on having more variety and more vegetables. Our host was really quite agreeable."

If we'd only known. It is one thing to feel gratitude for whatever we are given, quite another to manage the system so we are given more to be grateful for!

Dessert was the best part of dinner. I devoured the *profiterie* (creampuffs) topped with hazelnut ice cream and ladles of warm chocolate sauce. Gary chose a pear poached in red wine, with ice cream and caramel sauce on the side.

Thursday, October 17, 2002. Aubrac to Saint-Chély-d'Aubrac. 8 kilometers (5 miles).

We left Gary's backpack with the two suitcases in order to lessen the stress on his left foot. Then we squeezed a few extra items into the Bunny Bag. We would take turns carrying it.

It was a foggy, cool, rainy morning. We walked a short distance out of town on the road, then turned off to the left, next to a cross we could barely make out through the mist. The GR led through semi-shaded woodlands, then across stepping stones over a stream. There were bright red and purple berries everywhere, tree branches hanging heavy with them, bushes dripping with them. We weren't sure if they were edible but they were colorful. Gone was the arid, windswept Aubrac plateau with its vistas extending for miles. In its place were dense forests and steep hiking trails.

Our slick, leaf-strewn lane went downhill, lined on either side with nettles and ferns. Holly trees, with glistening, sharp leaves, rose twelve feet high, interspersed with towering oak trees. Underneath the soggy mat of golden leaves were jagged black rocks. The trail was treacherous. Our guidebook indicated we would drop 500 meters (1640 feet) in eight kilometers (five miles). And drop we did, slipping and sliding as we went.

During a break in the rain we took the bunnies out and starting arranging them for a photo shoot. As I posed Honey Bunny and

Rustle Ears beside some particularly lovely roses, Gary asked, "Just what do you plan to tell people when they ask what we're doing?"

I replied smugly, "We'll tell them we're making a picture book for our grandchild, Max. A book called *Bunnies in France.*"

"Do you think they'll believe you?"

"Why not? Besides, why do we care what anybody thinks?" I replied, with false bravado.

That was one of the lessons the bunnies offered us. Why *did* we care what anybody else thought? After all, we would never see again most of the people we encountered on the Chemin.

The cold drizzle increased in intensity as we struggled down a particularly perilous trail into Saint-Chély-d'Aubrac. Shivering and chilled, we arrived at the Hôtel-Restaurant de la Vallée, the only open hotel. Since we had walked such a short distance, it was only late morning.

After urging us to leave our dripping rain gear at the door, Madame showed us to our room. Fuzzy, ridged wallpaper covered the walls of the small room, presumably disguising layers of cracked

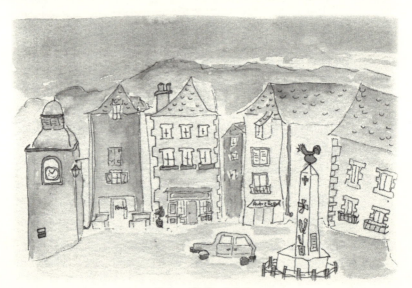

Saint-Chély-d'Aubrac

plaster. The room was tiny and cold, but at least the greeting had been warm.

After changing clothes we tried unsuccessfully to clean the mud off our raingear. Then we went down to the bar, where Madame served us hot tea and cocoa. A number of duffle bags were piled by the front door; each bore the tag, "La Pèlerine" (The Pilgrim). Apparently a group of hikers—or pilgrims?—had had their bags delivered to the hotel, or perhaps they were waiting to be picked up.

Eventually Madame decided the proper time for lunch had arrived, and she picked up two leather-bound menus and led us into the dining room. We were the only ones there. We chose a pureed vegetable soup, served by Madame from a large metal tureen, and a large salad of fresh lettuce, walnuts, country ham, and Roquefort cheese. *Aligot* was listed on the menu, and I noticed various preparations using duck (duck breast, duck wings, *confit de canard)* and walnuts (walnut aperitif, walnut cookies, walnuts in salad). The cuisine had changed with the countryside.

After lunch we went for a walk around town, even though it was drizzling. That seemed better than huddling together for warmth in our cold room. Suddenly a fire alarm blasted out over the rooftops. Volunteers streamed out of buildings and three vehicles roared up the street and out of sight. A bit unnerved, we waited under the eaves of a nearby shop, wondering what would happen next. Nothing did. So we continued our exploration.

The town looked medieval and undoubtedly was. Several-storied grey granite and volcanic stone buildings, their heavy wooden shutters closed against the cold, lined the narrow streets. We visited the well-cared-for communal *gîte*. Perhaps we should stay in one, I thought, but then again, maybe not: I didn't think they had private bedrooms or private bathrooms.

Private *gîtes* we understood, thanks to our journey with Collette and Danielle, but we weren't sure what the proper etiquette was in a communal *gîte*. I noticed a number of signs listing rules and regulations, but I wasn't sure what they all meant. Suddenly I better understood Collette and Marie's concerns about walking the Spanish Camino.

We talked with a Swiss couple traveling with their teenage children, who were staying at the *gîte*. This was their way of taking a healthy, inexpensive family vacation. The woman confided that when the fire alarm went off she thought it was something she had done. When we told her that the fire brigade had headed out of town, she was relieved. We weren't the only ones unsure how things worked in a foreign land.

We visited a fifteenth-century church with a statue of Saint Roch situated to the left of the altar. On the ceiling above, a Baroque gold-and-white head of God peers out of fluffy white plaster clouds. A motion-sensitive light turned on as we approached; the golden "sunbeams" shooting out from behind God's head glittered in the beam. We lit candles of gratitude and sat quietly, listening to the rain beating against the roof.

Just as we arrived back at our hotel, a group of ten dripping hikers tromped into the bar, their muddy shoes making a mess on the tile floor. The noise level rose precipitously. They rummaged through the duffle bags and claimed their own, hefting them up on their shoulders or hauling them along the floor. In a few minutes they had disappeared into their rooms.

I showed Madame my copy of *Miam Miam Dodo* and asked her where to stay in Saint-Côme-d'Olt. She offered to call the Hôtel-Restaurant des Voyageurs and make arrangements for us. A few minutes later she returned and nodded; we had a room. Just as important, we had successfully made arrangements for the first time without Collette.

Madame also agreed to transfer our bags. In the morning she would add our suitcases to the stack of duffle bags by the front door, and a local taxi would transport them to the next stop. The group of ten was walking to Estaing, a distance of more than twenty-one kilometers. We, however, intended to walk only as far as Saint-Côme-d'Olt, a mere sixteen kilometers away.

Wanting to thank Madame for her help, we patronized her bar, drinking mugs of hot chocolate. A drenched young woman entered the hotel and asked if the rowdy group of ten was staying there. When informed that they were, she looked distressed. She would only stay at the hotel if Madame could assure her that her room would be quiet. Unsatisfied with Madame's response, she decided to take a cab to Estaing.

The challenges of the Chemin: rain, cold, slippery trails, raucous hikers. The latter was one reason we never slept in the Spanish *refugios*. They were notoriously noisy, filled with snoring pilgrims and early risers. Hard-core pilgrims carried earplugs and either enjoyed the boisterous camaraderie or managed to ignore it.

One by one the members of the hiking entourage reappeared, ranging in age from mid thirties to early fifties, equally divided between men and women. They ordered beer at the bar, retreated to the lounge, and began conversing loudly. I watched several flirtatious exchanges.

What, I pondered, would the heavyset Swiss woman at Chanaleilles think of them? Probably she would declare they were having entirely too much fun. I wondered whether they would consider themselves pilgrims or excursionists on a holiday. The British woman we had met would probably have found them a confirmation of her vague theory that secular life and the sacred intermingled on the Chemin. But then, it always had. Preachers warned medieval pilgrims against the distractions of the road, and a popular saying had been, "Go a pilgrim, return a whore."

I thought about the drenched young woman who took the taxi to Estaing because she wanted a good night's sleep. We all had our priorities. Gary and I wanted a private room and a private bathroom. I wanted to make sure I had enough food (I had some low-blood-sugar problems) so we carried extra supplies. Privacy and nutrition were my bottom lines. And Gary's bottom line? I wasn't sure.

At dinner time the dining room, like the hotel, was nearly full. A middle-aged couple walked stiffly and wearily over to a nearby table. Definitely pilgrims. I nodded in greeting; they nodded back. The man had socks on but no shoes. Had he lightened his pack by not carrying a change of footwear?

Our dinner began with shredded carrots, hard-boiled eggs, tomatoes, garden-fresh lettuce, and a local specialty: a fried parsley, breadcrumb, and egg fritter. This was followed by a fried pork cutlet, a grilled broccoli-cheese-egg soufflé, and buttered noodles served with half a grilled tomato. Next came a cheese tray that included *bleu d'Auvergne,* Laguiole, and St Nectaire. Dessert was a home-made myrtle tart with raspberry sauce on the side. The myrtles were smaller, sweeter, and more delicate than blueberries.

While we ate, Gary and I made plans. The next day we would walk sixteen kilometers; the following day we had a choice of either six or seventeen kilometers. I leaned toward the latter but agreed that we should wait a day before deciding.

For me, walking two hours and relaxing the rest of the day was boring. I had nothing to read and the small towns offer a limited number of interesting sights. Although Gary managed to nap in the chilly hotel rooms, I couldn't. I needed to find some place to be alone, but I still hadn't figured out how.

Friday, October 18, 2002. Saint-Chély-d'Aubrac to Saint-Côme-d'Olt. 16 – 17 kilometers (10 – 10.5 miles).

Madame had assured us the weather would be pleasant but the weather continued cold and rainy. Gary strapped on his backpack again, and we put our two suitcases next to the duffle bags and gave Madame money for their transport. Would the driver remember to leave them at Saint-Côme? I took a deep breath and let go of attach-ment to outcome.

Our path led us through town to an old bridge over the Boralde River. A sixteenth-century cross with a pilgrim sculpted at the base reminded me that we were following a path that had been trod for centuries—a millennium—and that we were, indeed, "walking in the footsteps of our ancestors."

That phrase was popular on the Spanish Camino when I first walked it, twenty years before. I had always protested silently, "But they weren't my ancestors," since mine were, as far as I knew, Russian Jews, except for Hinda, my Turkish Jewish great-grandmother, for whom I was named. They had never stepped foot on the Camino.

Suddenly, however, I understood the phrase in a different way: those whose footsteps we followed weren't necessarily our genealogical ancestors. I was walking in the footsteps of people who followed a spiritual path—whatever spiritual path that might be. Some of them had been Jewish and Christian mystics; some had been Sufis; some had been alchemists and kabbalists. They, too, had followed the Way of Saint James, for various complex and mysterious motives. They were my ancestors on this journey.

The day felt magical as we walked through mist-blurred chestnut and evergreen forests. At one point we followed a broad, gold-and-rusty-red, leaf-strewn path through the woods; huge trees loomed overhead. I could imagine fairies peeking out from behind tree trunks. We greeted other pilgrims as they passed us by: the Swiss family of four, a German couple, a few of the hiking group. We, in turn, passed the middle-aged French couple we had seen at dinner at the hotel.

Placing one foot in front of the other, hour after hour, might sound tedious, but every step was a new step and every moment was saturated with sensory input: the sight of the landscape, the sound of the trees rustling in the breeze or birds chirping or feet striking the trail, the smell of damp soil or tannic leaves, the feel of raindrops or sunshine or a chill breeze on my face. There were intense tastes as well, a square of bitter chocolate dissolving in my mouth, a tart, juicy orange segment sliding down my throat.

Some days I had to struggle for every kilometer; other days I felt invigorated. Some days—for example, when we had walked with the athletic German pilgrims from the Ferme des Gentianes—we managed four kilometers an hour. Other days we managed less than three. Rather than struggling against "what is," I tried to appreciate *whatever* is—including my experience with cancer.

I wished we had purchased some fruit that morning. As soon as that thought crossed my mind, I noticed an apple orchard. Fallen apples dotted our path. I picked one up, filled with gratitude for the synchronicities of the Chemin. Our needs were, indeed, being met.

We spent the day clambering up and down rocky, slippery trails, some of them running with water. At one point, dense forest encroached on one side of the Chemin; fenced grazing land spread out on the other. Twining ivy covered the fence posts and the muffled sound of cowbells clanged through the light mist. We took pictures of the bunnies sitting on the weathered posts, staring at the rain-dappled cows in the fields.

Some of the fields were covered with rusty red, green, and yellow ferns and brambles. Moss practically dripped from the damp stone walls of the farmhouses. Fallen acorns and chestnuts crunched underfoot. Pointy-leafed holly trees thrust their branches between less-defended trees. The rain started, stopped, and started again.

It was past lunchtime but we waited until the rain stopped before pulling our meager supplies out of my fanny pack. While we ate, the middle-aged French couple that we had passed overtook us. They nodded. Once we began walking again, we caught up with them. With a friendly wave and an exchange of greetings, we passed them by. We were playing a sort of Chemin hopscotch.

Although I felt stiff that morning, by midday I felt great. I had a sense of propulsion when I strode uphill, a feeling that if I went too slowly I would lose momentum. It was a marvelous feeling. I felt strong. I felt healthy.

With a contented sigh I told myself, "This is as good as it gets!"

But I also felt an occasional twinge of sadness and worry. The cancer surgery flitted across my mind and back again, trying to lodge in my conscious awareness and fester. Was this "as good as it gets" and would it be a steep downhill slide from here? I picked up a stone and left it, along with thoughts about cancer, on a wayside cross.

A few kilometers from Saint-Côme the GR crossed a country highway. Should we take the highway or stay on the GR? We decided to keep to the easier, "traditional" path of the GR, not that it necessarily was; after all, the GR was as much a modern construction as the highway. Shortly after we made our decision, our trail headed abruptly uphill. You never know what lies ahead.

We had walked out of the Aubrac and into the Valley of the Lot. "Olt" is the old name for the river Lot, hence the name of our next stopping point, Saint-Côme-d'Olt. As we entered the town, the middle-aged French couple was ahead of us.

A sign proclaimed that Saint-Côme was one of the "Plus beaux villages de France"—a tourism classification that meant it was one of the "most beautiful French villages." That sounded promising. At the Hôtel-Restaurant Voyageur, Madame led us upstairs to a small room with flowery wallpaper and a tiny bathroom. The radiator was on. The room was delightfully warm.

Although we had walked ten miles in the rain we felt energized. Instead of resting we explored the town, using a tourist brochure to plan our route. Through some fluke of fortune or a prescient eye towards future tourism, the walled medieval center of Saint-Côme has survived nearly unchanged. The State has classified it as a national historic monument.

Two concentric streets lined with two- and three-story stone houses protect the inner core, entered through three remaining portals. I imagined the warlike atmosphere that had made such fortification necessary. A number of the fifteenth- and sixteenth-century buildings display plaques describing their original use and date of construction. Centuries of retouched mortar drip over the pale beige and grey building stones, giving the houses a dappled appearance that contrasts with the steeply pitched black schist roofs.

Nestled in the center are a turreted castle and the sixteenth-century Église de Saint-Côme-et-Saint-Damien. Its Renaissance doors are elaborately carved with fifteen medallions, a whimsical variety of imaginary beasts and faces. Precisely 365 forged iron rivets complete the design. The tenth-century Chapel of the Penitents with its twisted bell tower adjoins the church. High on one wall is a siren-mermaid carving, her split tail stretching up either side of her torso.

Alluring and seductive, this fishy female is filled with mystery. According to church doctrine, the siren-mermaid symbolizes the sin of lust. I wondered if the split-tailed female was a variant of the Sheela-na-Gig†, a figurative carving of a naked woman (often skeletal in appearance) squatting with knees apart, one or both hands

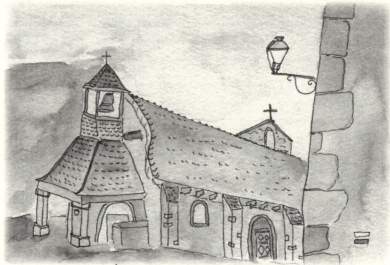

Église (Church), Saint-Côme-d'Olt

spreading wide her exaggerated vulva. Her wide-open vulva is the same shape as the *vesica piscis*, the double-pointed oval, the mandorla, which we had seen before.

Sheela-na-Gigs were carved on Irish, British, and continental European churches built before the sixteenth century; some still remain, though most have been destroyed. The Sheela's true origins are unknown and her meaning controversial. One person told me, "She represents where we came from and where we're going."

Some scholars think she is an ancient good-luck or apotropaic (ward-off-evil) symbol; others think she represents fertility. Still other scholars think the Sheela is more modern and that her off-putting appearance is the Church's effort to discourage lust. Whatever the Sheela-na-Gig or the siren originally signified, the church has embued both symbols of the feminine with a distinctly negative meaning.

We went into a *tabac* to buy some postcards. As the name implied, the shop sold tobacco—along with postcards, stamps, and an assortment of curios and tourist items. The music system was playing "I Just Called to Say I Love You," and Gary and I broke into song and dance, holding hands and looking lovingly into each other's eyes. The clerk enjoyed the show immensely—and so did we.

As Gary and I strolled around town, the fragrant Patisserie Saint-Jacques beckoned to us. The bakery was redolent with the aromas of fresh-baked breads and espresso. Racks along the back walls displayed an array of specialty breads, and glass-fronted cabinets presented a tempting assortment of cookies and pastries. We treated ourselves to hot chocolate, topped with whipped cream, and *tuilles*, curved, wafer-thin almond cookies named after the roof tiles they resembled. I asked the clerk if she had a stamp for our credentials; she did indeed—a stamp with Saint Jacques.

Munching cookies and sipping hot chocolate, we stared out the window. The middle-aged French couple walked by and I waved at them. They came in and placed their order at the counter. The woman spoke very precisely and walked slightly haltingly. Early Parkinson's, I wondered? Would I rather have Parkinson's than cancer? Definitely not.

My ex-husband, John (Jesse's father), had died in 1997 from metastasized melanoma. John had gone to a cancer support group for a few months, until he became too ill. He told me that when people discussed their cancer and their treatment (chemo, radiation, surgery, or combinations thereof), no one wanted to exchange *their* kind of cancer and its treatment for someone else's. This preference probably had some psychological explanation, such as "Stockholm Syndrome" (identifying with one's captors), or maybe it was because the cancer treatment was like an intense hazing initiation: the more you suffered the more attached you became to the experience. Or perhaps it was as simple as preferring "the devil you know instead of the one you don't."

Suddenly the hot chocolate, cookies, and my earlier sadness all came together in a surge of anxiety. I worried that my current diet (sugar, bread, and chocolate), along with not taking my usual supplements, meant I was setting myself up for a recurrence of cancer.

I told myself that French people ate like this all the time and *they* didn't all have cancer. I tried to convince myself that the exercise I was getting on a daily basis stimulated my lymphatic system enough to counteract any negative impact from my diet. Besides, I felt healthier and stronger every day. Didn't that count for something? But the anxiety remained. After all, I didn't know why I had gotten cancer, so how could I know how to avoid a recurrence?

I remembered a mantra a yoga teacher had shared with our class: "I am whole, I am holy, I am healed." From my mouth to God's ears, I whispered, remembering another expression someone had taught me.

The couple finished ordering and came to sit with us. After introductions, I asked them how they had reached town before us.

"We stayed on the highway instead of taking the GR."

Gary asked, "Did it go uphill and downhill a lot?"

The man shook his head. "It was an easy route."

With a sigh, I realized that I could never be sure in advance which way would be best.

Though language difficulties loomed large, we managed to share some personal information with Michelle and Jean Susani, who lived near Marseilles. We also learned we were staying at the same hotel. Finished with our indulgent refreshments, we said goodbye for a while.

While Gary and I wandered back to the hotel, we again discussed how far to go the next day. Should we walk six kilometers to Espalion or seventeen to Estaing? I wanted to walk to Estaing—I felt *good* walking—but Gary was hesitant. His ankle hurt and the bump on top of his left instep had returned. I suggested we leave the backpack behind, walk as far as felt comfortable, and then call a taxi to fetch our bags and bring them to wherever we were staying. The problem with this plan, however, was that the next inn might be full if we arrived without reservations. After more conversation we decided to have faith that we could reach Estaing. We could always change our minds.

Back at the hotel, I showed Madame the entry in *Miam Miam Dodo* and she called the Auberge Saint-Fleuret to make reservations. No problem, she indicated with a smile.

That evening Michelle and shoeless Jean were seated at the same table with us. We were the only people in the huge dining room, which was also used for banquets, judging by the large quantity of plates and wine glasses in the cabinets that lined one wall. The Susanis explained what the *menu* choices were, so we tried a few new items, including *fromage blanc*, a soft white cheese served with marmalade.

They asked where we were staying the next night, so I showed them *Miam Miam Dodo*, which they hadn't known about. I pointed to the entry for the *auberge* in Estaing and Jean indicated they would like to stay there as well. He went to make a phone call and returned looking pleased. He had made reservations.

It looked as if we had new companions on the Chemin. We appeared to be congenial, although it was difficult to communicate about anything other than lodging and food. We seemed to walk about the same distance each day. I had enjoyed the few days Gary and I had traveled without companions, setting our own pace, but I would enjoy company as well. Whatever happened was perfect.

Saturday, October 19, 2002. Saint-Côme-d'Olt to Estaing. 17 kilometers (10.5 miles).

The mattress at the Ferme des Gentianes had been so hard that my hips hurt; the bed at Saint-Côme was so soft that my back ached. Tired from not sleeping well, it took me a while to get ready for the day.

When we went down to breakfast, we learned that the Susanis had already left. Apparently they would be hotel companions, not walking companions. We paid for the taxi driver (Madame's husband) to transport our two suitcases and the backpack. Gary's foot still hurt so I carried the Bunny Bag.

Instead of taking the high-altitude GR variant that led up the hillside to the Vierge de Vermus, a large statue of the Virgin of Vermus, and to an impressive view over the Lot, we took the flat, low-impact country lane that ran beside the placid Lot.

The landscape had changed remarkably in just a few days of walking. On one side of us were steep bluffs; on the other, a flat, fertile river valley. We were walking through the Lot Valley, a rich agricultural area filled with cornfields and orchards.

Our immediate goal was the Église de Saint-Hilarian de Perse, an eleventh- or twelfth-century Romanesque church we had been told was a "must see," five kilometers from Saint-Côme and one kilometer before the town of Espalion. Although our guidebook indicated the church was often locked, we hoped for the best.

In 1998 the Chemin from Saint-Côme to Estaing was declared a UNESCO World Patrimony, just as the entire Camino de Santiago in Spain had been designated. The honor carried with it the likelihood of European Union (EU)† financial assistance, enhanced visibility, and increased tourism. Secular and religious goals walk side by side along the Way of Saint James. They always have. The Camino was originally established in the Middle Ages in part to repopulate northern Spain, decimated during the Reconquest; and the churches that vied for pilgrims' attention did so not just for pilgrims' souls but also for their donations.

After the UNESCO designation, travel—spiritual and touristic—had increased dramatically on the Camino, and many Spaniards had been able to establish commercially viable hostels, bars, restaurants, pilgrimage *refugios,* and other shops. I presumed the designation would have the same effect in France.

The day was overcast and cool, a pleasant relief after the rain we had encountered for the past few days. We walked briskly, enjoying the fresh morning air.

Espalion appeared in the distance, but before reaching the town we took a gravel road to the left, leading to the Église de Perse. The dusky-rose sandstone church stood on a slight rise at the edge of a wheat field. A former priory† and pilgrims' stopping place, it was dedicated to the martyred Saint Hilarian, whom the Saracens had beheaded at this scenic spot.

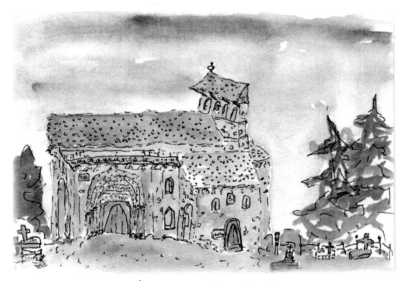

Église de Perse (Perse Church)

We walked past a picnic area and cemetery, then approached the imposing south doorway. The richly carved tympanum is divided horizontally in half. Two figures, each surrounded by a circle, are carved at the top of the tympanum. The figure on the left side (the sun) holds a sheaf of grain; the figure on the right has a crescent moon behind its head. Between them, three interconnecting circles with wavy rays shoot down onto the heads of the eleven figures below; in the center, a nose-diving dove represents the Holy Spirit descending at Pentecost. In the lower half of the tympanum the charming Last Judgment scene includes a wide-open mouth that spews forth monsters. The style of the carving reminded me of the tympanum at Conques. They are, indeed related.

The front door was locked, but we noticed a small sign and what looked like a doorbell. "Press here to enter," I translated. We pushed the bell and the heavy wooden door creaked open, a high-tech "Open Sesame."

As soon as I stepped inside the church, I felt an enormous energetic buzz. We walked around admiring the carved capitals (including battling knights and two birds sipping out of a chalice) and the bright red, yellow, and blue medieval frescoes that still adorned the vaults and upper walls of the chapel. I grew increasingly disoriented.

I tried without much success to focus on an exhibit of drawings made by the local school children. Posters described the history of the church and its relationship to the pilgrimage. The church, located on the original Chemin de Saint-Jacques, had served as the parish church until 1472, when another church replaced it. One poster showed nearby churches that shared the pilgrimage theme. A carving of a pilgrim eating bread can be seen at the church at Saint-Urcize; the church at Laguiole has a carving of Saint Jacques on its door.

An elderly grey-haired man approached us and started telling us in careful French about the church, the frescoes, and the recently installed electric door opener. I tried to concentrate, but I felt very confused and light-headed. After he led us outside, I immediately felt better.

He pointed toward the Adoration of the Magi, each of the three kings surrounded by a stone archway, carved high on the outside wall above the south portal. There were also two Virgins in Majesty with large hands. The Virgins on their thrones resembled the wooden Madonnas we had seen in Saugues and Chanaleilles. And why shouldn't they resemble each other? The popular artistic style of the time would have been quite similar; only the materials were different.

We thanked our guide and offered him some Euros, which he accepted. Then we walked back through the cemetery. When two pilgrims sitting at the picnic bench saw us, they asked if we had gotten inside the church. We explained about the electric button and they hurried to try it out.

Re-energized by our sightseeing excursion, we followed the GR into Espalion. With a population of 4500, it is a big city for this Aveyron region. It seemed like a metropolis after all the tiny villages we had passed through. A massive Renaissance château looms over the town, built on the banks of the river Lot.

We visited two museums—the folk-art Musée Joseph Vaylet and the underwater diving museum, the Musée de Scaphandre— located in the erstwhile Église de Saint-Jean. Why, we wondered, would a deep-sea-diving museum be located so far from the sea? The answer was simple: in 1864 two Espalionnais (residents of Espalion) invented a self-contained breathing apparatus and other deep-sea-diving equipment. Their invention inspired Jules Verne's *20,000 Leagues Under the Sea*.

We wandered through the folk-art museum, intrigued by the exhibits. There are wooden sabots with four-inch-high spikes for walking through forests carpeted with prickly chestnut burrs. One display includes a man's nightshirt from the nineteenth century (or perhaps it was even more recent) that features a large embroidered slit for his penis. Either the rural French were quite modest or their bedrooms were too cold to undress more completely, even for sex. (Given the rooms we had stayed in, I presumed the latter was the reason.) The nightshirt hangs on the wall in a sleeping alcove that includes a surprisingly short bed and a baby's cradle.

Gary and I continued down the main street and crossed a thirteenth-century stone bridge. Old stone tannery houses line the opposite side; each has steps leading down to the Lot, steps that end in a limestone platform. Medieval craftspeople knelt on the rough stone ledges while they washed animal skins in the river, rinsing off the toxic tanning chemicals.

We ate lunch at the Brasserie de la Marché (Market). Gary and I had the *plat du jour* (*menu* of the day): *aligot*, bread, wine, and our choice of stuffed cabbage or sausage. Overfed but well rested, we continued down the GR 65, following a grassy path alongside the Lot.

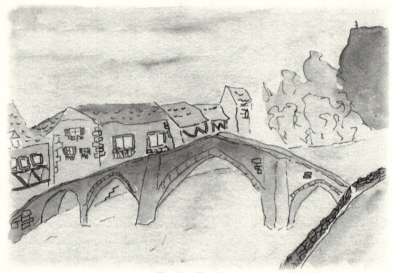

Bridge, Espalion

A kilometer later, still walking through the stretched-out town, we encountered Michelle seated on a low stone wall, rubbing her foot. A large blister covered the top of her swollen middle toe. Her Band-Aid had come loose and she had no replacement. I offered her a piece of stretchy, gel-lined tubing designed to protect and cushion toes. Grateful, she slipped it over her painful digit.

We walked together for several kilometers through fields of grapevine and a grove of boxwood to the next "must-see" spot, the pale-pink stone Église de Saint-Pierre-de-Bessuéjouls. Although the church is not on the main highway, the GR 65 leads directly to it. The site had been inhabited since Gallic times and the church is one of the oldest on the Chemin. Its eleventh-century bell tower contains a ninth-century altar. The rest of the church is more modern, dating to the sixteenth century. We knew that, like Saint-Hilarian, it was often locked.

The door was indeed locked, but this time we knew to look for an electric button. We pushed it and the heavy wooden door swung open. Ignoring the relatively modern church (after all, it was only 400 years old) and leaving the Susanis behind, we headed up the steep, narrow staircase that leads to the bell tower. After climbing

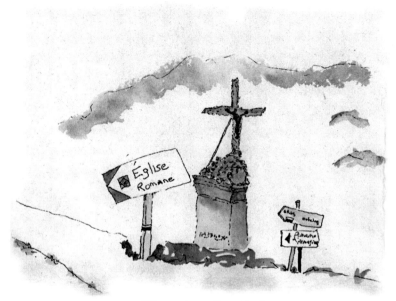

Waymarker to Bessuéjouls

the twisting, turning steps in near darkness, I saw a glimmer of light pouring through an open doorway.

Eagerly, I stepped out of obscurity into light. The stone walls are decorated with a carved border of intricate Celtic-style knots. I wondered if the knotwork preserves a distant aesthetic memory of previous inhabitants.

One side of the pink sandstone altar features Saint Michael pinning down a dragon with a spear, an action that has several possible symbolic interpretations. When pagan sites were converted to Christian shrines, Saint Michael was often called on to subjugate the previous spirituality. Some scholars think the dragon symbolizes the Earth-centered Goddess religions, others that it stands for the telluric (underground) water currents, which, in a Gaian† analogy to human capillaries, flow inside the body of Mother Earth.

Other scholars think the speared dragon represents the conquest of earthly vice and desire. All these theories share the idea that Christianity has triumphed over something, even if they don't agree on what. Since it is a spear, not a sword, thrust into the dragon's mouth, the gesture seems to indicate subjection but not death.

Saint Michael is also associated with the sun, the south, and fire, so perhaps the spear in the dragon's maw represents bringing together the energies of the sun, heat, and light with those of the earth. So many layers of meaning coexisting.

The Archangel Gabriel is carved on the opposite side of the altar. A banner spans his chest, but the inscription has disappeared long ago. Several capitals are decorated with unusual motifs. One shows nude figures peering out from behind large leaves. Is this a stylistic reference to the Green Man†, the vegetal image so popular in medieval European art, often portrayed as a face with tendrils and leaves coming out of his mouth?

Another column shows two centaurs facing away from each other, surmounted by a split-tailed siren-mermaid. If the siren represents a transmutation of the female generative organs, did the centaurs represent the animal-like nature of masculine sexuality? Or were they a reference to Sagittarius? So much remains a mystery.

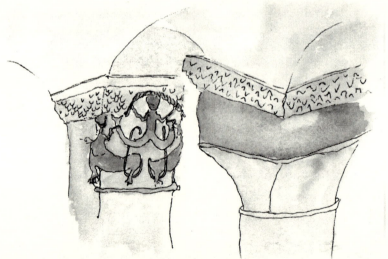

Siren-mermaid, Église de Saint-Pierre-de-Bessuéjouls
(Saint-Pierre-de-Bessuéjouls Church)

Jean stepped through the doorway, followed by Michelle and several other pilgrims. He put down his backpack, pulled out a 35-mm camera with a very impressive lens, and began checking the light with an exposure meter. Camera equipment filled most of his pack. No wonder he only had one pair of shoes, the hiking boots he was wearing on the Chemin.

I wondered aloud why the chapel of Saint Michael was on the second story, but no one seemed to know. One pilgrim pointed out that chapels dedicated to Saint Michael were often built on high places—on the top of hills, for example. In Carnac, Brittany, the chapel of Saint Michael was constructed on top of a megalithic burial mound, and in Le Puy, Saint-Michel-d'Aiguilhe perches on top of a volcanic plug. In both cases, Christianity had taken over a pagan site and claimed it for its own. Saint-Julien-de-Brioude, a Romanesque church near Le Puy-en-Velay with wonderfully preserved frescoes, also has a chapel of Saint Michael on the upper story. Perhaps putting the chapel up high was a concrete way of demonstrating who had dominion over whom.

After saying goodbye to the Susanis, who remained behind taking photos, we strolled up the tree-shaded lane to a small bar and sat down. Just when we had decided no one was going to serve us, a robust, red-faced man appeared, wiping his hands on his overalls. Judging by the grime, he had been working in the garden. We ordered bottled water and he went to fetch it.

After opening the bottles for us, he asked if we had visited the church. We nodded. Soon he was telling us, in pidgin French, about the church tower. It was Mozarabic, he declared, and originally had been a minaret.

What an unlikely concept, I thought. But when we looked at the church again, Gary and I both agreed that perhaps it might have been. After all, Muslim Saracens had martyred Saint Hilarian just a few miles away. Moorish craftsmen, who had built the cathedral in Le Puy, had carved a Kufic inscription honoring Allah on the front of the cathedral doors. Since they were Muslim, they must have worshipped in a mosque.

Did our host know why the chapel is on the second story? He shook his head. I wondered whether putting Saint Michael on top of whatever was below was a way of Christianizing the mosque—if, indeed, it had ever been one.

Folk wisdom, like folk etymology, could either reveal or obscure, and sometimes it did both at the same time. None of the material I had read suggested that this church was once a mosque. Besides, the chapel of Saint Michael in the Romanesque Église de Saint-Julien-de-Brioude is also on the upper story, and no one suggests that that church had been a mosque.

We returned to the main road and crossed over a bridge, then zigzagged steeply uphill. Soon the GR became a stony track that crisscrossed the country road. Eventually we followed a dirt trail on top of an undulating ridge, the bucolic countryside spreading out below.

The GR was relatively level for a while, but then we climbed steeply uphill again on a stony track that resembled steps cut into the side of the hill. It led us through the woods before it descended to a foliage-lined lane that paralleled the winding main road. Trees and the Lot separated us from the highway and its traffic. It was a pleasant, quiet stroll.

In the distance I saw dark grey roofs nestled in a gap between heavily forested hills. The towers of the fifteenth-century château of the Counts of Estaing and the church thrust up high above the town. Leaving the GR behind, we crossed a multi-arched Gothic-style bridge over the Lot and entered another one of the "Plus beaux villages de France."

We asked directions to the Auberge Saint-Fleuret, named after the patron saint of the town. The inn, we were informed, was on the rue François d'Estaing, the narrow main street that ran at a right angle to the river. The street was lined with *boulangeries, patisseries†, épiceries,* and a variety of specialty stores offering handmade jewelry, pottery, antiques, candies, and pastries. Despite Gary's impatience, I lingered in front of the inviting window displays.

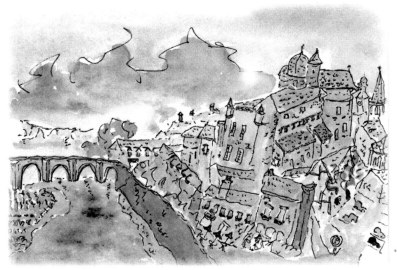

Estaing

Our hotel was in a somewhat decrepit stone building across from the Town Hall. I hoped the rooms would not be as dilapidated as the exterior. With some misgivings, we climbed a wide flight of shabby stairs into the lobby. Dark wood, elegant wallpaper in blue and gold, and amber lighting greeted us.

The owner and chef, Monsieur Gilles Moreau, came out of the kitchen when he heard our voices. With a welcoming smile, he took a large, old-fashioned key from a wooden plaque on the wall and led us up another flight of stairs. With a flourish he opened the door to our room. Recently renovated, it sported orange-sherbet-colored plaster walls, a blue and yellow Provençal bedspread and matching upholstered headboard. An electric heater was attached to the wall, warming the room to just the right temperature. The well-appointed bathroom featured towel warmers, electric heat, and a hair dryer (ideal for drying damp underwear). I sat down on the edge of the bed; the foam mattress gave a little, just enough.

Suddenly I wept. It was such a relief: a warm, attractive room with a decent mattress. I had had no idea how much I missed such simple comforts. I had thought I sincerely felt "gratitude, gratitude" for whatever life brings—but in truth, I had not felt thankful for some of our previous lodgings.

After I wiped the tears from my face and blew my nose, we went downstairs to inquire about our luggage. Monsieur Moreau called our previous hotel to check. With a reassuring nod he explained that it would arrive at the *auberge* by 5:00 p.m. I would have liked to change clothes before exploring the town, but I wasn't going to complain.

After washing up we headed to the nearby *syndicat d'initiative*, the small-town equivalent of a large-town tourist office. Brochures and flyers extolled the delights of Estaing. One even described it as "une perle dans un écrin." According to my tiny French/English dictionary, that meant "a pearl in a case," which I presumed meant I had incorrectly translated the phrase. Nobody in the *syndicat* spoke English so there was no one to ask.

In summer Estaing illuminates the château and bridge in the evenings and hosts a free-style kayak festival; in the second weekend of September there is a lavish medieval spectacle; and in July, Saint Fleuret's feast day is celebrated with an elaborate procession that includes over 150 characters representing holy personages and the more notable members of the famous d'Estaing family.

The brochures assert that the local d'Estaing wine is quite good and that artisan products include trout, mushrooms, sheep cheese, tripe, *confit*, *foie gras*, honey, and a kind of brioche called *fouace*, a specialty of the Auvergne—which we had already sampled in Nasbinals. In addition, numerous hiking trails, including the famous GR 65 and the Chemin de Saint-Jacques, surround the town, as do beautiful villages and lovely vistas. I began to regret we were only spending one night in Estaing.

I also learned that Estaing is approximately forty kilometers (25 miles) from Rodez, the town where we had stayed the night we arrived from the US. It didn't seem possible that we could be so close to a place that seemed so far away—a part of our pre-pilgrimage life. Distance is not only measured in miles.

Following one of the tours described in a brochure, we walked up the small knoll to the château and church complex. The château is now a convent; tours are available but we had missed the last one.

I noticed that a small shop in the courtyard was still open, so we went inside. It was a posh jewelry shop—indicative of Estaing's popularity in the proper season. The affable clerk showed us various jewel-studded crosses, including the cross of Estaing, named after the famous family that had once owned the château, and something glittering and expensive that he called "the circle of Tristan." We all knew we weren't going to buy anything, but he was quite amiable. Perhaps he was bored since it was off-season.

The church, located at the top of a tall flight of stairs, was our next stop. Mass was just finishing, so we waited before entering. We lit candles of gratitude and sat awhile in the stillness of sacred space.

Then Gary and I wandered through the twisting streets of Estaing, following signs leading to the Hospitalité Saint-Jacques. *Miam Miam Dodo* said that it provided friendly pilgrimage accommodation. We walked in and up a flight of stairs. Enticing aromas drifted through an open door; we peered inside. Three people were cutting vegetables for soup. They invited us in and, when they realized we spoke English but little French, they selected Michel to converse with us.

Our host led us to a nearby table and suggested that we sit down. He got us something to drink and then told us that the Hospitalité Saint-Jacques had been founded ten years before by a devout family dedicated to providing true Christian hospitality to pilgrims on the Way. Over the years the community had grown to include volunteers from all over France and Spain. The organization reminded me of the Spanish *refugios*, but those were usually run by lay confraternities or by municipalities, and weren't so overtly religious. Like the Hospitalité, however, volunteers staffed the *refugios*.

When Michel learned that Gary was a retired music professor, he picked up his guitar and began strumming. In solidarity we sang

John Denver and Beatles tunes. Soon the room was filled with the multi-textured sound of different accents singing English lyrics. We sipped our tea and waited for whatever would happen next. Michel inquired whether we wanted to stay there for the night. Perhaps we would attend the evening worship service? Politely, we refused and excused ourselves: dinner was waiting for us and we had other engagements.

We hurried through the darkened streets to our relatively luxurious *auberge*. The Susanis were already seated by the time we arrived. We nodded at each other and she pointed to her foot with a smile. The toe-tube had done the trick.

The *menus* looked enticing. After some indecision, I ordered a puff-pastry appetizer, followed by roasted lamb and a cheese platter and dessert. Gary chose a salad, poached fish, and a cheese platter.

Madame served each course with great attention to detail, turning the plate "just so" to best display the offering. Each plate was elegantly arranged. The pastry was crisp and light, the roast lamb tender and delicately spiced, the fish moist and aromatic. Dessert was memorable: an exquisite, warm chocolate tart. Monsieur Moreau was a master chef.

While we indulged in an after-dinner espresso, Jean approached our table and asked to borrow *Miam Miam Dodo*. After looking at a few pages he asked where we were staying the following night. We hadn't decided. They planned to walk sixteen kilometers to Golinhac where, according to the guidebook, only the communal *gîte* was open this late in the season. Jean offered to make reservations for all of us and we gratefully accepted. He left to make the phone call and soon returned, looking a little worried. He explained that he had made reservations for accommodation and dinner, but it wasn't clear if we would have private rooms. No matter, we reassured him, and thanked him.

Gratitude for angels, whether human or otherwise: Monsieur Thomas at the Église de Perse for giving us a tour; the man at the bar across from the Église de Saint-Pierre for solving (perhaps) the puzzle of the chapel of Saint Michael; me (I, too, could be an angel) for helping Michelle with the toe tube and providing the Susanis with information on where to stay; and the Susanis for making reserva-tions for us. Perhaps I was crediting angelic intervention for what was simply human kindness and attention. Nonetheless, looking for angels made me more attentive to the interconnected miracles of daily life.

Sunday, October 20, 2002. Estaing to Golinhac. 17 kilometers (10.5 miles) up and down steep hills.

Dreams flitted in and out of memory when I awoke. Something about needing different boots. Trying on a pair of ankle-high green Mephisto boots. Green. The color of Muhammad.

I'd dreamt about a green home a few nights before. Puzzled, I lay in bed trying to recall details, but they faded away like early morning fog. With a shiver, I got up and started my day.

Breakfast was a basket filled with two diminutive croissants and two tiny *pain de chocolate;* another basket with fresh, miniature ba-guettes; and an assortment of delicious homemade marmalades and jams. The fragrance of the still-warm pastries scented the air. I was trying to abstain from chocolate, but how could I refuse such entic-ing offerings?

On the way out of town we bought a freshly baked *pain de levant a l'ancienne*—sourdough bread baked in the wood-burning oven at the back of the *boulangerie*. I couldn't resist tearing off a piece to taste it; it was crusty on the outside, chewy and tangy on the inside. At another store we purchased a bulging-ripe disk of local goat cheese and fruit.

Confident that we had enough lunch supplies, we crossed back over the bridge to rejoin the GR 65. We endured a stiff uphill climb on a narrow footpath through the woods, occasionally crossing over a country road's hairpin turns. Pausing frequently to catch our breath, we climbed up and out of the Valley of the Lot. Soon we were on a high ridge. Dairy cattle grazed in the fields on either side.

Several hours later we caught up with the Susanis. Her knee was acting up so they were walking slowly. I commented on how difficult the ascent had been and she looked surprised.

It was a beautiful, sunny, breezy day and Gary and I both felt strong. Up and down, up and down through evergreen, chestnut, and oak forests. We stopped often, playfully posing Honey Bunny and Rustle Ears for photos beside a water pump by the side of the road or nestling in grape vines or sitting beside orange-topped mushrooms. We posed them on rocks next to our soon-to-be-consumed lunch. We posed them with oak leaves demurely covering their laps, and we posed them on the base of a lichen-covered stone cross. We posed them balancing on the branches of a twenty-foot-tall holly tree. Photos are supposed to be more engaging if they have people in them, so why not bunnies?

I still felt a bit self-conscious about traveling with plush animals, even though Collette and other pilgrims were quite taken with them. They added a significant dimension to my experience of the Chemin. They had important lessons to teach me about being playful and trusting, like a child who doesn't worry about the future. I realized that one could interpret our human-bunny interactions as pure fantasy, an escape from reality. But I preferred to think they were activities of the imaginal realm, which is quite different from the imaginary. The imaginal realm is where we explore our creativity and begin to bring our ideas into manifestation.

Besides, the bunnies were proof of the importance of synchronicity—of the interconnected web of existence. They had tried to warn me that my uterus had cancer—or at least that is the meaning I gave to their unexpected appearance in my life.

At one point, a GR 65 sign indicated that it was one hour and thirty minutes on foot to Golinhac. Much to my surprise, we made it in just that amount of time.

Every day we looked at each other and said, "This is as good as it gets." It was a variant of our leitmotif, "gratitude, gratitude for all that life brings." And every day *was* as good as it gets, although sometimes that awareness slipped away.

The expression could have had an ironic tinge to it—*This* is as good as it gets?—but I meant it straight-on. This day was filled with gorgeous views and amusing bunny photos; the day before we had had a marvelous dinner and slept in a comfortable bed. We wouldn't have appreciated it quite as much if the mattress in Saint-Côme had been more comfortable or if the meal at the Ferme des Gentianes had been tastier, but each of those days had been perfect as well, even if I hadn't realized it at the time. And each day gave new meaning to the next.

We arrived in the early afternoon at the communal *gîte d'etape* at Golinhac. The *gîte* is located in Les Chalets de Saint-Jacques, a recreation complex that includes campgrounds, a pool, laundry, individual cabins, a bar, and two communal *gîtes d'étape*, with twenty-one beds. The complex looked like it could be quite animated during summer but everything, except one of the *gîtes*, was closed. Our luggage waited outside the locked café/bar.

Two middle-aged women had arrived before us and were huddled over their hot tea in the dining room. They had claimed the small room with two beds. Jean had tried to reserve two rooms but, according to the sign-up sheet, only one room was reserved for the four of us. At the far end of the main level were several large communal bathrooms with showers and toilet stalls. None of the toilets had seats.

Wearily, we hauled our suitcases and the backpack up a steep flight of stairs to the second floor. Room Two had two bunk beds, one for each couple. We found another empty room at the end of the hall, with four beds and one bunk bed. Perhaps the Susanis could sleep there. Or perhaps we should. We weren't sure what to do. After much discussion, we settled into Room Two and claimed both bottom beds, figuring that if we had to move later to one set of bunk beds, we would.

It was too chilly to relax in the *gîte* so we went out to explore the town. All the shops were closed. Although *Miam Miam Dodo* indicated that the chalets, the restaurant, the *boulangerie*, and the *épicerie* were open until November, they weren't. It felt eerie to be in this isolated little village on the top of a mountain with no one else around except for the two taciturn women in the *gîte*.

The church was open. Paging through the *livre d'Or* I saw Akira's unmistakable note in Japanese. He had been there two days earlier. Gary and I lit candles.

"Gratitude for today and gratitude for tomorrow," I said, "Whatever it brings."

"Gratitude for all that we share," Gary added, blowing out the match.

Returning to the *gîte*, we found that the Susanis had arrived and settled into the other room. We hoped that arrangement was all right with them and that nobody else would have to join them. It was difficult to know what to do and even harder to explain.

While we rested on our separate bunk beds, Gary and I struggled to make a plan for the following day. Conques was only 21.5 kilometers away, but that distance included hiking up and down steep hills and deep valleys.

I realized I was in no hurry to arrive. In fact, I wasn't *ready* to arrive. I didn't want the pilgrimage to end. Once again I contemplated walking beyond Conques, extending our pilgrimage for a few more days. After all, fortune or fate had given me a copy of Raju's guidebook at the Ferme des Gentianes. Surely that was a sign, wasn't it? I broached the topic to Gary.

"We could keep walking to Figeac, you know."

"How far is that?"

"About fifty kilometers past Conques. We would have to walk twenty, then ten, then twenty kilometers. It would only take three more days. We have lots of time before my appointment with Dr Penoel."

Gary thought about it, and then shook his head. "I'm ready to become a tourist."

"I'm not."

"Maybe I'll feel differently later, but right now I don't want to walk any farther than Conques. We'll be coming back next spring to continue the Chemin, so what difference does it make?"

"I guess you're right. After all, we will be coming back." How could I argue? My beloved had been willing to go this far with me, so I was willing to agree to go no farther.

We tentatively decided to walk twelve kilometers to Sénergues where, according to *Miam Miam Dodo*, we could find accommodations; the following day we would continue to Conques. That would prolong our pilgrimage without prolonging the distance. It was a good compromise.

While we finalized our plans, the wind began to howl. We were at the top of a mountain that reminded me of the daunting pass at O Cebreiro, the gateway to Galicia on the Spanish Camino. Golinhac was only at an altitude of 650 meters (2100 feet) and O Cebreiro was at 1350 meters (4400 feet), but the howling concerned me.

Gary lay down to take a nap and fell asleep immediately, but I couldn't. The room was cold, even though the radiator was on. I wrote in my journal, trying to record details of our pilgrimage before I forgot them. Now I took our pilgrim life for granted, but I knew that when we were back in the US, this life would seem like a dream.

> *Our pilgrimage schedule: We go to sleep around 9:30 p.m., as soon as we finish eating. It is autumn, so it gets dark somewhere between 8:00 and 9:00 p.m. Ordinarily, going to sleep on a full stomach would give Gary acid reflux, but on the Chemin this doesn't happen. Perhaps all the exercise makes a difference for both of us: I feel healthier than I have ever felt before.*

> *We sleep through the night, then rise around 7:30 a.m., wash up and pack, and eat breakfast around 8:30 a.m. We start out around 9:30 or 10:00 a.m. We are in no hurry since we are not walking long distances and the days are not hot. (On the Spanish Camino in summer, we would start walking before daybreak to avoid the devastating heat.) Sometimes we arrive at our destination by 12:30 p.m. Today, a long uphill climb, we arrived by 2:00 p.m. We can walk much further and with less effort than when we began, thirteen days ago.*

I am finding this pilgrimage a surprisingly outward-focused journey, full of problem-solving exercises. There are, of course, plenty of opportunities to simply be present: present to the sound of tree branches creaking in the breeze, twigs crackling underfoot as we walk, the squishy sound of our boots on wet fallen leaves, the clack of our metal-tipped hiking staffs on the road. Present to the smells of cow manure, pine trees, tannin in rotting leaves, to the fragrance of Sunday dinner wafting out of the open window of a farmhouse by the side of the road. Present to chickens cackling and dogs barking, to fresh vegetables growing in a garden behind a house, to roses, marigolds, dahlias, and various unknown flowers blooming gaily in yards or along fences.

But even being present feels like "doing," not like "being." So many new smells, sights, and tactile impressions assail me each day, every step, that sometimes I feel overwhelmed.

Going on pilgrimage frees one from work obligations and societal expectations, providing time and space for interior exploration. Walking through sacred space, visiting holy places, participating in an ancient ritual process creates a vehicle for spiritual exploration. But it is very different from going on a retreat. There is a distinct advantage to being located in one place—to being a cloistered monk or nun—rather than traveling to a new place every day and walking all day to get there. One can be present to what is outside or present to what is inside. I long for more of the latter. Perhaps with lots of practice I can learn to do both.

Occasionally thoughts about the cancer surgery (now I distance myself from it by referring to it as "the" not "my") arrive like unwanted guests and I start to worry. Medical newsletters expound about proper nutrition and supplements, both of which I am ignoring on this journey. I feel healthier, however, than I have ever felt. Surely that counts for something.

*I tell myself not to worry, to have faith. I am grateful
to be alive, alive and walking with my beloved Gary. As
Collette said when we first met her, "After cancer, life seems
so sweet!"*

The cold, fierce wind blew harder, whipping the branches of the
trees and rattling the windowpanes. Gary woke up with a start.

At 7:30 p.m. we went to the café/bar for dinner. Although it was
just a few buildings away, the blustery wind chilled us in moments.
Shivering, we pushed open the door. The warm, bright room was full
of old men smoking and drinking.

The six of us from the *gîte* sat at one large table. The Susanis
told us that they were walking to Conques the next day. Did we
want them to make reservations for us at the Accueil Abbaye Sainte
Foy? Gary and I shook our heads. We planned to walk only as far as
Sénergues. The Susanis nodded. It would be a parting of the ways
for us.

The woman next to me had an *Año Santo* 1999 badge pinned on
her jacket, which meant she had gone to Compostela during the last
Holy Year. Eager to learn about her experience I smiled at her and
enthusiastically tried to explain that I, too, had walked the Camino
de Santiago. She wasn't interested. I tried again but she ignored me,
turning to her friend across the table and beginning another conversation. I had been snubbed.

My French was quite limited but it was good enough to talk
about the pilgrimage if the other person made half an effort. I knew
an assortment of nouns, gerunds, and adverbs (Where? When? How
much? Rain? *Fromage?* The weather?) that I could string together to
form a question. People were usually willing to answer me at length,
and I could understand much of what they said. Not this time.

Soon the Susanis and the two ladies were in animated conversation, making no effort to include us. There was no reason why they
should. I was surrounded by a babble of voices speaking a language I

barely understood. It wasn't the first time this had happened on the Chemin but this time I found it deeply distressing.

Dinner consisted of a thick, bland-but-filling lentil, cheese, and bread soup, followed by grilled pork cutlets covered with tomato sauce, with rice served on the side. Dessert was *fromage blanc* with sticky apricot marmalade poured on top. Gary and I ate in silence while I tried to understand our companions' conversation and why I felt so disturbed. One reason was that we had relied on others to make arrangements for us—whether it was Collette, the innkeepers, or the Susanis—and now we would have to manage on our own. Never mind that we had managed before we met these folks. It wasn't the situation, it was the significance I was giving to it.

I consulted *Miam Miam Dodo* again; the only shelter in Sénergues was a *gîte d'etape* with dorm rooms. Suddenly it felt daunting to make reservations and to get our luggage transported off this wind-blasted mountaintop. Besides, I didn't want to sleep in a bunk bed, particularly not in a room that I would have to share with others. I wanted privacy and a private bath. I wanted to snuggle in bed with Gary.

I was suddenly weary of trying to figure things out. I glanced at Gary. He looked exhausted. To make matters worse, the Susanis had reminded us that because tomorrow was Monday, all the grocery stores would be closed. How would we find food? The more we listened to the wind beating against the rattling windows, the more nervous we became. In Colorado that kind of wind meant the weather had turned. Snow was coming.

We were alone. Nobody wanted to talk with us. Everything had worked out perfectly for nearly two weeks, but I started to panic anyway.

I had thought I would confidently recommend the Chemin to someone who spoke very little French, but suddenly I had second thoughts. Like a balloon that had been punctured, I was instantly deflated.

While our companions carried on their exclusive conversation, Gary and I had one of our own.

"It's time to finish the pilgrimage. I don't want another night like this," Gary declared.

I nodded, disheartened. "I guess you're right."

"Let's get to Conques tomorrow. We can make it. It'll be our last day."

"Okay."

Gary took the cell phone over to a marginally quieter corner of the café and called the Hôtel Saint-Jacques in Conques to make reservations for the next day. He knew someone there would speak enough English for him to communicate his needs. He requested a *gran lit*. The first person he spoke with replied, "twin beds only," and hung up. He tried again. This time when he asked for a *gran lit*, a different voice at the other end of the phone replied, "But of course!"

We were still left with the challenge of transporting our luggage. A sign in the *gite* advertised taxi service to Conques but I hadn't written down the number. We went up to the bar and Gary struggled in French to ask about a taxi.

The bartender replied in Cockney English, "No problem!"

"You speak English?" Gary asked in disbelief.

"Spent a fair amount of time in England, I have," he replied.

We both heaved a huge sigh of relief. Our angel had appeared when we most needed it.

"Can you make us sandwiches for tomorrow?" I asked hopefully.

"Fraid not. I only have enough bread for tonight. Tomorrow's Monday and shops are closed."

Seeing my concern he added, "You'll be able to buy bread in Espeyrac, the next town on the Chemin. It's only eight and one-half kilometers away."

He pulled a card out of a drawer, dialed a number, and had a lengthy conversation, which culminated in our leaving money with him to pay the taxi driver. He told us to leave the luggage outside the bar in the morning.

"Outside the bar? But won't it be closed?" I asked.

"That's why you leave it outside," he replied.

That was easy for him to say, I thought. It wasn't *his* possessions that were being left in front of a locked building.

Our new plan was to walk to Conques the next day. If the weather was truly dreadful, we would stop at Espeyrac or Sénergues and stay there, or we would take a taxi to Conques and return the next day to finish walking the Chemin. It was a desperate plan, but we suddenly felt desperate—desperate and illogical. For some inexplicable reason we had lost our confidence.

Oh ye of little faith, I told myself. How quickly I had lost faith, the roots still shallow and easily uprooted in a storm. And how quickly faith had been restored. And lost. And restored again. Things always worked out. We'd been saying that all along, but when it had been put to the test we had suddenly panicked. All that we needed was provided for us. We were held in God's hands. Gratitude, gratitude, for all that life brings, I told myself, including an opportunity to test my green, sprouting faith.

Monday, October 21, 2002. Golinhac to Conques. 21 kilometers (13 miles).

I woke up several times during the night, grabbed my flashlight, and hurried down the long flight of stairs to the unheated bathroom at the end of the hall. Finally I gave up trying to sleep. This was our last day on the Chemin. Our frantic emergency fall-back plans of the previous night made no sense in the renewing light of dawn. I knew we would walk to Conques, no matter what the weather was like.

I lay in bed listening to the battering wind and saying prayers of thanksgiving for all that we had experienced, including this frigid bedroom. Gratitude for all the opportunities for learning to trust. Gratitude for all the angels that had come our way and for the chance to be angels to others. Gratitude for being whole, holy, healed, and healthy. Gratitude for not having blisters. Gratitude that the knob on top of Gary's instep has improved and that his right ankle doesn't hurt as much. Gratitude for today and tomorrow, whatever it brings.

Our intention had been to get to Conques in three weeks or less and we would make it in two. This very day we would return to Conques, arrange to rent a car, perhaps do some sightseeing, and relax. We had earned it.

Breakfast was sparse. The manager of the *gîte* had forgotten to bring milk and the bread was dry and days-old. I took a piece, then tossed it in the wastebasket. Then I remembered the stale roll I'd been given at the pilgrims' blessing in Conques. At the time, I had thought there might come a time when I would be grateful to have it. Repentant, I reclaimed the stale piece of bread.

We left before the Susanis came down to breakfast. As we walked past the war memorial in town and down a grassy lane, I realized I had never gotten their address. We would probably never see them again and had no way to contact each other, but that's how it was on the Chemin. You met people and you left them behind or they left you. It was like walking a labyrinth: we were all on the same path, and for a while our journeys had coincided. But the labyrinth is a convoluted spiral, so there are times when one person turns one way and someone else turns another.

Gary hoisted on the fanny pack and we stepped outside, expecting winter. The wind was still blowing but it was surprisingly warm outside. Clouds flew quickly by. All the fear of the night before was for naught. This was France, not Colorado.

We followed the GR, a mixture of grassy lanes and country roads. Soon we headed uphill through the forest, the trail covered with chestnuts and acorns—which, I discovered, were slippery when wet. Much of the time we walked downhill on a country road. In the distance we saw Espeyrac, the town with the open *boulangerie*.

No such luck. All shops were closed. I was determined not to give up. We came to an open hôtel-restaurant, but no one appeared to be on duty. A bunch of duffle bags with "La Pèlerine" tags waited by the front door, so I knew someone must be there.

I strode through the corridors calling out, "Bonjour!"

At last an old woman dressed in black waved at me. She was deaf and hadn't been able to hear me. With a nod, she leaned out the window and started calling to someone. She was our first angel of the day.

Soon a young woman appeared and asked what we wanted.

"Avez-vous pain?" I asked, hopefully.

She shook her head.

I tried a different tack. "Avez-vous sandwich?"

This time she nodded. She gestured for Gary and me to follow her into the bar and she pointed at the blackboard menu. "Fromage? Saucisson?"

"Fromage," we both replied.

She went into another room and soon reappeared with two large plates and two very large slices of cheese sandwiched between thick chewy bread. We disposed of them quickly.

Just as we were getting ready to leave, Michelle and Jean walked in. Our paths had coincided again. We happily greeted each other with kisses on both cheeks. They also ordered something to eat and sat down at a nearby table. After a brief exchange, we said goodbye and started back on the Chemin.

After crossing a footbridge over the river and walking up and down several other hills for three and one-half kilometers, we reached Sénergues. It was a small town but large enough to have a *supérette*—and it was open. We purchased chocolate, bananas, croissants, raisins, and goat cheese, enough food to get us through the uncertainties of several days, not just this one.

It was my turn to carry the fanny pack, so we put the bunnies in the plastic grocery bag, along with the groceries, in order to lighten the weight. As we walked through town we passed the Domaine de Sénos *gîte*, which looked quite inviting. I realized, belatedly, that *Miam Miam Dodo* had awarded it a "little flower." We could have stayed there if we hadn't gotten into such a fright the night before.

We started uphill again and suddenly I couldn't walk another step. I collapsed by the side of the road and cried. Maybe it was lack of sleep. Maybe it was because I had had no breakfast and had then eaten a large amount of cheese and bread. Maybe it was because I didn't want the pilgrimage to end.

Gary and I debated turning around and staying at the Domaine de Sénos but decided to continue. Gary fastened the fanny pack around his waist, then helped me up the trail into the woods. Up, up, up we went until we were deep into the forest. When we found a tree stump by the side of the road, I sat down and rested. Taking our supplies out of the plastic bag, we made lunch. Soon I felt revived and we started back on the Chemin. My energy level was as mercurial as my mood had been the night before.

The GR followed a country road that wound its way up and down through forest and field. Soon a large white cow trotted up the lane ahead of us. Every so often she bellowed and groaned, swinging her head toward the meadow to her right. A bull returned her call and followed her on the other side of the fence. We walked behind for a while and then carefully passed her by.

At the top of the hill two people were working in a field. We ran over to tell them that the cow was loose and they hurried back down the road. This time we had been the angels.

We came to an unmarked intersection and didn't know which way to turn. We started walking in one direction but within 100 meters a woman drove by and stopped. Leaning out the car window she waved at us and said, "Don't go that way—it's the wrong direction!" She was the second angel of the day.

A little while later, Gary suddenly crumpled by the side of the road, unable to continue. This time I felt strong enough to carry the fanny pack. After a short rest, we started up again. We walked silently, conserving energy, following the original medieval pilgrimage route that ran along the ridge and then descended to Conques, a mere three and one-half kilometers away in a deep gorge of the Dourdou River.

En route we stopped at the roadside chapel of Saint Marcel. Over the door, three scallop shells in a stained glass window commemorate the Chemin. Inside the small chapel we admired the statue of Saint Roch, attired like a medieval pilgrim, wearing a broad-brimmed hat, a cloak decorated with scallop shells, and holding a pilgrim's staff and water gourd in one hand.

When we emerged outdoors, rain was falling. Soon the GR turned into a slippery, rocky footpath. Just before the going got steeper, a large sign advertised the Accueil Abbaye Sainte-Foy. In French, English, and German, the placard told us everything the friars thought we needed to know about Conques:

> Pilgrims, and hikers, Sainte Foy welcomes you to Conques.
>
> This young (twelve-year-old) Christian martyr bore witness to her faith in Agen, where she was decapitated in AD 303. Her mortal remains arrived in Conques in 866 and were the very reason why the abbey church was built, with its famous tympanum in which our Savior offers us the Cross, Heaven, the damnation we must avoid, and the need for conversion.
>
> The Abbey's reception center, situated behind the church and run by our Norbertine Friars, offers board and lodging to suit all tastes.

We continued walking through a forest filled with moss- and lichen-covered trees. Millions of pilgrims' footsteps had worn down the stones on the path until it was treacherous when wet, a precipitous downhill trail. Slick moss coated the stones on either side of the trail.

We slithered and slid two kilometers down to the asphalt lane below as the rain poured down. A villager strolling down the road protected herself with a big umbrella, but the rain didn't matter to us. We had arrived in Conques. We had completed the first stage of our pilgrimage on the Chemin, although our pilgrimage through cancer had just begun.

The asphalt lane led us past the tourist office at the edge of town, so we stopped on our way to our hotel. Our thoughts had quickly turned towards tourism. We blithely assumed we could pick up a rental car in Rodez the next day, but no rental cars were available within several days and several hundred kilometers. We gave up and headed into town to the Accuiel Abbaye Sainte-Foy to get a stamp for our credentials. We had come full circle in a little over two weeks. Actually, it wasn't a circle, it was a spiral. Although we had returned to where we began, we were greatly changed by our journey.

And then we went to the church, where we lit candles before the statue of Saint Jacques. Gratitude, gratitude, for a safe journey, gratitude for all that we shared. Gratitude to Sainte Foy, that sweet, faith-filled young girl, for such a fantastic send-off just two weeks ago.

We made a vow to return the following May and walk the next 200 - 300 kilometers, assuming that I was still healthy enough to walk. I made another vow, this one silent, to live each day in gratitude, whatever it brings.

We walked into the nave to sit on one of the benches—and there was Akira! He ran over and hugged us. He had arrived on Saturday and was staying until Wednesday in a room at the Accueil. He told us he attended prayers at night and in the morning.

When Gary told Akira he had left the pilgrim's staff on the bridge, Akira related the rest of the story. Two Swiss women had arrived in Conques with the staff, which they had picked up at the bridge. Akira told them that it had been his for a brief time and then he formally gave it to them.

We invited Akira to join us for dinner and he agreed. Then he returned to his meditations. Just as we were leaving the church the Susanis walked in. More hugs and kisses. This time we exchanged addresses before saying goodbye.

At last we checked into our hotel. Our luggage had already arrived. Our room was on the third floor, with a beautiful view, and we had a private bathroom complete with bathtub. The staff had moved two beds together to make a *gran lit*. Now we understand why the first clerk had said "no" and the second had said "yes." There was a crack between the beds and they had separate sheets and blankets, but it didn't matter. Life was good.

I called Dad to tell him we had arrived. He was delighted. The bunnies were slightly bedraggled from posing for pictures on barbed wire fences and holly trees; they needed a bath but that could wait. The next day we would buy the scallop-shell fossil in the rock shop next to the church, assuming it was still available. Somehow, I knew it would be.

Lying on the bed I looked out the window at the mist rising in the valley. In the distance I could barely make out the Chapelle Sainte-Foy, perched high on a hillside one and one-half kilometers away. Next year we would walk up to that chapel as we continued our pilgrimage. I wondered what next year would bring, but it was a wondering filled not with anxiety but with curiosity. After all, whatever happened, I was held in God's hands. I was part of the interconnected web of life.

INTERLUDE

Eventually we were able to rent a car in Albi, but to get there we had to take an early morning school bus and connect with a long-distance bus. We grumbled at the inconvenience. How easily we had shifted from pilgrims on a sacred journey to impatient tourists.

I had mistakenly assumed that since we hadn't finished the Chemin—we were only pausing part-way to our goal—we would stay in pilgrimage mode longer. Without constant vigilance, old habits reassert themselves. I had much more practice with the old habits than with the new.

Gary and I drove off to explore the Cathar country in southern France while we waited for my appointment with Dr Penoel. My one-day visit with the intense doctor turned into several and concluded with the stern recommendation that I should return soon for a week or preferably a month, to get the full benefit of his work. I didn't know whether to be relieved or frightened.

In late October we returned home. Gradually life returned to normal, although "normal" had a different meaning now than it had had before cancer.

In December, six months after my operation, I had another Pap test. It came back abnormal.

I was terrified.

Dr. Williams tried to reassure us. "I really don't think it's anything to worry about. I'll run more tests on the sample to see if you have HPV, a virus that puts you at high risk for cervical cancer. But I think the abnormal result is because your cervical scar tissue is still healing. I've seen this happen before."

Gary and I held hands tightly. We were badly shaken.

Dr. Williams spoke calmly. "Take it easy, relax, and don't worry. We'll wait a while and then retest you."

We nodded in agreement, but all the time I was thinking, "Don't worry? Easy for *her* to say—it wasn't her test result. How could I not worry? I've had another abnormal Pap smear!"

True, it wasn't as bad as the one that had led to my hysterectomy six months earlier, but it was still abnormal. I knew that uterine cancer could metastasize to the lungs, but if that's what this was, why did it show up on the Pap smear? Had I developed another kind of cancer?

I reminded myself I was exactly the same person I had been before learning about the lab results. I felt healthy and there was no reason to feel sick just because of some words. Besides, Dr. Williams thought the test results were inaccurate. Nonetheless, suddenly it was difficult to believe that everything was as good as it gets, that things were perfect. I knew this was an opportunity to trust in whatever life brings, but at that moment trust felt impossible.

After the shock wore off I struggled to find a way to transform the disturbing test results into something positive. I started looking again at how I was living my life. I didn't blame myself for the abnormal Pap test; instead, I was determined to view it as a challenge and an opportunity.

What did I still need to change? What inner truth was still being muffled? What soul-level needs were still being ignored? What message was hidden within the apparently negative news? What supplements did I need to take? What could I do to make myself emotionally and physically healthier? I didn't know why I had gotten cancer in the first place, but I did know I could always improve how I lived my life.

A few weeks later I confided to my acupuncturist, "You know, I have never felt at ease in our house. If it were up to me I'd be out of there in a flash!"

"Do you know what you just said?" she asked.

I shook my head, so she repeated it.

"I said *that?*"

"You did."

I went home and told Gary, and he said, "If that's how you feel, we'll sell the house. We've done everything we could to make the house comfortable for you since we bought it four years ago, but if it doesn't work, it just doesn't work."

We went to our counselor and I told her that I had said, "If it were up to me...."

She looked at me quizzically. "Well, whom else *would* it be up to but you?"

Lesson learned. Or at any rate, *another* lesson learned.

We interviewed realtors and chose one who was excited about selling our home. Even though the market was excruciatingly slow (houses were averaging six months to sell), our house sold in a week. All of a sudden we had to find somewhere else to live. Fast. And we did.

My next Pap test was normal.

We made plans to return to the pilgrimage road in May 2003, a few weeks after the closing date on our new house. The house needed major remodeling, so we turned the project over to a contractor who would work on it while we walked the Chemin. We planned to be in France for five weeks and come back in early June to move in.

Our intention was to walk approximately 300 kilometers (nearly 186 miles), from Conques to Condom, a place picked arbitrarily by Gary and certainly not for its evocative name. Collette and Danielle planned to join us for a week. They would start walking a week before we did and meet us in Conques.

This time we decided to take only Honey Bunny. Two bunnies had taken up too much space in the fanny pack; besides, Honey Bunny seemed much more "enlivened" than Rustle Ears, who tended to simply sit silently and stoically on his broad, flat bottom. We gave Rustle Ears to our grandson, Max, who seemed to appreciate him.

We planned to take one backpack, my large fanny pack, and no suitcases; that way we could carry everything we needed and not have to rely on taxis or innkeepers to transport our baggage. Realizing how little material stuff we really need is an important exercise.

In the Middle Ages, that great Age of Pilgrimage, pilgrims started at home and travelled on foot or by horse or carriage until they reached the shrine that was their goal. They spent months on the road. Modern transportation, however, enables people to make their pilgrimages in stages, fitting in a few weeks of travel during the summer or a few days during a long holiday break.

I had viewed this modern multi-stage way of making a pilgrimage as an excursion, not a sacred journey. Liminality was too brief, "time out" too short. I believed that walking the Camino (and the Chemin) was transformative because it enabled one to spend an extended amount of time outside one's normal status and occupation, outside of one's usual social context and responsibilities, traveling through sacred space and time. That's when real change could occur. It was ironic, therefore, that my pilgrimage was unavoidably taking place in relatively short stages.

What I had thought was regrettable, however, turned into a meaningful lesson. By making the pilgrimage in stages I felt like I was still on the pilgrimage even though I was living in Boulder, Colorado. It became part of my daily thoughts and hopes, part of my daily prayers. Each day was filled with a sense of expectation as I looked forward to returning to the Chemin and walking another stage of our pilgrimage of gratitude.

May 2003 Pilgrimage

Sunday, May 4, 2003: Back to France.

Six months after we finished the first stage of our pilgrimage, we were going back to France. I had thought about the Chemin every day, eager to return. At last that day arrived.

The airport shuttle arrived and we hopped in. When the driver overheard us talking about the pilgrimage, he turned to us with a bemused expression. Several of his friends who were living in an Indian ashram were going to walk the final hundred miles of the Camino the following week. The woman sitting next to me, a professor at Yale University, expressed fascination and suggested we might work together on a book combining geology and pilgrimage. We exchanged business cards. Synchronicities of the Chemin—or were they just coincidences? I preferred the former: it made life more meaningful.

Monday, May 5, 2003. Arriving in France.

Our flight left two hours late and arrived just as late, but thanks to $55.00 in cab fare we arrived at the Gare Montparnasse just before the TGV pulled out of the train station. After a lulling ride to Toulouse, we transferred to the same slow train we had taken last October. As it chugged towards Rodez I dozed off. In that mist-filled place between wake and sleep, I had the following waking dream—or was it a waking vision?

The train's automatic door suddenly sprang open, then closed.

I asked, "Who's there?"

A sonorous voice replied, "I will be with you on your journey."

I had an "interior vision" of a bearded man wearing a brown cloak and holding a staff. "Who are you?" I asked.

"Saint James."

"But I don't even believe in you!" I exclaimed. "Couldn't you be the Archangel Raphael or Michael? Not that I believe in them either, but..."

He replied, "What's the matter, I'm not good enough for you?"

"No, it's not that," I apologized. "I'm just surprised to see you, that's all."

The automatic door opened again and, jolted awake, I jokingly told Gary, "That's Saint James, leaving."

Gary looked puzzled, so I explained. He still looked puzzled. So was I. It was one thing to speak metaphorically of Saint James's presence on the Chemin, quite another to have him pay me a visit.

We arrived in Rodez near midnight and Danielle, the taxi-driver from last year, was waiting to take us to the Hôtel de la Tour Maje. We greeted each other warmly and she asked whether we were returning to the Chemin. We said yes, and she shook her head in disbelief. I could hear her thinking, "These crazy Americans!"

We had wondered how we were going to reach Conques the next day without a car, but it occurred to me that Danielle could drive us there. She named a price; we agreed. All was effortlessly arranged. We were definitely "in the flow."

Christine, the desk clerk, also remembered us from last October and was pleased to see us again. Jetlagged and weary as we were, it was comforting to return to a familiar place and a familiar face. She even gave us the same room as last time, a quiet corner room with a view over the plaza. She swore it was just a coincidence.

Tuesday, May 6, 2003: Morning in Rodez; afternoon in Conques.

Gary discovered he hadn't brought liner socks. Although we had been thinking about the pilgrimage for months, we hadn't really prepared.

After eating too much at the lavish buffet breakfast, we asked Christine where we could find hiking equipment and homeopathics.

She smiled and gestured. "Around the corner."

Sure enough, just around the corner and up a side street was a shop that sold high-tech gear, including a wide choice of liner socks. Just a little further we found several pharmacies, each of which provided *homeopathique* as well as allopathic and *herboriste* (herbalist) medicines. The efficient, white-jacketed clerk made up a small plastic kit with six homeopathic containers and wrote on a piece of paper the appropriate use for each of them: flu, indigestion, muscle aches, heavy legs, headache, and diarrhea.

Our needs were being met. Once again I had the reassuring feeling of being held in God's hands. That was the most succinct way I could find to describe the loving support surrounding us, even though the phrase reminded me that the Biblical image of a male god had crept insidiously into my subconscious. In a different era, the image might have been that of a nurturing goddess.

After making our purchases, we hurried over to the thirteenth-century Cathédrale Notre-Dame. We entered the dark, cool sanctuary and I started to weep. So much had happened since our previous visit: we'd successfully completed the first part of the Chemin; I'd had an abnormal Pap smear followed by a normal one; I'd spoken my truth about our house and we'd sold it and bought another.

And there was more: a vacation in Mexico for massage training (Gary had taken it up after retirement and I went along to relax on the beach); a trip to San Diego for a book-signing for my 88-year-old father's latest book, *Where the Williwaw Blows,* a satiric novel about naval life in the Aleutians during WWII; a Sufi Order International retreat in California, where we both explored more deeply the relationship between the personal ego and the unlimited Source of which we are all a part.

It was as if I no longer had time to wait; I had to do it all now. One never knows how long one has to live, but in my case that hackneyed observation had immediate relevance. Live each day as if it were your last. No time to waste.

Hand in hand, Gary and I strolled over to the candle rack by the door and purchased a handful of long white tapers. Then we walked around the church looking for a sacred image to which we felt attracted. This time we chose a life-size marble statue of John the Baptist baptizing Jesus and a large oil painting of Mary dressed as a housewife, standing on a crescent moon. One of her bare feet delicately pressed down on the head of a fire-spitting dragon. Once again I saw the crescent-moon symbol of the Goddess and the dragon-serpent symbol of telluric currents, materialism, and/or earth-centered religions. The encoded messages were there for those who knew, whether their knowledge came from books or through secret initiation, to interpret however they chose.

"Gratitude for today and gratitude for tomorrow," we affirmed as we lit the candles and placed them between the splayed prongs on the black metal stand. "Gratitude for health—at least I *think* I'm healthy," I prayed silently, wondering if I would ever be sure that I was free *from* cancer. Free *from* cancer, free *of* cancer—what a subtle difference existed between those two words: the first suggested escape, the second suggested healing.

I was aware that now I hedged my bets, wary of being taken by surprise again. My euphoria, my enormous relief at finding the cancer early, had faded as I realized that my health status would remain a question mark for four more years. If the cancer didn't metastasize (most likely to my lungs, since I no longer had a uterus) within five years after surgery, my statistical risk level would return to zero and I could rejoin the population pool of "normal" human beings. Although the immediate threat was over, I still had a long uncertain slog ahead.

How hard it was to "keep the faith." Could I ever cross back over that great divide between those who have had cancer and those who haven't? Would a calendar date really serve as a bridge? I doubted it. There was no going back; there was only going forward.

Shaking myself out of my musings, I lit another candle. Gratitude for being back in France. Gratitude that we would soon be walking the Chemin again.

We left a small bag stuffed with French travel guides and airline comfort items like inflatable neck pillows at the hotel with Christine. We were always getting rid of things, even though this time we were only carrying one large fanny pack and one backpack filled with necessities, including our rain gear and umbrellas, extra shoes, clothes, cosmetics, electric toothbrushes, our cell phone, and two chargers. Just how much was I willing to do without, I wondered? Not as much as I had thought.

We promised Christine we would retrieve the bag in approximately two weeks. She wished us "Bon voyage." On the Spanish Camino, people wish each other "Buen Camino," but we were in France and "good journey" was close enough.

We ate lunch at the Aussie pub next to the hotel and waited for Danielle to pick us up. She arrived on time and forty-five minutes later she dropped us off near the abbey church in Conques, right in front of another Danielle—our pilgrim companion, who just happened to be strolling down the street. A few moments later, Collette walked around a corner. More serendipity—or was it synchronicity? I cautioned myself against reading too much meaning into events; after all, Conques was a tiny village. But it was much more satisfying to think that events were meaningful, not random—including having cancer.

Delighted to see each other, we kissed on both cheeks and then once more for good measure. I felt as if we had parted company the day before, but it had been over six months.

"Où est le lapin?" Collette asked eagerly.

With a flourish, Gary pulled Honey Bunny out of the bag. Collette gave her a big hug and then commented on her new necklace and her lack of clothes. We explained that we had left her sweater behind since it was springtime.

Honey Bunny was turning into quite a material girl, acquiring ear clips, ankle bracelets, and necklaces from our friends and the staff at our dentist's office. I had pointed out to Honey Bunny that "you can't take it with you," but she had replied, "Exactly! That's why I want it all now!"

While cuddling Honey Bunny, Collette described their week-long journey from Ferme des Gentianes to Conques. Not surprisingly, they lost their way several times, including one harrowing day of walking on railroad tracks and climbing over barbed wire fences. Collette hadn't yet had cataract surgery so she still couldn't see well, but Danielle continued to rely on her to guide them.

"So what's the plan for tomorrow?" I asked Collette.

A month earlier Collette had asked us if she should plan our walk together, and we had eagerly given her carte blanche. How easily we fell into the same pattern as Danielle. We had a rationale, however: it was better to have Collette make the arrangements because she spoke French and was in France.

"Tomorrow we walk to Livinhac-le-Haut. That's twenty-four kilometers."

Gary and I chorused in disbelief: "Twenty-four kilometers?"

Collette smiled and nodded.

The previous year we had usually walked only fifteen to sixteen kilometers, except for the last day to Conques when, spurred on by panic, we had managed twenty-one. Collette and Danielle had already walked for a week so maybe they were ready for a forced march, but we weren't. We had been too busy to get in shape before boarding the plane to France. Already I was regretting my previous priorities.

Seeing our consternation, Collette explained that it would be a tough first day but it was the only plan that made sense, given the subsequent six days. She had made arrangements that depended on our walking that distance but if we weren't happy with it…. Her voice dropped and she looked at the ground. I took a deep breath and assured her that it would be all right. We exchanged cheery smiles all around; ours were admittedly forced.

That settled, we checked into the Accueil Abbaye Sainte Foy, the large building located just behind the abbey church. Collette had reserved us a single room with two beds and a private bathroom, and it was austere but attractive. We agreed to meet them for dinner in the abbey.

We said, "A bientôt—see you soon!" and exchanged more kisses.

Then Gary and I sat down on the narrow beds and looked at each other in dismay.

"I can't walk twenty-four kilometers!" I proclaimed.

"What are the alternatives?"

"Maybe we can hire a taxi in Conques and meet Collette and Danielle twelve kilometers down the road. We could start walking from there."

"Or we could start walking with them and, if we can't make the distance, call a taxi. After all, we have a cell phone."

I nodded. "That's a better plan. That way we begin in faith, trusting that we can walk the distance. And we keep the faith that we will be able to get a taxi if we need one."

"Sounds like a plan."

After unpacking a few belongings—how much less there was to unpack—we went sightseeing. We walked across the yard to the church, approaching it from behind. As we drew near, I suddenly entered a "thin place" where the veil between past and present, this world and some other dimension, was strangely transparent. I felt the presence of centuries-past worshippers who had marched in procession on the same path we were following. I shook myself, but the experience did not go away.

We passed several empty sarcophagi lying beside the wall of the church and I could "see" the bodies that had lain within. It was as if an image appeared in my mind's eye, an image superimposed over the consensual reality of vacant stone coffins. When we entered the church, my strange double vision continued. I "saw" people standing in the empty nave. This, I knew, was what the interior of the church looked like in medieval times, before benches were added.

What I "saw" seemed real. It was quite peculiar, especially since I wasn't given to visions—despite Saint James's unexpected appearance on the train. Rather than feeling disturbed, I decided to observe without judgment or reaction both what I "saw" and what I felt about seeing it. I was intrigued, puzzled, surprised—and grateful for whatever was expanding my normal consciousness to include a broader reality.

Soon the vision faded and I was in only one time and one place—the present, filled with memories of last year's pilgrimage and my cancer surgery. I began crying again, weeping for all that Gary and I had been through together, for all the gifts and graces we had received, for all the unexpected opportunities, including all the hard-learned lessons. Sniffling, I lit a candle before the statue of Saint James. And then another. Gratitude, gratitude, for all that life brings.

After departing the church in silence, we strolled around town, revisiting familiar shops and monuments. This time there was no feast day of Sainte Foy to fill Conques with masses of devotees, but the streets were crowded, packed with tourists and school children on excursion. The store where we had bought the scallop shell fossils the year before had not yet opened for the season, but a number of other shops were doing a thriving business.

In one gift shop filled with tempting jewelry displays, I purchased a small silver scallop-shell pin to fasten next to the peace pin on my purse. After my vision of Saint James on the train, I felt the urge to proclaim my connection with the saint and the pilgrimage.

Then we visited a local pastry shop fragrant with fresh-baked goods. Announcing to Gary that it was important to sample local specialties, I bought a bag of *conquaises,* a sugarcoated cookie made out of shortbread dough and ground walnuts.

Gary looked at me with measured disapproval. I knew he was thinking: "Wheat? Sugar? She's into it already?" I was, after all, still struggling with my dietary regime and had gained weight since the previous year. The forbidden foods I had eaten on the Chemin out of desperation had turned into an ongoing source of comfort once I was home. Surely one cookie wouldn't hurt, would it? Besides, I promised Gary that I would share them with Danielle and Collette—and with him.

We returned to the church for vespers, the early evening prayer service held around 5:00 p.m. The word "vespers" derives from the Old French for "evensong," which in turn derives from Venus, the evening star. The sacred Feminine was present in the prayer cycle of the Church, unbeknownst to most worshippers and many priests.

The church was nearly empty since most of the visitors to Conques were filling the shops, not the pews. A scattering of pilgrims sat near the altar.

Then it was dinnertime. Hurrying back to the *accueil*, we met Collette and Danielle and found seats together at a long trestle table. Some fifty people were eating together in the communal dining room: pilgrims, excursionists, and church groups on retreat. Youth volunteers placed overflowing platters on the tables.

Dinner included pork *rillettes†* (a minced and well-seasoned meat spread, a bit like pâté), moist, chewy bread, cauliflower au gratin, stuffed veal roll, chocolate pudding, and fruit. I sighed, realizing that once again I was being presented with the opportunity to control my diet—or not. It was a lesson I was slow to learn despite many opportunities to practice. Part of me rebelled, thinking, "You might die soon, so why not enjoy yourself?" Another part responded, "You might die sooner if you do!"

After we had finished eating, our hosts led us in the pilgrims' song, "Ultreya."

> "Ultre-ïa! Ultre-ïa!
> Et sus eïa, Deus adjuva nos!"

"Onwards, always upwards, God help us," I whispered to myself.

The dining room filled with fifty ardent voices calling on God to aid us all as we went upward and ever onward, both as pilgrims walking across the geography of the land and as souls struggling across the geography of the soul.

After dinner we attended the evening Compline service, followed by another pilgrims' blessing ceremony. The previous October twelve pilgrims had stepped forward; this time there were also twelve, including the four of us. Last year I had been eager to receive all the blessings I could as I recovered from cancer and embarked for the first time on the French Chemin. How well I remembered, as I eagerly participated in the sacred rite once again.

When the priest raised his hands in blessing, I saw his fingers surrounded with a golden aura of etheric energy. My "double" vision had returned.

The service ended and we were again presented with a stale roll and a booklet of the Gospel of Mark. This time I knew there would indeed be times when I wished I had the rock-hard piece of bread to gnaw on.

Bright yellow spotlights suddenly illuminated the upstairs gallery; simultaneously an organ recital began. The evening tourist program had begun. Grateful for the unexpected opportunity, we bought tickets for a tour.

Along with several dozen others, we climbed the steep, worn stone steps to the gallery (the arcaded upper story over the side aisles, which opens onto the nave). I knew that carvings of Green Men, split-legged siren-mermaids, and hoof-footed figures adorn some of the 250 capitals in the church; perhaps I would find some of them in the gallery.

We and several others gradually fell far behind the guide despite her impatient gestures for us to stay with the group. Since she spoke rapid French, what was the point of listening? Setting our own pace, we admired the elaborately carved capitals and the milk-colored glass windows. For the first time I had a close-up view of Pierre Soulages' abstract glass; the glass strips change color with the shifting external light. They look nothing like the thirteenth-century stained-glass windows I admired in Chartres Cathedral. The light filtering through the jewel-like colors of those windows (including the unique "Chartres blue") supposedly helps heal and enhance the spiritual experience of people inside the church. Perhaps the medieval stained glass works in a similar way to infra-red and ultra-violet radiation; their different vibrational levels affect living beings in distinct ways.

Someone explained to me that Soulages' windows are intended to subtly reflect the external world rather than add their own colors to the interior. Last year I had found the windows unappealing, probably because of my expectations of what stained glass *should* look like. Rather than experiencing the windows for what they were, I had focused on what they weren't: they weren't colorful. This time I saw them with more unbiased eyes. The artist's intention had been to create windows that complement the austerity of the bare stone abbey walls. He had succeeded.

Wednesday, May 7, 2003. Conques to Livinhac-le-Haut. 24 kilometers (15 miles).

With great trepidation we left Conques on a cool, overcast morning to begin walking twenty-four kilometers. Our hiking sticks tapped rhythmically on the uneven stone pavement as we strode down the rue Charlemagne, the medieval pilgrimage route that still leads pilgrims out of town and towards Santiago de Compostela, some 1300 kilometers (815 miles) down the road. I fancied I heard the echoing tramp of millions of pilgrims' feet that had passed this way before us. We were following in their footsteps. They had made it—at least most of them had—so we could too.

Conques is located on the side of a deeply wooded gorge of the Dourdou River, a tributary of the Lot. Last year Gary and I had slipped and slid our way into the gorge; this year we had to climb out. We marched across the highway, over a bridge that crossed the Dourdou, and then began to ascend the trail, which leads straight up the side of the gorge. It was so steep that in some places stone steps had been carved into the hillside. I had to stop every few meters and take deep breaths. My legs felt as if they were on fire. Gary explained that my leg muscles were not getting enough oxygen, so I should breathe deeper, but that was hard to do since I was out of breath.

After an excruciating half hour we reached the Chapelle Sainte-Foy. The year before, I had seen the tiny chapel from our hotel room window; it had looked unreachable, although it was only one and one-half kilometers from Conques. Built beside a spring whose healing waters, according to legend, brought relief from eye complaints—as did prayers to Sainte Foy—it was the site of a local pilgrimage. After my visionary experiences of the last two days, I realized that one's vision could be affected in many ways, not all of which were physical.

Gradually the route became less steep, though it was still quite intense. The pain in my legs diminished as my body began to relearn the rhythm of the Chemin. Seven weary kilometers farther, we encountered a pair of pilgrims stretched out in the shade in front of the Chapelle Saint-Roch. At first we saw only one of them, a woman lying on her back, hair and neck covered with a blue kerchief, a floppy, black Oregon Pacific hat pulled over her eyes. One leg was crossed over the other bent knee.

She heard us coming and abruptly sat up.

We greeted her, and she said "Hello" in a harsh voice, then called out, "You talkin', Bubba?"

A spectral figure rose from the ground behind her. Lean, grey-haired, "Bubba" smiled at us from his nesting place. "Hello," he said.

We introduced ourselves. Susie and Bubba obviously were Americans, but I couldn't figure out where Susie came from. There was something odd about her accent, as well as the quality of her voice. In response to our questions, Susie, who did most of the talking, told us she had walked the Chemin six times: once all the way to Santiago, the other times to towns along the route in France. "Bubba" or Rick, as he was also called, had walked it seven times.

I was curious what drew her to the Camino. She explained in her grating voice, "It's great exercise and a great way to lose weight. Why, last year when I got off the plane to start walking, my backpack bumped against my butt, that's how heavy I was! I lost thirty pounds, no time."

"How did you do that?" I asked in amazement, since I had gained weight on the Chemin last October.

"Back home I eat out with friends, we drink, have dessert, you know, the usual. Here, I pretty much follow Bubba's lead and eat real healthy."

"But I still don't get it. Why do you walk the Camino? I mean, you could go for a long walk in the US and lose weight, if that's your only motive."

"Well, it's pretty here and there are interesting places to stay and eat from point A to B. You just don't find that back home."

Collette and Danielle listened to our conversation in silence, furtively exchanging looks of disapproval. Equally full of judgment, seeing Susie and Rick not only through my eyes but also through those of our French companions, I found myself thinking that Susie was the worst kind of stereotypical American: abrasive and superficial. I made no attempt to be an impartial observer.

"What about you, Rick?" I asked.

"I go for the reasons most pilgrims go. To think about my life, to get away from my daily routine. I'm sure all pilgrims find time on the Camino to contemplate their lives."

Not necessarily, I thought, judging by (there I was, judging again) Susie's rationale for the journey.

"How did you two meet?"

Susie explained that they had met at a travel lecture. Rick had walked the Chemin and suggested she join him the next time. The first time they walked together they didn't get along, so they split up somewhere in France and Susie had continued to Santiago alone. Over time they had learned to travel together, sometimes staying together, sometimes separately.

"We're good walking companions but bad roommates," Susie explained.

They both carried large backpacks, and Bubba pulled a green plaid, two-wheeled shopping cart behind him. It was laden with provisions that met his strict dietary requirements: WASA crackers, fresh carrots, and rice to cook for breakfast.

I thought it absurd for Bubba to haul all that food, although the previous year I had understood Akira's need to do so. I had even admired his perseverance. "Judge not less ye be judged," a tiny voice whispered in my ear. I ignored it.

I asked, "How difficult is it to pull that shopping cart?"

"Not bad. I've done it for six years."

Susie added, "Sometimes we split up because Bubba has to stay on paved roads with his cart." She continued, "Usually there aren't many Americans on the road. Come to think of it, there've been more recently."

"Has the Chemin changed much since you started walking it?" I asked.

She nodded emphatically. "We didn't used to have to make reservations to find a place to stay. Now we gotta plan in advance. It's kinda getting spoiled."

I wondered what she thought of the Spanish Camino, which in recent years has become much more crowded and commercialized than the Chemin. Some pilgrims refer to this popularity as the "MacDonaldization" of the Camino. But I didn't ask. Instead, I inquired cautiously, "Where are you from?"

"You mean the way I talk? People think I'm from the South, but I'm not. I've got a speech impediment that wasn't corrected when I was young. 'Lazy English,' they call it."

Chagrined, I realized I was judging Susie by the quality of her voice and her motivations, and Bubba by his choice of luggage—which actually was quite a brilliant solution to a difficult challenge. I had noticed the censuring looks Collette and Danielle gave them and had shared their censure. Although I might be making slow but steady progress on the physical Chemin I was definitely slipping backward on being nonjudgmental. At least I realized it this time, which was a sign of progress. Rather than just circling around to do the same old thing in the same old way, I was spiraling around and doing the same old thing—but from a slightly more aware perspective.

We said a falsely hearty "Goodbye" and, eager to escape, walked over to the nearby chapel, whispering catty unpleasantries. Then we admired the modern stained-glass windows, vibrant with swirling colors that form abstract patterns and at least one human figure: a crucified Christ with a glorious orange sunburst behind his outstretched arms. By the time we left the chapel Bubba and Susie had walked on.

Our country road led us past green meadows filled with yellow and white flowers, tranquilly grazing black-and-white cattle, and pastel-colored houses, sometimes covered with pale salmon, quiet peach, or soft yellow stucco. Our good spirits were quickly restored. Occasionally we sang songs together as we walked along, just as we had the previous year.

At one point we got a little lost. "A little lost" meant we knew we had only recently strayed from the path. It happens often enough in life: you're not completely lost but you realize that, one step at a time, you've gotten slightly off track. Lost is lost, but "a little lost" is easier to correct.

We knew we had to head downhill to Livinhac-le-Haut, but Raju's guidebook was confusing. We had probably missed the white and red blazons of the GR 65 while exchanging judgmental remarks about Susie and Bubba.

We continued down a narrow lane in an unnamed village, wondering where we were. Suddenly a couple appeared out of nowhere who volunteered to show us the way back to the Chemin. Gratefully, we followed them up the street and down another one to the main road, arriving opposite a modern bridge over the Lot. With a wave of their hands, our angels disappeared from sight.

With many rest stops we managed, despite my misgivings, to walk twenty-four kilometers to our *chambres d'hôtes,* the Magnanerie (Silkworm Farm). A high stone wall with a large, double-door entry surrounded the Magnanerie; a scallop shell adorned one of the solid plank doors. Inside were several nineteenth-century stone buildings, a stone tower, and an extensive yard full of mature trees and garden furniture. A sign on the front door of the *chambres d'hôtes* said that our host, Monsieur Robertson, would return at 5:00 p.m.

We entered and saw eight or ten shoeless pilgrims waiting resignedly in the large kitchen-dining area. Taking off our boots, we left them at the side of an odoriferous heap. Everyone was exhausted, eager to wash and rest, but we would have to wait an hour. In other words, we were being given the opportunity to practice patience.

After several nearly fruitless attempts to make conversation with our fellow pilgrims or hikers—everyone was too tired to talk— I examined the spacious room. Tins of British tea decorated a high wooden display shelf, which made me wonder whether Monsieur Robertson's surname was evidence of a WW II marriage between a British soldier and a French demoiselle. That was the origin of Alan Anderson's surname. He was my Basque friend in Saint-Jean-Pied-de-Port who had saved me from disaster on the Camino in 1982. But perhaps Monsieur Robertson's name went back much further, to one of several prior and less-welcome English invasions. Or maybe he was an English-speaking émigré. How wonderful it would be not to have to struggle to make ourselves understood!

Flyers on a large bulletin board announced taxi services, luggage transport, church services, and other *gites* further down the Chemin. A handwritten note from Monsieur Robertson requested help. The gossip among the pilgrims (too tired to talk but not too tired to gossip) was that he was recently divorced and needed assistance to run the place. I remembered Monsieur Grossouvre and his two failed marriages. Maybe running a *gîte* placed excessive stress on marital relationships.

At last Monsieur Robertson bustled in with several overflowing bags of groceries. Tomorrow's breakfast, I wondered? He greeted us all, then checked the registration list and assigned us our rooms. He didn't speak English but it didn't matter. Sign language and good will sufficed, aided by Collette, of course.

Danielle and Collette, and Gary and I, had private rooms, each with two beds, in the loft above the dining room. We climbed up the spiral staircase to examine our rooms, attractively furnished with antique furniture, relatively firm mattresses, and stacks of books in several languages. The shared bathroom, complete with modern shower, toilet, and electric heater, was located at the end of the hall. Gary and I sank into the comfortable beds and were almost instantly asleep.

A few hours later the four of us followed Monsieur Robertson's suggestion and strolled over to the Restaurant L'Ambiance, located next to a bridge over the Lot.

The robust, florid-faced owner/chef greeted us at the door. Arms crossed over his ample chest he exclaimed (in French), "No reservation? Well then, no table!"

Collette became quite upset but he was adamant—and then he laughed. It was all in jest. It took a while, however, for him to calm her down. Chuckling to himself, he led us over to a table near a window and presented us with the evening *menu*. Before long, the parking lot was full of cars. Tourists, repeat customers, and pilgrims came in and were seated at nearby tables. We nodded to the latter in recognition of our shared community.

I favored the more expensive *menu* with four courses (appetizer, main course, cheese, and dessert), but Collette and Danielle preferred the three-course *menu* (without dessert and with less interesting entrees). Collette indicated with a somewhat downcast glance that ordering a diverse number of courses would disrupt the dinner service. Since I wanted to respect the nuances of French etiquette I went with the majority.

We fortified ourselves for dinner by drinking glasses of Ratafia, a popular local liqueur made from brandy infused with walnuts, although it is customarily made from wine infused with bitter almonds, cherry kernels, or other fruits—or from Armagnac, bitter orange juice, orange zest, and simple sugar syrup.

This auspicious beginning was followed by melon and ham soup, *joue de boeuf* (beef cheeks) slow-cooked in cider, and moist, chewy, crisp-crusted bread. Dinner finished with a flourish, a tray of local *fromages*, including *cabécouʄ de vache* (little round disks made of cow's milk) that were light as a cloud.

Only two days on the Chemin and I had already thrown dietary discretion to the winds. You only live once and we were in France, the land of excellent dining. I had decided to enjoy myself. My nagging concern about whether dietary indiscretion would lead to a recurrence of cancer had lost out to rationalization.

After more byplay with the owner-chef and his elderly mother, who was the cashier, we waddled back to our home for that night on the Chemin.

Thursday, May 8, 2003. Livinhac-le-Haut to La Cassagnole. More than 24 kilometers (15 miles), but we hitchhiked and took a taxi for half the distance.

In the morning I watched a green plaid grocery cart descending the tower stairs. Bubba had spent the night in a small room on the second floor. Susie had slept somewhere else.

Much to our surprise, Collette's arrangements called for another grueling twenty-four-kilometer day. In addition, she had failed to inform us that our route would bypass the town of Figeac, a town on the Chemin that I had hoped to visit. I presumed there must be a good reason for this plan—perhaps it shortened the overall distance—but twenty-four kilometers certainly didn't seem short. I wondered again if Collette had been overly ambitious but, after all, we had survived the previous day.

We had been grateful when Collette offered to make all the arrangements. We had placed ourselves in her hands without hesitation, without asking to approve her decisions. It was our responsibility if we weren't happy with the results.

The overcast day warmed up as we walked along, and soon the weather was delightful. Honey Bunny hopped out of her bag and Gary wedged her under a strap on the side of his backpack. A fresh breeze, green rolling hills, wildflowers—it was a perfect day for walking the Chemin. Wooden cross-shaped signposts indicated the direction of the GR 65 and often showed the distance to nearby towns.

Six kilometers from Livinhac we reached the hillside village of Montredon. As we walked through town, we found ourselves in the middle of a funeral procession. According to printed announcements posted on houses, an elderly woman had passed on. The woman's relatives, friends, and fellow villagers were walking en masse behind a hearse heading away from the church and toward a cemetery on the outskirts of the village. We followed a respectful distance behind them until our path diverged from theirs.

Further along the trail I saw a sign, dated 1998, on a telephone pole, declaring in English as well as French,

> Under the international convention of cultural and natural heritage, the Pilgrim Ways across France to Santiago de Compostela have been placed on the UNESCO World Heritage List in order to protect them for the benefit of the whole of humanity. Through Montredon, Felzins, Saint-Félix, and Saint-Jean-Mirabel, toward Figeac, the path forms part of

the Puy-en-Velay Pilgrim Way used by countless pilgrims ever since medieval times.

A road-weary pilgrim had scrawled in black marker below the sign, "It's a long way to Santiago." It was indeed: 1266 kilometers (787 miles). We were glad we only had 503 kilometers (313 miles), more or less, to go.

As we walked down the road we passed a number of identical cast-aluminum crosses erected on large cement pedestals by the side of the road. They resembled miniature trees with cast-aluminum bark; twining metal vines and flowers and a disproportionally tiny Christ completed the design. Pebbles and stones were piled on top of the cement base. Like the cuisine and the landscape, the roadside crosses changed as we walked from one region to another.

After a fair amount of "upping and downing" we reached the Chapelle de Guirande, a Romanesque chapel dedicated to Sainte Madeleine, its interior decorated with late-fourteenth-century murals. Unfortunately, it was locked, and we peered through the barred windows without success. No matter. A lovely picnic area beckoned across from the chapel, so we took out our cheese, bread, and fruit, sat down at a table, and began eating.

After an ample rest we started back down the road. We followed Raju's guidebook, which suggested staying on the D2 highway to avoid the often-boggy GR and to shorten the route by three kilometers.

I am directionally challenged but I was certain we were going the wrong way. Even though I normally rely on Gary's excellent navigational skills, I asked him repeatedly if we were going in the right direction. He kept saying yes. Finally he began muttering to himself. He couldn't track our path on the topo-map.

Seeing his uncertainty, I declared assertively, "This can't be right."

Nobody believed me. After all, I get confused the moment I walk out of a hotel in a strange city, so how could I possibly know we were going the wrong direction? Then I saw a steeple poking up from a nearby hillside village.

"Look," I said, pointing triumphantly toward the church. "That's Montredon, the village we walked through a few hours earlier. Somehow we got turned around."

Danielle once observed that the Chemin teaches you humility: you think you can do something but you find out you can't. She was right. Sometimes, however, you learn that you can do something you thought you couldn't. I learned another lesson as well: It was easier to follow someone else's lead than my own intuition, but that didn't mean it was best.

Gary was exhausted and Danielle's knee hurt a great deal. We had only covered at most twelve kilometers, but we had walked twenty-four the day before. The effect was cumulative. Worn out and frustrated, we tried to decide what to do. Going back to the chapel and continuing on in the correct direction was one alternative, but we were too tired.

After much debate, we agreed to hitchhike. The details weren't clear to me, but just then a car drove by, we stuck out our thumbs, and it stopped in front of us. Gratitude, gratitude.

Despite Gary's protests, Collette and I insisted that he and Danielle climb into the back seat, along with all our packs. We agreed to meet at Saint-Félix, approximately eight kilometers away. I presumed Collette and I would walk to Saint-Félix since we were no longer burdened with my fanny pack and Collette's backpack, but just then another car drove by. We stuck out our thumbs again and within minutes we were speeding along to Saint-Félix. That had been Collette's plan all along. She knew it would be easier for two pilgrims to catch a ride than four.

Ten minutes later the driver dropped us off in the tiny hamlet, next to Danielle and Gary, who were sitting by the side of the road resting against a cool stone wall. Collette wanted to continue walking from there, but I knew Danielle and Gary were worn out, so I suggested we call a cab.

Collette pursed her lips and Danielle informed me that we wouldn't have much luck. It was a "red letter day"— WW II Armistice Day—and most taxi drivers, like everyone else, were on holiday. Besides, we didn't have a phone number. Not willing to admit defeat, I looked in *Miam Miam Dodo* and found a number for the tourist office in Figeac. We telephoned; they were open; they gave us a phone number; Collette called; and the taxi driver agreed to pick us up. Another angel? Perhaps.

A young American couple stopped to talk with us. They were quite sad because they were ending their pilgrimage at Figeac, fourteen kilometers away, and then returning home. Somewhat embarrassed, they explained that this day and this day only they had used Transbagage to transport their bags so that they could walk a longer distance. We didn't mention that we had hitchhiked to Saint-Félix.

Saint-Félix's claim to fame rests on its eleventh-century Romanesque church dedicated to Saint Radegonde. While we waited for the taxi we admired the delightfully naïf Adam, Eve, and serpent carved on the tympanum above the main portal. Adam and Eve are nearly naked. They have one hand covering their genitals, the other hand reaching for the forbidden fruit. Adam sports a pointed patriarchal beard and cap; Eve has tiny pendulous breasts and large protruding buttocks. Between them a sinuous snake winds around a minimalist Tree of Knowledge. Each of its five drooping branches ends in a sphere. The serpent holds in its mouth the same globe that Eve is holding in her hand.

What exactly the forbidden fruit was has been greatly debated, since it isn't named in Genesis. It might have been a fig, a pomegranate, or a tamarind since there were no apples in the Holy Land at that time. The Christian association of the apple with the Tree of Knowledge of Good and Evil was made much later, probably when

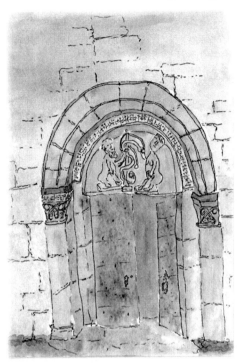

Tympanum, Saint-Félix

medieval monks noted that the Latin word, *malum*, means both apple and sin.

But this connection was not just a harmless play on words. For millennia the apple had been associated with Venus and the Earth-centered religions. Slice it crosswise and the seeds form a five-pointed pentagram. The number five is frequently associated with the Sacred Feminine and with the four elements (air, fire, water, and earth) and Spirit. Hidden beneath the seemingly innocuous association of apple and sin was an attempt to demonize the Feminine.

Even the serpent has been perverted. Before Christianity, the serpent was associated with rebirth (it sheds its skin), wisdom, and the Goddess. Although some Gnostic Christians interpreted the snake in Genesis as wisdom, in most Judeo-Christian interpretations, the snake was sinister. Even the word "sinister," which refers to the left, distaff, or feminine side of the body, became associated with something underhanded or evil. Although the tympanum is charming, the message is clear: the apple, the Feminine, and the serpent are linked together with sin.

The Tree of Knowledge is not unique to Judaism or Christianity. Similar trees appear in many other religions and cultures—including a tree guarded by a serpent, found on ancient Sumerian seals. The Buddha achieved enlightenment under the Bodhi tree; in Norse mythology, Odin hung for nine days on Yggdrasil, a giant ash tree that links the underworld, this world, and the realm of the Gods, in order to acquire knowledge. The powerful symbol of the World Tree or *axis mundi* is found around the world, but it usually represents the sacred link between this world and the next rather than Adam and Eve's fall from grace.

We waited a long time for our taxi driver. With a smile he slung our bags into the trunk and explained he had been at a holiday gathering. Soon he transported us effortlessly over numerous hills, skirting the town of Figeac, and dropped us off outside of La Cassagnole at Le Relais Saint-Jacques, our stopping place for the night.

The *relais* resembled a fanciful Middle Earth hobbit town: a group of stone buildings with tile roofs nestling in the midst of sweet-smelling herb and flower gardens, shaded by huge trees. Bright red geraniums bloomed in flowerpots scattered along the meandering stone-lined paths that connected the different buildings. No wonder the *relais* had been awarded a "little flower" accolade by *Miam Miam Dodo*. Priority for rooms was given to "non-motorized" visitors—those arriving on foot.

While we waited to register, I saw many of the pilgrims we had encountered on the Chemin during the last few days. Most of them looked even more exhausted than we were. They must have walked the entire distance.

A tough, middle-aged Swiss man exclaimed, "Dur chemin!" as he wiped his sweaty brow with a stained bandanna. He explained that he and his companion had been lost and tromped up and down hills for hours.

Our rooms were in the building at the far end of the herb garden. We left our boots inside the front door and hurried across the cold tile floor to our room, "Samarkand." Next door was "Prague."

Our room featured a large bed and a private bathroom. What a pleasure! Despite previous assurances by our hostess, there was no heat in the room, but we had plenty of blankets, a private shower, and a bed to snuggle in. Gratitude, gratitude for the bounty of the Chemin, for rides freely offered, a taxi when we needed it, and a comfortable place for the night.

Gary stretched out on the bed and fell asleep while I did laundry. There was a row of clotheslines on the hill above the herb garden, and I wanted to take advantage of this unexpected luxury before it started to rain.

While I hung up our clothes I thought about the lessons the Chemin had offered that day. Humility: you can't necessarily do as much as you want to. Bounty: the people who had picked us up when we were hitchhiking and the taxi driver who hadn't levied a holiday surcharge. Gratitude: the lovely countryside, the sweet scent of irises, the sight of acacia trees bursting with white blossoms, rides when we needed them, a *gîte* filled with beauty and fragrance, and both time and energy to enjoy my surroundings.

I preferred to forget how judgmental we had been of Susie and Bubba—but that, too, was another lesson of the Chemin.

Done with my washerwoman tasks I walked down the fragrant, flower-lined path to the communal kitchen. A couple sat at a table talking and drinking beer while a woman in her mid 30s did cleanup chores at the sink. Assorted canned goods were stacked on shelves, and the refrigerator was stocked with beer and cold drinks, all available for purchase. I must have looked puzzled, so the woman at the sink explained in English that everything ran on the honor system. There was a "kitty" (a small box with a slit in it) above the refrigerator, where one deposited money.

Soon Thérèse and I were deep in conversation. She'd heard via the pilgrim telegraph that an American expert was walking the Chemin. When she realized that was me, she was delighted.

Thérèse was an MA student in religious studies at Caen University; the tentative title of her thesis was "Compostela or the Reenchanted Way." At the *relais* she was conducting fieldwork with interviews and questionnaires. Her hypothesis was that a central motive for the pilgrimage was the desire for magic and mystery. She also placed great importance on "the gift," a theory of the French anthropologist Marcel Mauss. This concept refers to the exchange of something other than money, such as friendship or relationship.

Thérèse believed that companionship and community were also central to the modern Chemin but varied by nationality. She had observed that when pilgrims offered food or a gift to other pilgrims, the French pilgrims wouldn't accept it because they expected something would be asked in exchange. She had also noticed that French pilgrims complained about paying more for the canned goods in the *relais* pantry than if they had bought them at a supermarket. They seemed oblivious to the fact that someone else had to buy the supplies, bring them to this isolated location, and wait for possible reimbursement. Thérèse hypothesized that perhaps because of these French tendencies, relationship and community on the Chemin became opportunities to break free from cultural constraints.

Agreeing to continue our conversation later, I put money in the kitty in exchange for a cold beer for Gary. It had begun to sprinkle so I dashed over to the clothesline, gathered up the still-damp laundry, and headed back to our room. I hoped the socks and underwear would dry overnight but it wasn't likely; the radiator was still not warm, so it would do no good to spread damp laundry on it.

Collette informed us that her friend Mimi, who lived in nearby Faycelles, was going to join us for dinner at the *relais*. The next day the four of us would go to Faycelles with Mimi, then drive back to Figeac for lunch.

When I looked at the guidebook I discovered that we could have walked from our *relais* to Faycelles since it was on the Chemin, but (as I already knew) we had missed Figeac, since the *relais* was southwest of it. I also realized that Collette had chosen to walk the scenic GR 651† through the deep-cut Vallée du Célé rather than follow the more historic GR 65. Apparently we were going to be tourists, not pilgrims, for a while, whether I liked it or not.

We had placed ourselves in Collette's hands; better we should have placed ourselves in God's. But who knows: perhaps they were the same.

While we waited for Collette's friend Mimi, the *traiteur* drove up in a van and lugged heavy, foil-covered pans into the large dining room. By the time Mimi arrived, much of the food was gone.

Friday, May 9, 2004. The Relais at La Cassagnole to Figeac to Corn by car, then by foot to Espagnac-Sainte-Eulalie. 7 kilometers (4.3 miles).

Breakfast was the standard assortment of bread, toast, jam, coffee, tea, hot milk, and packaged cocoa mix. Nearly everyone had left by the time we got to the dining room: we had slept late since we only had a short distance to walk that day.

While we waited for Mimi to arrive, we filled out Thérèse's pilgrimage questionnaires. I appreciated having the opportunity to reflect on what the Chemin had taught me. What came to mind was: trust, patience, faith, humility, gratitude, and simplicity—at least some of the time. Collette wrote: a willingness to do without, to endure hardships, to leave comforts behind.

Thérèse and I discussed pilgrimage some more and promised to stay in touch by email. I still wasn't convinced that reciprocity was the central motivation for walking the Chemin but I realized we all have our pet theories. Mine is that in our secularized, disenchanted world, people hunger for a meaningful connection with the sacred. They are starved for spiritual sustenance even if they are physically well fed.

Because many people are disconnected from, disinterested in, or distrustful of organized religion, they have to create their own relationship with the holy. In increasing numbers, people are doing so by going on pilgrimage, a time-honored ritual process that requires no intermediary and provides the opportunity for people to learn personalized lessons—to make their own meaning out of their varied experiences on the Chemin.

At last Mimi arrived and, squashed into her tiny car, we drove over a winding country road to her home in Faycelles, a bastide† town. Both the French and English built fortified towns during the Hundred Years' War† (1337 - 1453), a sporadic conflict that pitted the English against the eventually successful French.

The bastide towns were planned settlements based on a grid with a central market square and fortified perimeters, quite unlike most medieval towns, which were a hodgepodge maze of streets developed over centuries. Bastides are most commonly found in southwestern France in what had been disputed frontier areas. Nearly 300 have survived, and many are part of an organized tourist route.

While Mimi and Collette visited, Gary and I wandered aimlessly around the town. I felt deflated, irritated, unsettled. We had shifted from being pilgrims to being tourists, and I didn't like it. It was one thing to go sightseeing or visiting when the opportunity arose, quite another to arrange our journey for those purposes.

Several hours later we headed to Figeac. It took us longer to find a parking place than it did to drive there. During a quick walking tour of Figeac's medieval center, I was impressed with the attractive half-timbered buildings that lined the narrow, twisting lanes. Mimi explained that the town had undergone massive urban renewal in the last fifteen years. Some local wit had proclaimed, "Figeac looks better now than it ever did—even in the Middle Ages!"

The French may have won the Hundred Years' War but the English were returning in droves because housing was much less expensive in rural France than in Britain. This latest invasion appeared to be peaceful, although some French people complained about the soaring cost of property, the marked-up prices, and English imports taking up too much shelf space in local stores.

Gary went to a Laundromat to finish drying our clothes while I went to buy socks. My feet felt just a little crunched in my boots, so I hoped to find thinner socks. I found a shoe store that sold an assortment but they were all cotton, which I didn't want. I asked the clerk for something else, and she informed me that I was quite absurd not to want cotton and I knew nothing at all about socks.

My French wasn't good but I understood exactly what she was saying. Soon my face started to flush. I thought to myself, "In the States a sales clerk would never be so rude. They're trained to pretend the customer is always right." In the States I would have marched out of the store and found another one. In Figeac, however, my choices were limited. Muttering unhappily, I purchased two pair.

We ate lunch at La Puce a l'Orieille (The Flea in the Ear), located in a restored medieval building complete with uneven tile floors and a bathroom at the top of a narrow, winding wood staircase. I suppose that was the only place they could put it; after all, in the Middle Ages there wouldn't have been a bathroom.

We chose the $18.00 *menu*—or rather, everyone else did so I went along. As usual, I would have preferred a different *menu* that included more regional specialties. However, Collette and Danielle again made it clear that it would be better if we ordered from the same *menu* with the same number of courses—and they wanted fewer, not more. I vowed that if we ever returned, I would order whatever I wanted.

Lunch began with a deliciously fresh *salade composée* consisting of walnuts, preserved duck breast, bacon, curly endive, lettuce, and sliced green apples, followed by our choice of chicken *confit* or quail with raisin sauce. Our third course was chocolate mousse with golden raisins and rum sauce or prunes cooked in spiced wine.

While waiting for dessert, I paged through *Miam Miam Dodo* and saw that a variant of the GR led from Figeac to Rocamadour, forty-two kilometers to the northwest. Gary and I had visited Rocamadour by car several years before. A wealthy pilgrimage site since the Middle Ages, Rocamadour had been sacked several times and nearly destroyed during the Wars of Religion. It was heavily reconstructed in the nineteenth century, turning it into a kind of religious Disneyland that draws as many as 1.5 million visitors a year, thanks in part to the widely venerated Black Madonna of Rocamadour.

She is a dark, walnut statue without elegant embroidered robes—without any covering of any kind. Her face is serene, her body emaciated though heavy-breasted. Her forearms form part of the throne on which she sits. A jeweled, golden diadem, identical to the one worn by the infant Jesus perched on her unyielding lap, and a gold collar are her only ornaments. Since the Middle Ages, pilgrims have traveled great distances to pray for miracles in the votive-filled Chapel of Notre-Dame.

While we finished our delicious desserts in Figeac I was far away, fantasizing about walking to Rocamadour. Realistically, walking the Chemin was difficult enough for us, so an excursion to Rocamadour was not sensible. Nonetheless I hoped that someday we would walk there. I wanted to be a real pilgrim again, not an excursionist.

Late in the afternoon we squeezed back into Mimi's car. She drove us past Faycelles to the outskirts of Corn, where we would meet up with the northern variant of the Chemin, the GR 651. We said goodbye to Mimi and began walking seven kilometers to Espagnac-Sainte-Eulalie. The narrow country lane soon turned into a trail through the forest. The Célé ran quickly (its name comes from *celer*, which means "rapid") far below. Honey Bunny came out of hiding and sat on my shoulder bag.

Thick lichen hung from grandly spreading oak trees, and fields exploded with blue columbine and white and yellow wildflowers. The isolated, cream-colored stone farmhouses featured well-tended gardens, and roses filled the air with evocative perfume. Irises of different colors grew in clumps along the fences, each color with its own unique fragrance. The maroon-and-brown ones were spicy; the yellow reminded me of the scent of fresh-squeezed orange juice; the traditional purple ones smelled like candied violets.

After an hour and a half we reached a *gîte* that Collette thought was our stopping place but wasn't. An elderly couple was getting it ready for holiday residents who would stay a week or two. They assured us we were close to Espagnac-Sainte-Eulalie, which, according to them, was one of the most picturesque villages along the Célé.

It was. Grey-white stone buildings with sloping red-tile roofs clustered together near the riverbank. On the opposite side of the river, trees dotted a steep limestone bluff marked with extensive horizontal outcroppings of rough grey stone. We were in the land of the *causses*†, ancient eroding limestone plateaus that continued to Rocamadour, site of my lunchtime recollections.

Collette asked a passerby where the *gîte d'étape communal* was, and he pointed to the local government building. We went inside and met Marie, who escorted us to a renovated medieval gate-tower. The adjoining building served as the kitchen-dining area. These buildings were what remain of a once-important Augustine convent, Notre-Dame-du-Val-Paradis, founded in the twelfth century but greatly expanded in the next. It had met its demise during the Revolution. Marie explained that originally the tower had two gates at the base and a wall around it to keep men out of the priory.

We followed her up the newly constructed corkscrew staircase inside the tower. Each floor had been transformed into a guestroom with several bunk beds and a private bath. Our room, on the second floor, had an evocative view over the ruined convent to the cliffs beyond. Marie explained that we could rent towels and sheets, but we assured her we didn't need them. We had brought silk sleep sacks and microfiber travel towels.

Then Marie asked Collette if our group had paid in advance. A lengthy exchange followed, none of which we understood, but Collette and Danielle looked shocked, then sympathetic, then concerned. Seeing my curiosity, Collette explained that the local volunteer had absconded with the funds and Marie was trying to get everything sorted out.

After paying Marie what was owed and dropping our packs in our rooms, we went for a stroll around the hamlet. Although we had not walked far that day, Gary and I realized we felt weighed down by our packs. We began to plot a way to lighten our burdens by utilizing a luggage-transfer service at the next opportunity.

Espagnac-Sainte-Eulalie had once been a substantial medieval village with an important priory, but only a dozen houses and a sadly truncated church now remained. The church had managed to retain its slender bell tower, crowned with a latticework timbered chamber and a pointy octagonal roof.

Iridescent blue butterflies danced alongside as we strolled through the village. Climbing roses bloomed profusely on the stone walls, begging to be touched. Velvety red, they were bursting with fragrance. Maybe those butterflies and roses were angels too, I thought. After all, how did I know what angels looked like?

We stopped at a small bar and drank sodas. Then we asked where we could get our credentials stamped. With a wave of the hand, we were directed to a nearby building, where Dani graciously stamped them and gave each of us a signed postcard. Gary's said something like, "Walking in another's footsteps is a pleasure of the Chemin"; mine had a picture of the gilt altar painting in the church.

Our companions engaged Dani in animated conversation. Collette was quite proficient at that, demonstrating a sincere interest in almost everyone we met, whether it was a mushroom hunter or a pilgrim. After a while Dani recommended that we ask Madame Bonzani, whose house was just around the corner, for a tour of the church.

We rang the doorbell and at last a stocky, red-faced woman with short grey hair appeared and grumbled in French, "What do you want?" We explained and she gruffly agreed to take us on a tour the next morning.

As we headed back to our tower we admired a ten-foot-tall wooden statue of Saint James carved in 1993 by Roland Delsol, a one-armed sculptor from a nearby village. The local legend was that Delsol had had an accident, lost his arm, and took up sculpting, although he was not formally trained. (I later read that he did have artistic training, but the first version made a better story—and regardless, he still was one-armed.)

Since we had brought dinner provisions with us, we went to the kitchen-dining room, sliced up our cheese, bread, and chocolate, and shared a tin of pâté. Collette saw an announcement on the bulletin board that Espagnac's *table paysanne* (country cooking) restaurant offered baggage transfer, so after supper we found the restaurant and asked the proprietor whether she would take our baggage to Marcilhac-sur-Célé, approximately fifteen kilometers away. First she said no, then yes. We also arranged to have breakfast at the restaurant and Madame agreed to make us a picnic lunch.

Our needs were provided for. Maybe it was synchronicity, maybe it was just luck.

Saturday, May 10, Espagnac to Marcilhac-sur-Célé. 16 kilometers (10 miles).

Madame Bonzani was waiting impatiently for us after breakfast. She collected her fee, then provided us with an exceedingly knowledgeable history of the convent of Espagnac. She spoke French with a bit of Spanish thrown in for my benefit. Notre Dame de Vallée de Paradizo (Notre-Dame-du-Val-Paradis or Valparaiso) was begun in the twelfth century and expanded in the thirteenth. Its famous benefactor, Aymeric d'Hébrard of Carjac, became bishop of Coimbra in Portugal. At first I was surprised at how far he had traveled from France, but then I realized that wandering monks, medieval pilgrims, merchants, and Crusaders frequently traveled much farther.

I understood Madame to say that there was an ecclesiastic connection with Brazil, which would not be surprising, since Portugal colonized Brazil. At one time approximately 100 nuns lived in the convent, but after the French Revolution, none remained.

Inside the church, moss and ferns sprouted out of the crumbling tombs that lined the walls. The tomb of Bernade de Trian, wife of the knight Hugues de Caraillac-Brengues (who died in 1342), is remarkable for its exquisitely detailed stone effigy. Intricately carved flowers festoon her shoes, tiny buttons ornament her sleeves, and a stone facsimile of a treasured gold necklace adorns the effigy's neck. Bernade's sense of style lives on, long after her body has turned to dust.

Madame Bonzani told us about many features of the church that were no longer present, since so much had been destroyed. The unusual bell tower, which still survives, has eight sides and "8," she informed us, is the sign for infinity. She also told us a story about the origin of the Auvergne specialty *aligot*, which we had first tasted in Saint-Alban-sur-Limagnole the previous October. Her version involved politics and the history of the French language. Historically the southern French spoke Languedoc, where *d'oc* was "yes," while the northern French spoke Languedouie, where *oui* was "yes"—a distinction that can still be heard.

According to Madame, *aligot* had originally been *alicot,* a Languedoc word that meant "give me bread"—an important phrase for hungry pilgrims when they arrived at the abbeys and convents along the Chemin. And given bread they were, mixed with cheese. At some point after the discovery of the Americas and the importation of potatoes, pilgrims in the Aubrac were given potatoes instead of bread. Over time, *alicot* became *aligot,* which derived from the Languedouie expression *aliquo*—indicative of the linguistic and political victory of northern France over the south, as well as of the culinary influence of South America.

Waving goodbye to the charming little hamlet of Espagnac, we started back on the Chemin. Our route took us along the limestone *causse* across the river. Troglodyte houses were occasionally carved into the hillside and people still lived in some of them. I supposed they were cool in summer and hard to heat in winter.

The morning began quite auspiciously. We followed a narrow trail through the forest, the steep *causse* on one side, a sheer drop-off to the river on the other. Tree-covered limestone plateaus rose beside flat fertile farmland. Clusters of stone houses with steep *lauze* (limestone tile) roofs, or *lauze* and red tile roofs, dotted the hillsides. We walked past *caselles,* ancient dry-stone huts with beehive roofs, and meadows filled with flowers. After a while we realized that the meandering road in the valley below would have been easier to walk and might have been just as historically accurate. But we were on the hillside, far above the valley, and there was nowhere to go but forward. Ultreya.

I found it harder and harder to walk. The day warmed up to 75° - 80° F and the trail became very rocky, so I had to watch my footing. I was lightheaded and pale from a sudden drop in blood sugar. Danielle offered me an orange, which immediately helped.

While we carefully picked our way along our picturesque trail, both longer and more arduous than the road below, I pondered my health. I had expected that walking the Chemin would be easier this time than the last since I wasn't recovering from surgery, but instead it was harder. Because the weather was warmer? Because we were walking farther? All I knew was that the journey was surprisingly tough.

I pondered the impact of expectations. Without them, I would simply have experienced whatever I was experiencing, without comparing it to something I remembered as preferable. Last year on the Chemin, we had had no expectations and had felt gratitude for whatever the journey brought. At least, I thought we had.

Our path led back down into the Célé valley and to the village of Marcilhac-sur-Célé. Our three-star *chambres d'hôtes,* Les Tilleuls (lime trees), was a stately 200-year-old house nestled inside a private park. The eighty-two-year-old owner greeted us in the living room, reclining on a sofa. She was laid up with a bad case of phlebitis and had to rely on friends to help her run the B&B.

Madame Ménassol had moved to Marcilhac twenty-four years ago and had turned the house and park into a *gîte.* At one time the house had belonged to a famous nineteenth-century doctor who specialized in mental maladies. He created a foundation to help recovering women make the transition back into normal life and work. The high walls allowed the women to wander around the park in privacy, and perhaps its stately cypress and peaceful pond soothed them.

Susie, the loud American we had met a few days before, was right about the uniqueness of the Chemin: there wasn't anything like this in the States—inexpensive, charming, historic accommodations (a medieval tower, an nineteenth-century sanatorium), reached by walking from A to B. The Appalachian Trail and other American long-distance hiking routes rarely include historic places to stay, gourmet restaurants to eat in, and of course, are completely bereft of medieval architectural treasures.

We walked up an elegant wooden staircase to our second-floor room. Each room had a name. Ours was "Portrait," and the door plaque included a hand-painted bouquet of yellow and white flowers.

The bed was saggy; the plumbing minimal; but the windows were large and the view into the garden was charming. Gary commented that the 200-year-old building had 100-year-old wiring. I wondered if we were at risk for electrocution, but Gary assured me there was nothing inherently unsafe in the arrangement.

After a brief rest Gary and I strolled around Marcilhac, a popular tourist town with 250 inhabitants. We wandered over to the ruined Benedictine abbey, constructed between the ninth and fifteenth centuries. Once powerful, it had been pillaged during the Hundred Years' War, partially rebuilt, and then pillaged again during the Wars of Religion† (1562 - 1598), a struggle between French Catholics and Protestants (Huguenots). The French Revolution put an end to the abbey.

What once had been inside was now effectively outdoors, as the roof had disappeared long ago. We walked among decaying arches and columns with sculpted, weather-beaten capitals of various heights. They formed a mute and crumbling forest.

The church is noted for the charming eleventh-century tympanum on its south portal; the intricate carvings are eroded but still visible, protected by a slight overhang. Carved in a naïf style similar to that at Saint-Félix, Christ sits at the top, framed by the sun and moon; two angels below him hold instruments of the Passion; and Saints Peter and Paul stand below.

We ambled along the path that followed the river, stopping at one of the many picnic tables provided alongside. The Célé splashed swiftly along, tickling itself against the banks, sloshing against the boats tied up along the shore.

At a tiny grocery store we purchased a local guidebook and supplies for the next day, including yogurt and a package of granola patties. I also bought a little bag of a local specialty, *Caprices de Noix*, walnuts buried under a bitter-chocolate coating. Then we stopped by the Restaurant des Touristes, run by Madame Lagarrigue, where we had a drink and made reservations for dinner for four.

Madame explained to us that these days she only cooked for ramblers, cyclists, and equestrians who agreed to eat early (at 7:00 p.m.) because she and her husband were tired and not well. We were not offered a choice of *menus* but we saw her washing mounds of asparagus and fresh strawberries. Our mouths watered in anticipation.

When we arrived that evening, only a few tables were occupied. Dinner began with a huge platter of freshly steamed white asparagus drizzled with a delicate shallot vinaigrette. Danielle put a bit of the chewy country bread under her plate to keep the vinaigrette at one end. Next, Madame brought a platter of fragrant ripe melon slices. The main course was sautéed chicken breasts with mushrooms in cream sauce and delectable fried new potatoes, crisp outside and tender inside.

A carefully chosen selection of cheeses—Pyrenees, *cabécou*, and Cantal—accompanied by fresh strawberries drenched in sugar completed the meal. Danielle sprinkled pepper on the *cabécou* and a little wine on the strawberries to bring out their flavors. I was learning French tricks for enhancing even the simplest food.

Sunday, May 11, 2003. Marcilhac-sur-Célé to Cabrerets. 17 kilometers (10.5 miles).

In the morning Madame treated us to a feast at the long trestle table: homemade cakes, sweet breads, *confitures,* and yogurt. She sat at the far end of the table, unable to stand, so a neighbor served breakfast. Madame must have been well liked in the community, even if she was a relative newcomer, since without her friends' help she would have had to close her *chambres d'hôtes.*

Two French women also came down to breakfast. They were going to start walking the Chemin and would meet their husbands somewhere along the way.

Well fed, refreshed, and rested, we started back on the Chemin. Although the terrain was similar to that of the day before, I found walking easier; perhaps I had finally recovered. Chatting as we walked along, the kilometers passed quickly.

An establishment by the side of the river rented canoes and kayaks, and advertised ice cream and coffee. Eyeing the picnic tables shaded by canvas canopies, we wondered if we could eat our lunch there. The two proprietors welcomed us, explaining that they had just opened for the season and were happy to have customers. We savored sandwiches made of bread we had bought warm that morning, topping the thick slices with local Salers, a semi-hard, relatively mild cheese, ripe tomatoes, and a little dry *jambón Serrano* (a French version of Spanish-style dried ham).

Sitting by the swift-running river, munching our delicious meal, Gary and I looked at each other and smiled. "This is as good as it gets." And it was. Enjoying the moment, appreciating the bounty around us, sharing love and companionship—it didn't get any better than this.

I knew that was a tricky expression. In the movie *As Good As It Gets*, starring Jack Nicholson and Helen Hunt, "as good as it gets" meant "This is as good as it is going to get so take it or leave it." But I meant that every moment really is superlative. Sometimes it is difficult to remember that, and I tended to forget it when things were rough, but I was remembering it more often.

We dawdled over steaming cups of espresso, then continued on to Cabrerets. Although we had only walked seventeen kilometers, it felt like more than enough.

The town was nestled against the steep cliffs of the *causse;* the river ran below. Monsieur and Madame Bessac's *gîte/chamber d'hôtes* was uphill. Just when I thought I was done for the day, more was required. Another lesson of the Chemin. I took a deep breath. I could make it.

The building was surrounded by a small moat. I asked Madame Bessac, a Belgian who spoke excellent English, if it had been a mill house originally.

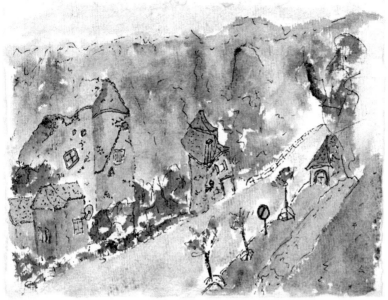

Cabrerets

"No," she replied. "My husband just thought it would be nice to have a moat."

Breakfast would be served in the main room on a table currently covered with laundry. The room was a combination breakfast room, laundry, tearoom, and library. Off to one side was a large cubicle; windows allowed whoever was inside to see what was happening in the main room while still maintaining isolation. Other rooms, probably family quarters, were marked "Private." The arrangements felt a bit haphazard and chaotic.

Even though Madame was quite friendly, she seemed a bit depressed. Maybe she was just overworked. She asked if we planned to visit the famous Grotte du Pech-Merle.

"Pech-Merle? Isn't that a famous cave with lots of prehistoric rock art?" I asked. Paleolithic art fascinated Gary and me.

"Indeed."

"How far is it from here?" I asked.

"Only four kilometers, but it is all uphill."

We looked at each other. We were too tired to walk there, but we really wanted to see the cave.

As if answering our unspoken desire, Madame offered, "I'll drive you there. It's only a five minute drive. Walking back down will be easy."

We thanked our angel of the day and agreed to meet downstairs in fifteen minutes.

On a corner table in the multi-use main room was a display of tourist brochures, including several describing Pech-Merle. According to one pamphlet, Pech-Merle ranks with Lascaux, Niaux, and Altamira as an exceptional legacy of prehistoric art. The famous French prehistorian Abbé Breuil praised it with the following words: "Pech-Merle cave is the Sistine Chapel of the Causses of the Lot district, one of the most beautiful monuments in Paleolithic pictorial art."

For a long time our so-called pilgrimage had been moving in fits and starts. I had found it hard to get into the flow and had objected to being a tourist. But now a ride to a wonderful cave, a short walk back, sounded perfect.

Collette and Danielle joined us, and we climbed into Madame's van and started up the hill. The narrow serpentine road to the cave was indeed steep. It would have taken us an hour or two to hike it, by which time Peche-Merle would have been closed.

We bought tickets at the entrance and wandered through the small museum while waiting for the next tour to begin. The cave had been known for centuries, but after two teenage explorers discovered the prehistoric art in 1922 it became of interest to more than just local residents. In 1923 a man-made entrance was constructed; later, developers installed electricity and built the reception area. We admired models and maps of interconnecting galleries while we eagerly waited to enter the cave.

Eventually our guided tour began. We walked down a tunnel carved through thirteen meters of stone, through a door that closed behind us, and into chilly darkness. When the guide switched on the electric lights, a collective gasp emanated from the group.

The first gallery is a stunning mix of geological formations and prehistoric art. A splendid black charcoal frieze of horses, bison, and mammoths spreads along one wall. Impressionistically drawn, sweeping downward lines depict hair, trunk, and tusk without a single wasted stroke. Red ferric-oxide splots are splattered on the wall and over some of the animals. A five-foot-long fish resembling a pike is dotted with red spots. What do they mean? Our guide, who spoke some English, shrugged his shoulders. Nobody knows.

The grotto contains more than eighty drawings, some of them more than 20,000 years old, of animals and humans, as well as hundreds of symbols, some painted, some engraved, including red dots and what we would call exclamation marks. Often the artists took advantage of natural outcroppings in the cave walls to add three-dimensionality to the paintings. Elegant, curvaceous, black-maned, black-spotted horses as large as ponies prance across one wall. One is partially superimposed on the other, giving a sense of depth.

Ghostly handprints formed by blowing black paint around the artist's hand frame the horses. The negative handprints seem like a kind of autograph or perhaps an attempt to personalize the art: "See, this is *my* handprint. I was here. I painted this. And I left this mark behind." But there is no way of knowing.

Deer, aurochs, and other animals stared out at us from walls, lit for a moment by artificial light. Was it sacrilegious for us to see these figures hidden deep within the earth? Was this a holy chamber, a private space for secret rituals? There is no way of knowing. After all, nobody knows why the drawings were made.

I wasn't sure whether Paleolithic art was the proper label for what we were seeing. Art, after all, is a category constructed by Western scholars to distinguish between something they consider

art and something they don't. Maybe the drawings were part of religious ceremonies having to do with hunting magic, or maybe they
were a way of recording important events.

To our eyes they are beautiful so we call them art, separating
them from utilitarian decoration in the same way we separate sacred
from profane. But perhaps Paleolithic people, like many surviving
indigenous cultures, didn't divide things that way.

What would it be like, I wondered, to live in a world where
instead of duality there is unity, where instead of separation there is
interdependence, an on-going flow uniting all aspects of life so that
everything is seen as sacred and perhaps everything is what we call
art?

In one gallery we came upon a poignant sight: a dozen footprints made by an adolescent boy crossing the bottom of a dry pool
12,000 years ago. Over time the calcite floor had consolidated, pet-
rifying the traces of his steps. There had been no tide, no wind, no
water to wipe away the impressions. 12,000 years later, evidence remains of a young boy who had walked alone in the darkness of the
cave. Perhaps he had carried a small stone oil lamp, but the cave was
immense and he was small. The direction of his footsteps shows he
went somewhere and then returned. What was he doing there by
himself? Was he participating in an initiation? In a dare? Was he a
pilgrim visiting a beloved shrine? We will never know.

We saw the cave painting once known as the Wounded Man,
with what were once thought to be lances sticking into his body.
Researchers have since decided that the marks are not spears going
in but lines going out. The same radiating man drawing has been
found forty kilometers away in the Grottes de Cougnac at Gourdon.
Did the same artist paint it, or was this a symbol shared by a larger
community? Regardless, what did the symbol mean?

The earth-mysteries researcher Paul Devereux has suggested
that shamanic journeying inspired this figure and many other Paleolithic symbols, including the red dots. Maybe so. Maybe the lines
going out of the figure represent energy.

Researchers have found many groupings of spots or dots that appear to be sacred numbers, including 3, 7, 13, and 28. I pointed out to our guide (who didn't seem to know) that thirteen was the number of lunar months in one year. One painting has thirteen black dots, so perhaps it is a lunar calendar.

The paintings also feature triangles, some of them red. Are they a reference to female genitalia, perhaps to the goddess? To menstruation? Scholars interpret a number of cave paintings, including stylized bison with pendulous breasts, as female, but there is no way to know.

Years before, I had seen a photo of a 25,000-year-old carving, the "Goddess of Laussel," found in the Perigord region. She holds a bison horn marked with thirteen hatch marks in her right hand, probably representing the lunar calendar. This figure also has a pronounced pubic triangle, not unlike the triangles decorating the walls at Pech-Merle. Is this evidence of a widespread goddess cult? Of shared artistic styles continuing over a period of at least 5,000 years? Probably so, but there is no way to prove it.

Pech-Merle is more than a gallery of ancient art and sacred symbols, however. It is also a two-million-year-old cave filled with stalactites and stalagmites, mineral curtains, cave pearls formed by calcite accretions over a bit of gravel or sand, a spinning "top" that was originally a cave pearl but because of its location was set spinning and eventually formed a flying-saucer shape, translucent cave onyx, and more, much more, including free-standing calcite disks, columns, and fistulas.

Our tour ended and we emerged, blinking, into the light and warmth of the above-ground world. We bought postcards and guidebooks at the museum shop, then ice cream cones from the nearby vendors. As we sat on benches under some shade trees, licking our dripping cones, we agreed that Pech-Merle has it all: geological wonders, ancient footprints, exquisite art—and an abiding sense of the sacred.

Pilgrims travel great distances to view saintly relics. We had just visited a different kind of sacred site: a cave adorned with the markings of our ancestors, including the 12,000-year-old footprints of a young boy walking alone in the dark.

The trail back down to Cabrerets was only a few kilometers long, but it was rocky and so steep that we wished we had brought our hiking staffs. Tiny wild orchids lined the path. We stopped often to take photographs and rest, enjoying an impressive view of the town below. The limestone cliff-face looked like a slightly askew layer cake, ornamented with bushes and frosted with trees.

Our trail took us past the thirteenth-century château of the Duc de Biron and the church, which was only open for mass, according to a sign posted on the locked door. Collette explained that the lack of staff made rural churches an easy target for theft.

When we arrived back at the *gîte* another pilgrim had just arrived. I handed her the Pech-Merle brochure and enthusiastically urged her to see the caves.

"I'm a pilgrim, not a tourist," she said huffily, and then tromped upstairs to the dorm.

I thought to myself: Even medieval pilgrims went sightseeing.

Following Madame's recommendation we ate at the Hôtel-Restaurant des Grottes, located on the banks of the Célé. A lovely terrace looked out on the river but it was too cool to eat outside, so we sat at a table in the near-empty dining room. This time I was determined to select the *menu* I wanted—and nobody disagreed. For $28.00 (including wine and café) we each enjoyed a multi-course meal of local specialties including *foie gras,* walnuts, and duck.

A group of pilgrims from our *gîte* came in and sat together at a large table. English was the language of choice for this mixed band of German, French, Belgian, English, and American pilgrims. We waved to each other in solidarity.

Danielle and Collette introduced us to the aperitif Fenelon, concocted from local red Cahors wine mixed with cassis and walnut liqueur. Named after the tutor of the young Louis XIV, it was dark red, not too sweet, delicious. The waiter brought a bowl of peanuts as an accompaniment. Once again I realized the advantage to traveling with French people: they knew what to order and received additional little offerings.

Dinner began with *foie gras de canard* (duck liver) prepared exceptionally well, according to Danielle, who explained the cooking process to us in minute detail. My main course was *aguillettes de canard grillade* (grilled back fillet of duck) with new potatoes, green beans, and grilled tomatoes topped with breadcrumbs. The others had *sandret̸ a la salamandre,* a perch-like fish drizzled with a green tarragon sauce. For dessert we had our choice of crème brûlée, apple tart with chocolate sauce, or walnut ice cream.

When she tasted the *foie gras,* Collette sighed happily and said, "Ah, 'l' infant Jesú en pantalon velour!'" Literally, "the baby Jesus in velvet pants."

Bewildered I asked, "What does that mean?"

"It means it is a lovely dish, a lifelong memory."

During dinner Collette asked us about English food expressions. For example, she declared that Danielle was a "bon coup de fourchette"—a "good stroke of the fork"—in other words, she had a healthy appetite. "Chow-hound" was the only comparable phrase I could think of, but calling Danielle a chow-hound didn't seem polite. Nor was I sure that calling Danielle a "bon coup de fourchette" was polite, but she hadn't seemed upset. The conversation degenerated from there, with numerous jokes about Susie and Bubba eating raw carrots.... It was quite risqué and everyone laughed a great deal.

Not everything was so cheerful, however. A general train strike was threatened for Tuesday, so Danielle and Collette informed us they had decided to catch the 12:30 p.m. train from Cahors to Paris on Monday—the next day—instead of on Wednesday, cutting our time together from a week to five days.

Suddenly, we had run out of time. No more singing English and French children's songs while we strolled through the forests; no more sharing our lives and journey. No more having Collette cuddle Honey Bunny and whisper tender French endearments into her floppy ears. I wanted to cry. Even though sometimes I had gotten weary of Collette and Danielle's chattering while we walked, I knew that I would miss their melodious voices.

Monday, May 12, 2003. Cabrerets to Cahors by bus.

Madame Bessac agreed to drive us to a nearby town to catch the morning bus to Cahors. As we rode along, I looked longingly at the stunning scenery we would not be walking through. Even though our pilgrimage had morphed into an excursion, it had never occurred to us to say "Bon Voyage" to Collette and Danielle and send them off on their own. We were on this journey together, at least until the end of the day.

We reached the bus stop an hour early. It was chilly and damp, with occasional splatters of rain, so we scurried down the road to a nearby hôtel-restaurant for shelter and hot chocolate. At last we boarded the bus, which rumbled and lurched to Cahors. En route we saw another "Most Beautiful Village in France" on a hillside across the river—Saint-Cirq-Lapopie, a perfectly preserved, fortified medieval village. It was on the GR 651, so if we ever returned, we would walk through it.

While Collette and Danielle confirmed their reservations at the train station in Cahors, Gary and I searched for a hotel. The guidebook recommended Hôtel Le Melchior, across from the train station. We asked to see the room, and a friendly young clerk led us upstairs. The hallway was smelly and dingy, the carpet stained and torn. The room reeked of stale cigarette smoke. We politely declined.

We hurried back to the train station to meet Danielle and Collette, but they were nowhere to be found. After fifteen minutes of frantic searching we reconnected at the fountain outside the station, near a large town map that showed hotel locations. We decided to try to stay at La Chartreuse, located at the edge of town next to the Lot River, which formed a big loop around Cahors. Collette called and made the reservation. She also made reservations for our next few nights on the Chemin.

Then we returned to the station and sat in the lunchroom drinking espresso and hot chocolate. We took a photo of Collette pretending to feed Honey Bunny. I wondered if she would miss us as much as she would miss Honey Bunny. In the photo Danielle is smiling at both of them. Although I thought Danielle was withdrawn, I suddenly realized that she actually smiled a lot.

An elderly woman sitting near us observed our interactions with Honey Bunny and asked condescendingly if we had returned to childhood.

Collette snapped, "I hope we never left!"

The woman was taken aback. After a moment's hesitation, she asked to make Honey Bunny's acquaintance. An entertaining exchange ensued.

Before leaving, Danielle invited us to her vacation house near Tours and Collette asked us to her home in Lille. We promised we would try to visit. Then, somewhat tearfully, we saw them off on the train.

I had enjoyed their companionship, but now Gary and I would be free to make our own choices about where to stay and how far to walk and when to stop for lunch—and even which *menu* to choose. Of course, we had always been free to do so. It wasn't Collette's fault that we acquiesced to her arrangements and then privately grumbled. It was one thing to accept what is, another thing to complain.

I did have a moment's discomfort about being without linguistic support, but it quickly passed. We would manage. We had managed before, even on that terrifying, panic-filled night on the mountaintop at Golinhac. This time I was determined to have faith that everything would work out. After all, it always did.

Gratitude for their friendship; gratitude for their assistance; gratitude for no longer compromising. And gratitude for another lesson of the Chemin: We had learned what it felt like to let someone else take charge of our pilgrimage—and our lives. It had been easy. But it hadn't been good.

We walked through town, across a large bridge, and around the horseshoe bend in the Lot to our hotel, La Chartreuse. Layla, the friendly receptionist, spoke English. I told her that "Layla" is the name of the absent beloved in "Majnun," a famous Middle Eastern story.

Majnun (said to have been a seventh-century Bedouin poet) fell in love with Layla, the most beautiful and perfect of all women. Forbidden to marry her, he went mad with longing. She married someone else and died young. He spent the rest of his life writing love poetry and wandering in the desert. The legend has become a metaphor describing the human longing for the absent Beloved—God. Layla seemed intrigued by the story but said it had nothing to do with her name.

Lovely Layla gave us a spacious room overlooking the river. Ducks drifted down the current and excursion boats tied up at a nearby dock. Peace and quiet—just what we needed. When I went back to the reception desk to thank her, I asked if she could help us transport Gary's backpack to Lascabanes, our next scheduled stop. The longer Gary carried it, the heavier it became. With a smile, she called Factage and arranged for them to pick it up in the morning. Would that all burdens could be so easily discarded.

Since it was lunchtime we went to the hotel's *gastronomique* restaurant, clearly *the* place to eat. Business people dined at several long tables. The men wore suits, as did the occasional woman. The chef came out periodically to shake hands with important guests. Although normally we ate a light lunch, this time we splurged. Gary had warm goat cheese in puff pastry for a first course; I had *rillettes* of goose and *foie gras*. Next he chose a mousse of *sandre* and salmon, while I selected lamb in garlic sauce. Cheese and a tempting selection of desserts followed.

Needing to walk off our meal, we strolled back into town to find a pharmacy selling Compeed, a skin protector with a tiny gel-like cushion in the middle. I had been fortunate to avoid blisters the year before. I didn't want to get any blisters on this journey, so I planned to take pre-emptive action and apply Compeed at the first sign of redness or discomfort.

Cahors is a relatively large town, population 21,000, the principal city in rural Quercy. Romans founded the town 2000 years ago, and some Roman ruins remain. Several bridges cross the river, including the dramatic fourteenth-century Pont Valentré at the west end of town, near our hotel. Touted to be the finest surviving fortified bridge in Europe, it boasts seven arches and three towers. The sculpture of a devil on one of the towers commemorates a legend about the bridge's builder and a pact he made with Satan—a variant of the Dr. Faustus story. Rumor has it the bridge tower was built over an ancient Roman shrine; perhaps that is what is really being commemorated by the sculpture.

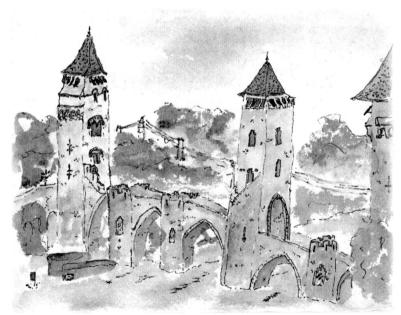

Bridge at Cahors

Later we ran into Susie, sipping espresso with an attractive young man with intense dark eyes. Susie gushed that she just loved Cahors. I asked about Bubba and she seemed evasive.

We headed over to the twelfth-century Cathédrale de Saint-Etienne, famous for having the largest church dome in France, probably modeled after Byzantine constructions. The walls in the Old Town were covered with graffiti; gangs of intoxicated, somewhat threatening men strolled the streets or clustered in corners. The acrid smell of urine drifted into the air. It was the first time I had felt unsafe on the Chemin.

Inside the cathedral, excessive renovations in the nineteenth and twentieth centuries resulted in garishly painted walls. What is not painted is covered with mold. It is a disturbing combination. I wanted to see a sculpture of a pilgrim in the cloisters but a helpful young man informed us that they were closed. He suggested we visit the Tourist Office to ask for information. When we lost our way, another helpful person led us to the bureau. The clerk explained that it wasn't tourist season yet so there were no visitations. Seeing our disappointment she suggested a Le Petit Train tour, due to depart in fifteen minutes from the other end of town, near our hotel.

We ran back along the tree-lined riverbank. Panting, we arrived just in time to buy tickets and find a seat. Soon the train was putt-putting up the road back into town. Serendipitously (or was it synchronicity?) a British couple sat behind us and soon we were carrying on an animated conversation.

We learned that the night before, Graham and Janet had stayed in an unpleasant hotel in another town, and they wondered if we had had better luck in Cahors. We had, and enthusiastically recommended La Chartreuse.

Sitting comfortably in Le Petit Train as it wound through the city streets, I realized that Cahors was a study in contrasts. Modern upscale buildings in the business center contrasted with run-down, desolate buildings and churches in the medieval section. Helpful citizens contrasted with vaguely threatening gangs of drunks. Judgment, judgment. It was so habitual that I hardly noticed the lens through which I saw the world.

Our train twisted its way through narrow streets, passing by various towers and the Arch of Diana, all that remains of the Roman municipal baths. Then Le Petit Train struggled up the hill outside of town to a scenic overlook: from the tree-covered limestone *causse* overlooking the city we could at last appreciate the huge cupola of the cathedral.

Gary felt feeble and chilled when we got back to the hotel, so we had an unfashionably early dinner. Given the restaurant's emphasis on truffles I decided I would give them another chance.

I ordered the truffle omelet. Judging by the exorbitant price, I presumed that this time I would finally have the real truffle experience, something that hitherto had escaped me, despite several attempts. The omelet arrived hot and runny with flecks of black sprinkled through the bright yellow eggs. I took a bite, hoping for an epiphany. There was none. The black truffle specks were crunchy and brittle. Concentrating intently I took another bite and noticed a faint, earthy taste. Once the omelet cooled off there was a bit more of what I identified as subtle truffle flavor, but who wanted to eat cold eggs?

I wondered once again why truffles were such an object of cultish devotion. Were they an acquired taste? A culinary example of "The Emperor's New Clothes"? Maybe my lack of appreciation was due to an uneducated palate. Or perhaps I lacked some important chemical taste processor.

Tuesday, May 13, 2003. Ride from Cahors to near Lascabanes. 23 kilometers (14 miles).

Gary felt better the next morning but I felt weak and shaky. I hoped eating breakfast would make me feel better. Graham and Janet, the Britons whom we had met on Le Petit Train, were sitting in the breakfast room at a table next to ours. They had taken our advice and were quite pleased.

While Gary ate, I felt worse and worse. I felt too sick to walk, so we decided to have Layla call a taxi to take us to Lascabanes. I had looked forward to setting our own pace, making our own plans now that Collette and Danielle had left us—but I hadn't expected our plans to look like this.

Graham and Janet overheard our conversation and he offered to drive us. Gratitude and faith resurged. We were being given the help we needed. Sometimes we were given the strength to walk; sometimes we were given a ride.

Leaving our backpack for Factage to deliver, we drove off to Lascabanes. Graham marveled at the narrow country road and confided that he had never driven in rural France. He was concerned about finding his way back, but we reassured him that the country lanes were numbered and he could follow the road signs back to Cahors.

After half an hour we saw a sign pointing to our *gite*, "L'Happy-cool-teur," a kilometer or so before Lascabanes, but Graham kept driving, intent on taking us to Lascabanes. He dropped us off at a small, deserted plaza. We thanked him effusively and promised to stay in touch.

Since it was still early in the day, we decided to find something to drink in town. No such luck. The stores and the communal *gite* were closed. The church, however, was open so we went inside. It was small, well cared for, and filled with weapon-wielding statues. An angel speared a fallen devil with wings; Joan of Arc brandished a sword; the Virgin Mary impaled a dragon; and Saint George attacked another one. Once again I wondered about the symbology: were the indigenous Earth religions being held down by the Church? The iconography was as puzzling to me as the Paleolithic cave art we had admired at Pech-Merle. I could imagine many meanings, but which of them were correct?

Since the shops were closed and we were thirsty, we made our way slowly back to L'Happy-cool-teur, our *chambres à la ferme* (farm bed-and-breakfast). We were in the region once known as the Quercy, where the houses are built of creamy limestone, often left unstuccoed, with tile roofs that are not as steeply slanted as where we were walking just a few days ago.

Some 800 meters (half a mile) down the road, then 50 meters on another country road, then 800 meters further, we arrived at a farm complete with geese, a rooster, a donkey, a grey-haired dog, a fruit orchard, and lots of flowers, including brilliant orange poppies and multi-colored clumps of iris.

Two pilgrims on horseback were saddling up as we arrived. They trotted back down the road as we waved. A slim, dark-haired woman and her young daughter were working in a field covered with orderly rows of mounded earth. Denise saw us and came over to greet us.

Sometimes *Miam Miam Dodo* indicated that inn proprietors spoke English but they really didn't. At this *chambres à la ferme* we didn't expect anyone to speak English but Denise was willing to try and we were grateful. She explained that she and Giles, her husband, were beekeepers as well as organic farmers, and he thought English-speaking travelers would have an easier time remembering their place if it sounded English—hence "L'Happy-cool-teur," a bilingual pun on *abeille culteur* (apiculture).

The family had been living in the south of France but they had wanted to raise their three children in a clean, organic environment. When they saw the advertisement for the farm three years before, they bought it. They were part of a contemporary movement that was not communal but did include barter and exchange, facilitated by networking organizations.

The guesthouse was a newly remodeled stone building with its own dining area and kitchen, two bedrooms, a bathroom, a fireplace, and a solar cell for generating hot water. Bottled organic fruit juices stocked the refrigerator, paid for on the honor system. Our backpack was already waiting for us.

We went out to the field to watch Denise and Sara, her three and one-half-year-old daughter, harvest the white asparagus hidden beneath the mounded soil. Sara was a chubby-faced little girl with dark hair cut in a bob with bangs. I brought Honey Bunny along. I thought Sara might enjoy playing with Honey Bunny but she pointedly ignored her. Sara was a very serious little girl.

At last Denise asked, "Is that a mascot?"

We hesitated a moment, then nodded.

They had planted the asparagus when they had bought the farm. This was the first year they have been able to harvest it. This year the crop required twenty to thirty days of work; next year it would require sixty. The asparagus would turn green if it poked through the soil because its chlorophyll would be activated by sunlight, so Denise had to cut the spears before they emerged. Using a long tool with a curved, spoon-like blade at the bottom, she dug into the mound every morning. She loosened the earth, judged how deep to go with the tool, and then cut the asparagus. It was an art not a science. Some of the severed spears were too thin, some quite large, and some were cut too short.

After she had harvested enough for the day, her husband cut each stem to a uniform length. They then sold them to a vendor who distributed them in markets around the region, making their small operation commercially viable. Since their farm was *biologique* (organic), they fit into a niche market and could charge more for their produce.

Giles transported their bees to different locales, depending on what was in bloom. Currently the bees were located near Moissac, buzzing around the sweet white acacia blossoms. Next Gilles would move the beehives to be close to certain mountain flowers.

"Is the honey *bio*?" I asked.

"Not exactly. We can't control the *bio* part with the bees, although we know how far they roam so we can control what the honey tastes like."

I pointed to the orchard. "Fruit trees?"

"*Noisette*—hazelnut. We planted them three years ago when we bought the farm. We'll be able to harvest them in six years."

I usually found it hard to plan a month in advance, or even a day in advance on the Chemin. I'd have made a lousy farmer.

The day was clammy and overcast, and suddenly I started to shiver uncontrollably. Gary looked at me with concern.

"A bientôt—See you soon," I said. We hurried to our room so I could lie down, but it was as cold inside as it had been outside, so I went back out and asked Denise about heating the bedroom.

She responded in disbelief, "You *heat* your bedrooms in the US?"

Chastened, I went back to the bedroom. Gary and I huddled together for warmth and I soon fell asleep.

While I slept, Gary called a *gite* in Montcuq to make reservations for the following night. The owners said they were not ready to open, but finally they agreed to let us stay.

An exhausted French couple arrived and settled into the other bedroom. Robert explained in a mixture of French and Spanish that Juliette had pain in her legs, perhaps shin splints. They were walking the Chemin in 250-kilometer (155-mile) segments because they only had two weeks' vacation each year. This year's journey was from Figeac to Condom.

While Gary massaged Juliette's legs, Robert told us that they had met the previous year on the Chemin and fallen in love. They tried to see each other every month or so, but he lived in northern France and she lived near Marseilles in the south. The long-distance relationship was difficult, but true love would win out, or so they hoped.

I put on several layers of clothes, tucked Honey Bunny under my arm, and went outside to the picnic table. It was warmer there than inside the unheated stone building. I started writing in my journal.

> *I haven't found a rhythm for this trip. What a revealing choice of words: trip instead of pilgrimage. Our trip has been broken up with taxi rides, social events, and sightseeing jaunts. Last year we started slowly and walked every day. It was a pilgrimage filled with gratitude.*

This year is different, or maybe I just don't remember how hard it was last year. We weren't in shape when we started and we still aren't, even though we've been walking for a week. I feel stiff and sore when I wake up and when I go to bed. It's hard to get going, hard to keep going. It's not just me; Gary's struggling too.

I hope we will be able to find our rhythm now that it's just the two of us. Assuming I feel better, tomorrow we will walk nine kilometers to Montcuq. I hope I can make it.

I need to figure out what's making it so hard for me to walk, so hard to keep going. I know I've been eating sugar, bread, buttery croissants, and chocolate. It's so hard to resist. Besides, what are the alternatives? And now I'm like an alcoholic who's fallen off the wagon. Last year I ate this way, so why should it be a problem this year? I know, I know. Last year was last year; this year is this year.

I worry about not feeling well and about my ankles swelling because I'm afraid they are indicators that I'll get cancer again. I worry that a cancer cell escaped during surgery and it might metastasize if I do the wrong thing. The problem is, I don't know what the wrong thing is.

A friend of mine told me, "There's no such thing as a root cause—looking for that is like trying to hit a moving target." I know she thought that would reassure me, but it didn't.

I'm finding it hard to live in trust, to let go of worry, to have faith that everything is perfect—even if I do have a recurrence of cancer. Whatever happened to the optimism I felt on the Chemin last fall?

Last year I was buoyed up with excitement and re-lief—the surgery was successful and a mere three months later I was walking across France! Thoughts of a recurrence never crossed my mind. Now, almost a year later, I have had an abnormal Pap test. I have to come to terms with the fact that the surgery was just the beginning.

I see ahead of me a long grey slog through uncertainty until four more years have passed—my five-years-after-surgery "magic milestone." But since my late ex-husband, John, died from a recurrence of melanoma eighteen years after his initial diagnosis and surgery—and eight years after his "magic milestone"—I doubt that I'll feel reassured even then.

I know that you never know what's going to happen, but most of the time you don't live with that awareness on a daily basis. It could feel liberating, but it doesn't.

Despite all the challenges, this springtime journey, trip, pilgrimage—whatever I call it—is beautiful. Each day we see a profusion of wildflowers, rosebushes exuberantly climbing up stone walls, clumps of irises blooming by the roadside. Fragrances are everywhere, as are fluttering butterflies and the incomprehensible conversations of birds. The sun doesn't set until 9:30 p.m., so there is plenty of daylight to enjoy it all.

Sara came to join me while I wrote in my journal. A bit hesitant, she started to play with Honey Bunny, looking at me with grave mistrust. Maybe seeing an adult playing with a plush bunny confused her. Sometimes it was confusing to me, too, but it made me feel good. Honey Bunny reminded me not to take things too seriously—though she seemed to be failing at the moment. Maybe it was a lot to ask of a plush bunny.

Gary awoke from his nap and came outside, so I put away my journal. We explored Denise and Gilles' shop, stocked with jars of honey, including acacia, chestnut, and lavender. They also sold home-made propolis extract, touted as a wonderful disinfectant, tonic, and antiseptic. Other products included royal jelly, beeswax candles, and a *bio* honey, nut, and egg-white nougat. Of course I had to try the candy. I also bought a small bottle of propolis.

Camino businesses trusted their patrons to a surprising degree—and vice versa. Transbagage and Factage transported bags on the Chemin, an arrangement based on mutual trust. Factage expected us to pay them on the last day of our planned itinerary, not daily. Granted, they had our bags, but presumably we could have absconded the final morning and not paid. We paid for our lodging in the morning before leaving instead of in the afternoon when we arrived. The "happy-cool-teur" shop was unlocked. At the Relais Saint-Jacques near Figeac canned goods and drinks were available on the honor system. Maybe people thought pilgrims were honest. Or maybe rural French customs were simply different.

Dinner was at 7:00 p.m. at Denise and Gilles' stone house, next door to the *gite*. The main room overflowed with kids' schoolbooks, jackets, and assorted paraphernalia. Fabric was tacked on the walls for decoration; clothes pegs were nailed into the walls. It was either a scene of barely manageable disorder or of exuberant family life, depending on your perspective.

We four pilgrims joined Denise, Gilles, and their three children (two teenagers and Sara) for dinner, eating at a large table in the combination kitchen-dining room. Dinner began with an omelet made with fresh white asparagus and eggs from their chickens; next Denise presented a casserole of bulgur wheat and carrots, with thick-sliced whole-grain bread served on the side. *Clafoutis*, a traditional custard and fruit tart, finished the meal. Instead of sugar there was honey to sweeten the coffee. I was surprised they served coffee, but I supposed some habits die hard.

At last I understood the baffling phrase, "épicerie bio restreinte," that accompanied their entry in *Miam Miam Dodo*. "Restricted organic" apparently meant vegetarian.

Wednesday, May 14, 2003. Lascabanes to Montcuq, 9 kilometers (5.5 miles).

I slept from 9:30 p.m. to 7:30 a.m. but I woke up tired and aching, perhaps because the room was so damp and cold. I wondered what *bio restreinte* surprises would await us at breakfast. It was quite tasty: honey to spread on dense multi-grain bread and homemade spice bread they had bartered for.

Denise told us about a shortcut to Montcuq, so we set out with renewed energy and a sense of adventure. Unfortunately she had failed to mention that the shortcut went up and over the hills. I thought about how only a few days earlier I had sincerely proclaimed, "This is as good as it gets!" Now the phrase held a faintly sardonic twist.

Eventually the trail got easier, or maybe we just got used to walking. We passed fields of rye sprinkled with bright orange poppies. For a while it would be cool, overcast, in the mid 60's F; then it would be sunny and warmer; then cool again. I took off layers and put them back on in an ineffective attempt to get comfortable. After scrambling down a steep, unpaved trail, we reached Montcuq. It had been a long nine kilometers.

When Gary made the reservation at Le Souleillou they told him the *gite* was at the entrance to Montcuq, but we didn't see it. Wearily we trudged through town until we reached the tourist office. A stylishly dressed (a hoop earring in one ear, collarless cotton shirt, handwoven vest) German in his mid 60s greeted us. Horst informed us in excellent English that Le Souleillou wasn't on the GR; it was on the highway that led into town.

Seeing how tired I was, Horst offered to give us a ride to the *gite*. He was our angel for the day. Thinking that this was a rare opportunity to learn about our environs, I mentioned that Cahors had seemed run down. Horst explained that Cahors had once been central to the region but had missed out on economic development opportunities. There were indeed many vagrants, but they were a problem elsewhere as well. They gravitate toward southern France because it is warmer.

After locking the tourist office, Horst led us to his van, a modern version of the magic carpet. In a few minutes we arrived effortlessly at Le Souleillou.

A decorative sign featuring a sunflower and lavender sprigs growing out of a scallop shell pointed the way to a building that was still being painted. The new *gite* wasn't officially open, but it was open enough for us to sleep there. The proprietors, Monsieur and Madame Lagane, were busy getting the place ready. Madame and a friend dusted new glassware and plates, then put them into a cupboard in the dining room. Madame smiled at us and asked if we wanted tea.

Monsieur Lagane came forward and shook our hands. He was a small, wiry man who resembled an Old Testament prophet: he had a big bushy beard, a high forehead, and a beak of a nose. His wife was a typical matronly French countrywoman, with a warm, welcoming smile.

As Jacques led us to our room on the second level, he told us that "Le Souleillou" is Occitan (Languedoc) for "an open area to dry things under the rafters"; apparently the language is still in use in Montcuq. We had to squeeze around a painter balancing precariously on a ladder on the winding cement staircase. How ironic. Our house in the US was being remodeled and we had left to avoid chemical exposure; now we were staying in a *gîte* that was being painted. I told myself that if I kept repeating my mantra of "gratitude, gratitude" I might remember to feel it more often.

Jacques explained that there were name plaques for the rooms but they hadn't had time to put them up. The *gîte* would have ten rooms, numerous bathrooms, and the capacity to sleep thirty people. One room would be handicap accessible. The laundry room would include several washers and dryers, and there would be facilities for camping and for horses.

We had been promised a large bed but that room was not yet ready, so we were given a room with two bunk beds. We would be the first to use the bright red blankets and sleep on the mattresses. The room was cold, however, and Gary and I wouldn't be able to snuggle together for warmth, so I stripped the blankets from the upper bunk beds.

The bathrooms and showers were located at each end of the hall. We freshened up, then went back downstairs. How quickly our exhaustion had faded once we arrived at our destination.

After proudly showing us the gleaming kitchen, the large dining room, and the laundry room, which we could use once they hung the door, Madame made us a pot of tea. They were supposed to open

May 20 but the demand had been so great that they had decided to open provisionally. This day was their debut, and already they had reservations for eight pilgrims.

As we drank tea I watched Madame and her friend bustling around, getting things set up, breaking a dish, sweeping it up, figuring out how to do it all for the first time. They were glowing with excitement. This might be a money-making operation—it had to be, of course—but it was also a gift of love for the Chemin.

Although Montcuq seemed like a nondescript backwater town in the middle of nowhere, that hadn't always been the case. The town had developed within a Roman *castrum* or fort. Located in a river valley, it was on a major thoroughfare linking Cahors with Agen— the town where Sainte Foy had lived and died so many centuries before. The donjon tower that pokes up over the roofs of the town is what remains of a twelfth-century castle that was torn down in the thirteenth century during the Albigensian Crusade (1209 – 1229, although Quéribus, the last Cathar stronghold, didn't fall until 1255).

This crusade (named after the town of Albi) was a state-and-church sponsored effort to decimate the Cathar sect that thrived in the independent southern part of France known as the Occitan. The Cathars' heretical views were the official reason behind the crusade, although politics and greed were undoubtedly more important motivations than saving souls. Just as history is written by the victors, so is heresy determined by which religious group is in power.

Montcuq belonged to the counts of Toulouse—powerful, wealthy nobles who were sympathetic to the Cathars and quite possibly were Cathars themselves. Hence the raid and subsequent destruction of Montcuq.

Scholars used to think that "Cathar" derived from the Greek *katharos*, which means "clean" and "pure"; now they are not so sure. Whether that is the correct etymology, that's what Cathars, who called themselves *Bons Hommes* and *Bonnes Femmes* (Good Men and

Good Women), strived to be. They believed in a simpler Christianity, a kind described in the Sermon on the Mount.

Guided by humble traveling teachers who stood in sharp contrast to the clergy of the avaricious and powerful Church of Rome, Cathar adherents included members of the nobility as well as many simple peasants and villagers. An identifiable sect by the twelfth century, Cathar beliefs spread throughout Europe, reaching from the Rhineland to France to northern Italy.

Based on a version of Gnostic dualism in which the created world was seen as inherently evil, Cathars believed that the real spiritual task was to have as little to do with the material world as possible. There were two kinds of Cathars. The vast majority were simple *credentes* or believers who tried to live good lives but knew that, since the world was evil, sin was inevitable. A much smaller number were *perfecti*, who lived ascetically and prayerfully and ministered to the believers. Cathar beliefs encouraged vegetarianism, equality between men and women, simplicity, pacifism, sexual abstinence, and freedom from Catholic sacraments, confession, and tithing. Before death, Cathars would take the *consolamentum,* a rite that combined absolution, baptismal regeneration, redemption and liberation of the soul, and ordination.

The Albigensian Crusade began in 1209, shortly after Pope Innocent III excommunicated Count Raymond VI of Toulouse for aiding and abetting the Cathars. In collusion with Philippe II of France, he then preached a formal crusade against the Cathars. Northern knights and nobles knew an opportunity for a feeding frenzy when they saw one. Thus began a crusade that was to last for almost half a century. Whatever its putative religious justification, the Albigensian Crusade was a power-hungry invasion of Occitania, where people spoke Languedoc, not Languedouie. Less than 10% of the people in the region were Cathars, but the brutal crusade united southern Catholics with the Cathars as they struggled unsuccessfully to fend off the invaders.

The city of Beziers was attacked in 1209. Roman Catholic residents were urged to leave but they stayed in solidarity with their Cathar neighbors. Arnaud-Amaury, the Cistercian abbot-commander and papal legate, was asked how the invading troops would be able to tell the Catholics from the Cathars. He purportedly replied, "Kill them all! God will know his own." He proudly reported to Innocent III that 20,000 people were tortured, mutilated, and slaughtered. Only 200 of them were Cathars.

Simon de Montfort, Seigneur de Montfort-l'Amaury, 5th Earl of Leicester (1160 – June 25, 1218), also known as Simon de Montfort the Elder, was the most well known and hated of the northern nobles who participated in the Albigensian Crusade. As part of the unrelenting campaign, he raided Montcuq in 1212. The town got off relatively easily. With the help of the Dominican-led Holy Inquisition, eighty-three residents were later convicted of heresy. Although the guilty were sometimes sentenced to a year or two of confinement "behind the wall," they were more often burned at the stake, frequently in large groups—a kind of communal heretic roast that often included a few Catholics as well.

Simon de Montfort grabbed for himself the properties of the count of Toulouse, including the town of Montcuq. Toulouse capitulated in 1229. A number of Cathar castles, owned by sympathizers if not by actual Cathars, eventually succumbed, including Montségur on March 16, 1244, after a ten-month siege. It took another seventy years for the crusade and the Inquisition to root out the remaining Cathars. The Inquisition continued for centuries after, spreading religious conformity and terror throughout Europe.

Montcuq suffered through numerous other wars as well, including the Hundred Years' War with the English and the Wars of Religion, during which Protestant Huguenots looted the town and set fire to the Église de Saint-Hilaire. The church was later rebuilt. What a sad, sordid history the town had witnessed, where religion was used as a bludgeon to bring death and destruction.

We walked back into town and sat at a café table next to a British family with squalling twin toddlers ensconced in high chairs. The obese mother kept shoving food into their gaping mouths. The tall, skinny father looked dazed. One child had learned to get attention by screaming and throwing a tantrum, which he did after he had ceased to be amused by the French fries his mother was stuffing into his mouth. The other child watched silently, then he, too, began to shriek. We exchanged wide-eyed glances with two women at a nearby table, a silent way of sharing our mutual horror at the scene.

The mother disappeared inside the restaurant, leaving the father to cope. As he wheeled the twins away in a stroller he hissed to himself, "Such *charming* children!"

After eating a mediocre lunch we stopped at a *tabac* and I looked at the postcards on display. I learned that the name "Montcuq" supposedly came from the Latin Montis Cuci, "Mount Cuckoo." When pronounced as Montcuq, without the final 'koo' of cuckoo, the word sounded like French for "my arse." This joke was the basis of a number of silly postcards.

We walked up to the top of the town to the Église de Saint-Hilaire and the 85-foot-tall, twelfth-century Tour Comtale, all that remains of the once-impressive castle and a visible reminder of the town's tumultuous past. The tower required too much effort to climb but the church was open. Grateful for shelter from the cold, we went inside and sang "Ultreya," then sat quietly on the wooden pews.

On the way back to the *gîte* we purchased a local goat cheese for lunch the next day and identified the *boulangerie* where we would buy bread. Back at the *gîte* our backpack (filled with dirty clothes) was wait-

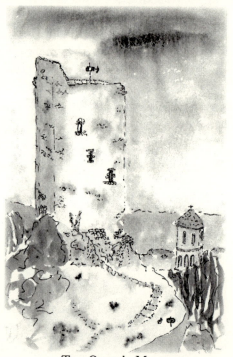

Tour Comtale, Montcuq

ing, so we started a load of laundry in the high-tech washing machine. A washing machine. What a luxury.

Madame invited us to pick fresh cherries from the trees in front of their home across the street. Juicy and sweet, fresh off the branch, they were delicious. Gratitude, gratitude, for all that life brings.

That evening's celebratory dinner began with Ratafia and crackers, followed by vegetables, noodles with mussels and shrimps, bread, and ice cream. Looking at my plate of noodles, I wondered how I could avoid eating wheat. The answer was: not easily, especially when I wasn't really trying.

Maybe my challenge on this pilgrimage was to move from self indulgence to respecting my body—treating it as a temple of God and nourishing it rather than feeding my appetite. But it was so hard. I remembered a quote by Frank A. Clark: "If you find a path with no obstacles, it probably doesn't lead anywhere." And another quote: "That's why they call it practice. You have to keep doing it." I was certainly being given enough opportunities.

A young Swiss pilgrim couple that had started the pilgrimage in Geneva ate tomato sauce on their noodles instead of seafood. Apparently they were strict vegetarians and determined to maintain their dietary regimes. She was extremely thin and so was he, though they ate several helpings.

They spoke English so I asked why they had started in Geneva. They looked at each other and shrugged. Maybe they didn't have words to explain, or maybe it was obvious. Or maybe they didn't want to tell a stranger.

Dinner conversation began in English but soon French became the language of choice. We talked briefly with a couple in their forties. Christopher was a pharmacist at a ski resort six months of the year; his partner, Sonia, lived near Lille. They wanted to be together more often, but they couldn't get work transfers.

Another French pilgrim, Jerome, listened silently before suddenly speaking in English. We talked enthusiastically, but he soon became engrossed in a conversation in rapid-fire French about esoteric Egypt and the pyramids. Although we couldn't understand much, it was good to share the communal meal and to be with fellow pilgrims on the Way.

Thursday, May 15, 2003. Montcuq to L'Aube Nouvelle (21 kilometers; 13 miles), near Durfort-Lacapelette. We walked 13 kilometers (8 miles) to Lauzerte, but then Gary's knee gave out and we took a taxi the remaining 8 kilometers (5 miles).

As we left town we stopped at the *boulangerie* and bought walnut bread and chewy almond cookies. "We need them for strength," I declared defiantly.

Since yesterday had been chilly I had dressed for cool weather; but the day quickly became hot—80° F—and sunny. Nonetheless, we felt energetic enough to take a one-kilometer detour to the hamlet of Rouilhac to admire remarkable twelfth-century frescoes on the subject of Original Sin. I felt like a real pilgrim, going out of my way to see a sacred site.

My energy and enthusiasm soon waned, however. We walked uphill, we walked downhill, we walked uphill again. It was hot. Everyone we encountered felt beaten down. The hardy Swiss pilgrim we've seen several times before on the Chemin rested under the shade of a tree. He nodded in greeting. At one point the trail was so steep that someone had tied a thick green rope from tree to tree. Even with that assistance, the path was difficult to ascend. It would be treacherous when wet.

We walked through oak forests, past vineyards and peach, pear, and apple orchards. We saw trees laden with plums (the source of the famous *pruneaux* products of the region), walnuts, and kiwis. Fields of sorghum, perhaps rye, wheat, and beans spread out before us. This was a region of diversified agriculture, including goat herds. It was beautiful, but the path was strenuous and the day was unpleasantly hot.

We saw a *buron* (a stone shepherd's hut), dug into a small grass-covered mound in the middle of a field. We also saw a new kind of GR marker that combined the red-and-white blazons of the GR 65 with the stylized scallop shell of the EU, along with the words

"Chemin de Compostelle." We were not just walking a long-distance hiking trail: we were on the Chemin. I felt like our pilgrimage had truly begun.

Now that I thought about it, I realized we hadn't seen any groups of hikers since before Conques, and even though we had had trouble feeling like we were making a pilgrimage, we had nonetheless assumed that the people we met on the Chemin were pilgrims. And they were. And so were we.

At a farmhouse at the top of one long uphill effort, a farm wife had set up a small table under an awning; she had left a row of plastic-wrapped *gateaux de noix* (walnut cakes) for sale. We bought two, leaving payment behind in a basket. Once again we experienced the trust inherent on the Chemin. Unfortunately, our trust proved to be misplaced: the cakes were so dry they were almost inedible. How quickly my trust felt violated.

I was on an emotional rollercoaster. One moment I told myself I could walk to Saint-Jean-Pied-de-Port; the next moment, after the brilliant sun came out, I was afraid that I couldn't walk another kilometer. A little devil whispered in my ear, "You don't have to keep walking! You deserve a rest. Sit back, relax." It wasn't a devil, of course, it was just a part of me trying to weaken my resolve.

My mood was as changeable as the weather. Yesterday I had been full of joy and happiness. Today I swung between gratitude and depression. Suddenly, again, our journey didn't feel like a pilgrimage. It had been a tough walk, with lots of rocky trails going up and down steep hillsides: the discomfort could have made it feel more like a pilgrimage if I believed there was virtue in suffering. I didn't. There was enough suffering in life, so why go looking for more? "Ultreya," I told myself disheartedly.

We walked fourteen kilometers before we quit at the bottom of the hill leading up to Lauzerte, a thirteenth-century bastide founded by the Count of Toulouse. Gary's right knee hurt too much for him to keep walking, so we stopped at the commercial zone on the outskirts of town, across from a supermarket. Two Canadian women we had seen earlier were waiting in the shade.

We called the Hôtel-Restaurant L'Aube Nouvelle, our lodging for the night, and asked them to pick us up. Although the guidebook indicated that someone at L'Aube Nouvelle spoke English, the male voice at the other end of the cell phone only spoke French. I understood him to say that he would call a taxi to pick us up.

We waited in the ever-decreasing shade outside a Moroccan import shop. Bored and tired of waiting, we eventually went inside and examined the wares. I struck up a language-challenged conversation with a friendly French-Moroccan man who was carrying in merchandise from his truck.

After an hour I began to worry that I had misunderstood the man at L'Aube Nouvelle. The young man called the hotel for me and reassured me that the taxi was on its way. He offered to give us a ride but we regretfully declined.

At last the taxi driver arrived and transported us eight kilometers on a long winding road to L'Aube Nouvelle. As we got out of the car, Gary realized he'd left his hiking staff behind at Lauzerte, so I drove back with the taxi driver, hoping it would be still be there. It was. The young man at the import shop had safeguarded it for us. Another angel.

A Belgian couple ran the slightly seedy L'Aube Nouvelle, an eighteenth-century stone mansion that had been turned into a hotel fifty years ago. Our tiny room had been awkwardly retrofitted with a bathroom in one corner of the room, a shower, and no closets. We had a clothes rack instead. However, we did have a *gran lit*. The room was warm, for which I was grateful; I looked forward to snuggling with Gary not out of necessity but out of affection.

The brochure for the hotel stated it was "situated between vineyards and prairie … listen to Mozart while sitting in the Tuscan garden." So we did. We sat in the shade of the garden, drinking espresso and eating an assortment of cakes. Other pilgrims stopped to get something cold to drink, rest for a while, and then walk on. It had been a strange, hard day. Everyone we talked to at L'Aube Nouvelle agreed.

While we relaxed in the garden I pulled out my journal and ruminated about the pilgrimage.

Last year, we had had no expectations. When we began walking we told ourselves, "If we can walk one mile, or two, or ten, we will be happy." Whether it was cold and rainy or sunny and breezy, I didn't complain. Whatever it was was perfect. I was grateful to be alive.

This time, I find it hard to be thankful for feeling weak and sick, for scorching hot days, for chilly hotel rooms. I'm still grateful I'm alive, but I find it difficult to have the same simple, heartfelt gratitude for whatever life brings.

Although last year I experienced a deep, abiding faith that I was held in God's hands, this year I feel a deep well of uncertainty opening in front of my feet. Last year I chose to make positive meaning out of events—from having Honey Bunny come into my life, to finding an apple when I was hungry. I saw synchronicity as proof of the interconnected web of existence. This year I feel disconnected, isolated, and just plain tired.

I know I'm still part of the interconnected web—I'm still held in God's hands—how could I be and then not *be? The only thing different is the way I'm choosing to look at things—the lens I'm looking through. But I'm having a very hard time putting on a pair of rose-colored glasses.*

The garden tables filled up so I put away my journal. Soon we were chatting with fellow pilgrims—Belgian, Swiss, German, and French—about US politics, about the Chemin, and especially about the Camino in Spain. It was quite a change to be able to have a fluent conversation in English with someone other than Gary. How language-challenged we were in comparison to these other pilgrims, many of whom spoke two or three languages fluently.

One man wanted to know whether the dogs in Spain were as dangerous as people say. Usually no, Gary replied, but then he recounted one terrifying experience in 1997 when we had startled a shepherd's dozing dog. It rose up, bristled, bared its teeth, and threatened to attack us. Gary and I backed away slowly while Gary pointed his hiking staff at the dog's nose, ready to defend us if needed.

A petite, blond-haired, middle-aged German woman asked, "Do you have to be able to speak Spanish?"

I replied, "No more than you have to speak French to walk the Chemin. It's important to be able to ask for a place to stay or for food, but if you take along a Spanish phrase book and a friendly attitude, you should be fine. Besides, in a pinch you can usually find someone who speaks French or German or even English. And that someone may be a fellow pilgrim."

The German woman's husband, a tall, lanky fellow, informed the group that Paulo Coelho (a Brazilian author whose book *The Pilgrimage* has quite a cult following) was very popular in Germany, as was the Spanish Camino, but Germans weren't very familiar with the French route.

We went down to dinner, which was heavy and disappointing, particularly given the prices we were paying. As we conversed with fellow diners, we learned that the middle-aged Belgian couple at a nearby table was using La Pèlerine Randonnées Pédestres to book their journey and transport their luggage, the same organization we had encountered the previous year on the Chemin. I borrowed their brochure and examined the itinerary. Some of the stages were unrealistically long and in Spain they skipped many kilometers. I wrote down the names of their lodgings on the Chemin for the next few nights.

Friday, May 16, 2003. L'Aube Nouvelle to Moissac. 14 kilometers (8.7 miles).

After an indifferent breakfast we walked one and one-half kilometers to Durfort-Lacapelette to buy groceries for lunch. The *boulangerie* clerk had nautical tattoos on his thick hairy arms and a bulbous red nose. He snarled at our feeble attempts to speak French.

On a whim I pulled Honey Bunny out of my pack and pretended to have her say "Allo!" and wave at the man. He looked quite startled and then laughed uproariously. He was in such a good mood that I even bought some thin, chewy almond *tuilles*.

We started out walking alone, but the German couple from the previous evening saw us coming and waited. Showing us the

GR topo-guide, they said they planned to take an easier, alternative route. They invited us to join them and we eagerly accepted.

Irma and Wilhelm lived near Munich. They were about Gary's age, in their mid-60s. Irma was petite, blond-haired, and energetic, her short legs pumping along to keep up with her husband's long ones. Wilhelm was well over six feet tall, thin, grey haired, with a small, well-kept moustache. Both of them carried large daypacks; Transbagage was transporting their backpacks.

Wilhelm was a retired business executive. They had lived in Vermont thirty years ago when his business had transferred him to the US for a few years. It was there that Irma had learned English. They also spoke French. Soon Irma and I were walking side by side, sharing life stories; Gary and Wilhelm walked together, probably talking about careers.

A farmer invited us to pick cherries from his trees, the boughs practically bending down to meet our eager hands. The cherries were sweet and juicy—even better than the cherries at the Le Souleillou. Gratitude, gratitude, for the bounty of the fruit trees, for interesting companions.

Irma plied me with questions about pilgrimage: what I thought it was, why people went, what it meant. Making the pilgrimage to Santiago was part of her quest to find a meaningful connection to Catholicism—her birth religion but one she had turned away from. We discussed whether it was possible to participate in a religion when you disagreed with its stand on birth control, celibate male clergy, and so forth. It was a difficult dilemma.

From the moment she learned about the Chemin, Irma had wanted to go on the pilgrimage. It was approximately 2800 kilometers (1700 miles) from their home to Santiago de Compostela. Wilhelm had protested, "Not me! Do it yourself. You're nuts!" Of course he wouldn't have let her go without him, but it took some convincing at first. They had bicycled from Munich to Le Puy the previous year. Then they had walked from Le Puy to Conques. This time they had started walking from Le Puy and planned to reach Roncesvalles, the first stop on the Spanish side of the Pyrenees.

We shared a pleasant walk on country roads, over gently rolling terrain. Our companions set a faster pace than we did but we were able to keep up with them. The weather ranged from warm to cool, sunny to rainy, but unlike the previous days it was delightful. Walking and talking with new friends shifted my attention from the weather and my exhaustion. Perhaps my fatigue had been more a mental state than a physical one.

We reached Moissac, a town of 12,000, in what seemed like no time at all. Ever since I first saw photos of the abbey church in Moissac, I had longed to visit it. Moissac was an important pilgrimage stop in the Middle Ages and it still is. The sculptured portal is a masterpiece of Romanesque sculpture, as are the famous cloisters. My eagerness to visit the church gave me a taste of what medieval pilgrims might have felt, arriving footsore after walking for weeks or months, but filled with joyful anticipation.

The street in front of the Église de Saint-Pierre was lined with sidewalk cafés and our attention was diverted from food for the soul to food for the body. Suddenly we realized how hungry we were. Our first restaurant meal with Wilhelm and Irma provided an opportunity to see if we could agree on where to eat. We did.

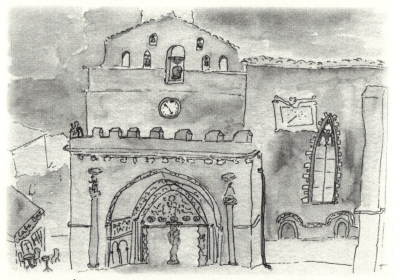

Église de Saint-Pierre (Saint-Pierre Church), Moissac

Wilhelm ordered an expensive *foie gras* dish; he was determined to savor as much of it as possible while in the heart of the *foie gras* region. I don't recall what I ordered since the church mesmerized me.

From the outdoor table where we sat, I could see the unusual scalloped door jambs of the church—a Moorish detail indicative of the artistic exchange between France and Spain. I admired from a distance the graceful, elongated figures carved on either side and on the column in the middle. Lunch could wait; I could wait no longer.

Leaving Gary and our new friends at the café, I walked over to the church. Miraculously, it had survived the ravages of war (Arabs, Normans, and Hungarians sacked it; Simon de Montfort pillaged the town in 1212 during the Albigensian Crusade; and during the Revolution the abbey-church was used as a gunpowder factory and soldiers' billet); modernization (it barely escaped being torn down to make way for the Toulouse-Bordeaux train line in the 1830s); and nature (Moissac was inundated by a massive flood of the Tarn in 1930, which destroyed much of the town). Fortunately the Église de Saint-Pierre has been designated a UNESCO World Patrimony site, which should assure its preservation for the immediate future.

The twelfth-century carvings I was admiring are remarkably well preserved, protected from the elements by the overhanging *clocher-porche* (bell-tower with porch), of which the scalloped south portal forms a part. A central column, called a trumeau†, divides the double entry doors, which are approximately twelve feet high. Over the doorway is a row of carved wheels; above that is the tympanum. Christ sits in judgment, holding the book of life in his left hand, his right raised in benediction. The ox, eagle, lion, and human symbols of the four Evangelists surround him.

An achingly beautiful prophet Jeremiah is sculpted on one side of the trumeau. His elongated body is draped in flowing stone robes that curve across his belly and fall in rhythmic folds against his legs. The sculptor delicately chiseled the curving tendrils that form Jeremiah's long beard, hair, and handlebar mustache. He stands on tiptoe, one leg crossed over the other, his head turning back to look behind him. His eyes look wistful. No wonder, given the centuries of mayhem and destruction he has witnessed from his vantage point in the middle of the scalloped portal.

There was much more to admire, but for the moment I was content to have seen the doorway up close. The church would still be there after lunch. I hurried back to our table and my excellent meal.

As soon as we finished eating we all strolled over to the church to admire the portal together and explore the interior. The church had been completely restored in the fifteenth and seventeenth centuries, and there were other, more recent renovations. The inside is painted in red and faded gold designs that seem artificial but are probably accurate, according to Irma, who studied art history. It is a mistake to assume that medieval churches were originally barren of colorful decoration—even the sculptures were often painted.

After making reservations to tour the cloisters later in the day, we set off to find the Hôtel-Restaurant du Luxembourg, located a distance from the old part of town. We agreed to meet in an hour, which gave us time to wash up and rest a bit.

As I lay on the bed I contemplated my inner turmoil. It had calmed for a little while at the church—it helped to be occupied—but it was now back in full force. In spite of the good weather and charming companions, my mood fluctuated. Suddenly a flash of sadness would sweep through me or I would feel irritated at Gary. I knew it had nothing to do with Gary. I was the one saddening myself; I was the one irritating myself. I was choosing to experience whatever was happening in a way that caused me discomfort and distress. But why?

Maybe I needed time alone. We'd been together 24/7 for months. Perhaps I was fretting about what I would do when we got back to the States. Gary was planning to do more genealogy research and massage training. What would I do? What did I *want* to do? I felt empty and tired, both physically and emotionally. I wanted to be of service in the world, but all I had done recently was recover from a cancer-related hysterectomy. I wanted to get on with my life, but how? Write a memoir about the Chemin?

Our counselor once said, "Watch out for the ego. It loves to create distance." And distance was what I felt every time I felt irritation at Gary. But why was I irritated? Because I felt at a loss about what to do with my life? Because I was worried about my health? My ankles were swollen: did that mean something? I was eating bread and sugar—and every day I woke up and did it again. With a sigh, I got up and washed my face.

We went back to the church with Wilhelm and Irma for the cloister tour. Unfortunately for me, it was in French. I tried to follow it for a while but soon gave up. According to the English-language guidebook, the cloisters include 116 columns and 76 capitals, 46 of which have carvings of Bible stories or lives of saints. We admired the double and single columns carved out of pink, green, and grey marble that alternate around the cloister perimeter. It served as a model for many other Romanesque cloisters.

Suddenly Wilhelm and Irma heard a familiar voice. It was an art history lecturer they knew from Munich. That chance meeting led us to discuss synchronicities. We shared stories, affirming our belief that more was at play than mere luck.

We ate dinner together at the hotel. The Belgian couple on the La Pèlerine program was staying there as well, as was a French couple we had seen at L'Aube Nouvelle. It was a pilgrims' mini-reunion. Dinner included an appetizer, a salad of vinaigrette-drenched beets and tomatoes, a choice of perch with white sauce and rice or beefsteak with new potatoes, and several different desserts, including fruit. I chose cherries. Even one healthy choice was a step in the right direction.

We discussed plans for the next day and agreed to travel together for a while. Irma made reservations at a *chambres d'hôtes* near

Saint-Vincent-l'Espinasse, making sure there was a room available for us and telling the proprietor that an American couple would be calling. It would have been more efficient for Irma to make reservations for all of us, but for whatever reasons, she preferred us to make our own.

Saturday, May 17, 2003. Moissac to Malause (12 kilometers [7.5 miles]), then by car to Saint-Vincent-l'Espinasse (5 kilometers [3 miles]) and Le Grenier du Levant.

That morning I did my meditation practice for the first time in two weeks, hoping it would help my low-level ennui and flashes of irritation. I told myself I simply hadn't had the time to do it before because we got up each morning, packed our bags, had breakfast, and started walking. But I knew that not having time was just an excuse. All that was required was a bit of willpower, a bit of determination. Not having time? What else did I have but time? And who was in charge of my time if not me?

We left Gary's backpack by the front door for Factage to pick up. It joined a pile of unlocked luggage and duffels. Learning to trust was a basic theme of my journey: trust that our possessions would be safe, trust that I would remain healthy—trust that no matter what happened it would not only be okay, it would be perfect. It was a lesson I had to learn one step at a time, one opportunity at a time. And then sometimes I had to start over again.

My learning curve reminded me again of a labyrinth walk: the meandering path turns this way and that, sometimes going in the opposite direction and heading away from the center, but it inevitably, eventually, reaches its goal.

We had a leisurely start with our new travel companions. First we went to the covered market in Moissac and strolled through the aisles, feasting our eyes and bellies on the attractive array of fruits and the impressive variety of *bio* (organic) products. We purchased a loaf of *bio* sesame bread and a bag of exquisitely sweet red cherries, several aged *cabécou* goat-cheese rounds, and homemade *bio* almond biscotti. We also bought a carton of bright red Mara de Bois wild strawberries that tasted like perfume. I use to think there were only two kinds of strawberries—ripe and unripe—but French markets offered half a dozen varieties, each with its particular fragrance, taste, shape, and use.

Wilhelm and Irma discovered a German vendor who owned a farm near Moissac, where he raised pigs and sheep and made German-style cured meats. While they purchased an assortment of sliced ham and sausages, Gary and I went to purchase a knee support for him. The pharmacy clerk measured his knee and selected the most effective elastic brace.

Then Irma and I searched for magnesium for muscle cramps. Irma spoke excellent French so I let her do the talking. (One of her intentions on the Chemin was to deepen her French fluency.) We bought regular magnesium tablets and *homeopathique* pellets, curious to see which was more effective.

On our way out of Moissac we took a minor detour to visit one of the oldest churches in France, the Église de Saint-Martin, also known as Saint-Ansbert. According to my guidebook it was built in the sixth or seventh century over the hypocaust (a plumbing system that uses hot air to heat from beneath the floor) of a Roman bath.

The entrance was locked, but someone had placed stepping stones against the door so you could look through a small window. I peered inside the church and barely made out some arches and possibly some frescoes. The rest of the interior appeared to be a wreck of crumbling stones. It was just one more decaying edifice in need of costly repair.

We had a choice of several routes, none of which was authentic since a major highway interrupted the historic Chemin. One route led up a ridge to impressive scenic views; the other was level. Without a moment's hesitation we took the low road south across a bridge over the river Tarn. We followed a towpath along the Canal des Deux Mers. Moissac lies on a lateral canal of the Garonne and on the Tarn, which flows into the Garonne about two miles below the town. Occasionally a long narrow canal boat wended its way up the canal, pausing at the locks.

"I've always thought that would be a nice way to take a vacation." I commented.

"Well," Irma replied, "We have friends who rented one for a vacation, and they said it was pretty boring. All they saw was the canal."

I looked at the relative height of the canal and the boat. She was right.

Our path was flat and shaded, the weather mild, and the conversation engrossing. The kilometers sped by. At one point we crossed the Garonne and found a place to sit by the side of the canal. We shared the cheese, meat, bread, and fruit we had purchased that morning. Convivial exchanges continued about who we were, our children, our personal histories. It was that halcyon time of "getting to know you, getting to know all about you…."—though it wasn't "all," of course, since we present edited versions of our life stories, both to ourselves and to others.

Irma saw Honey Bunny peeking out of my fanny pack. Despite my misgivings about letting Honey Bunny out of the bag, I had decided not to care what other people thought.

"Who is this?" Irma asked, her eyes open wide.

I handed Honey Bunny to Irma—or rather, she leapt from my hands into Irma's arms. With a contented smile Irma tucked the plush bunny under the waistband of her fanny pack. She had no hesitation about people seeing her with a "fuzzy kid." As we walked I explained about Honey Bunny and her part in my story—the first notable example of synchronicity on my journey through cancer. Irma nodded appreciatively and patted her on the head. Her long ears flopped forward, covering her bright brown eyes.

"She really likes to see where she's going," I said gently.

Irma rearranged her ears immediately.

By early afternoon the day had turned uncomfortably hot, but we had walked so quickly, energized by conversation and the Webers' faster pace, that we had already reached Malause. The proprietor of Le Grenier du Levant had told us to call from Malause for a ride. Still full of energy, Wilhelm wanted to walk the five kilometers to the B&B, which was located outside of Saint-Vincent-l'Espinasse. None of our maps showed the village, however, since it was off the GR. Regretfully Wilhelm agreed to take the ride.

Irma called Le Grenier on her cell phone and soon Monsieur Granier whisked us away to the *chambres et table d'hôte/gîte d'étape*, another multi-purpose establishment.

Le Grenier du Levant boasted several picturesque stone buildings, their exterior walls attractively draped with vines and flowers. Madame Annie greeted us when we arrived.

Despite her warm welcome, all was not as we expected. Although we had reserved two rooms, Madame Annie explained that several guests had decided to stay longer, so she had made different arrangements for us. Far from the GR and other accommodations, we had no choice but to agree.

We followed her into the main building, its cheery living room filled with rustic bric-a-brac. Annie led us up a spiral staircase to the second level and showed us our accommodations for the night: a bed on the open landing at the top of the stairs and a separate bedroom with a bathroom and toilet. The toilet was in a tiny cubicle just inside the bedroom.

We wouldn't mind sharing the toilet, would we? Annie asked rhetorically. We looked at each other a bit hesitantly but agreed. Wilhelm and Irma were given the bedroom, which had two beds, since that is what they had reserved; Gary and I got the landing since we had wanted to sleep together. We soon learned that the purported bed was a decrepit sleeper-sofa with an inadequate mattress and a footboard, which made it too short for Gary. He would have to sleep diagonally and I would have to sleep in whatever space was left.

Seeing our unhappy faces, Annie explained that no other arrangements were possible. At least we had a place to stay, I told
myself. Gratitude, gratitude.

Annie gave Gary and me towels and showed us the spacious
communal shower and bathroom on the main level, used by those
staying in the *gîte* accommodations. Since no one was there, we
would have the facilities to ourselves.

Annie was the epitome of graciousness while she deftly substituted marginal sleeping accommodations for what we had reserved.
I presumed that we would pay less.

When Annie learned that I spoke Spanish, she was delighted.
Although she had spent little time in Spain, she had a great affinity
for the language. Suddenly the language of choice was Spanish. I
enjoyed having an actual conversation with a French person instead
of stumbling along in marginal French. Neither Irma nor Wilhelm
spoke Spanish, and although Gary understood some of the conversation, it became an exchange between Madame and me.

Annie explained that large groups would come to Le Grenier
for lunch or dinner, for an ice cream and soda break during a long
day-hike, and to use the bathrooms. Since she was a practical businesswoman, she charged for the use of the facilities.

We went back outside to relax in the garden with Monsieur and
Madame Termes, two of the Graniers' friends. They had brought
samples of Armagnac (the local brandy) from their Domaine de la
Meigne in Manciet, located near the Chemin. Not only were we in
the land of *foie gras*, prunes, and walnuts, we were also in the land
of Armagnac, a region defined in 1909 as an AOC† (Appellation
d'Origine Contrôlée). Monsieur Termes offered us a sample of 1981
Armagnac. It was powerful stuff.

With expressive gestures that made translation unnecessary,
Louis showed us how to drink Armagnac. "First you have to appreciate the bouquet." He sniffed it. "Ahhh. Then you swirl it in your
mouth. Wait a few moments and it will open up."

We imitated him. The fragrance and the flavor did indeed expand.

He then told us a long complex story about the difference between Armagnac and Cognac. The gist was that Armagnac is "closer to the earth," less refined, not blended, and therefore more authentic—unlike the more pretentious Cognac, produced in another region of France.

Annie handed me a brochure, "Armagnac: The Best Brandy in the World." I learned that Armagnac is famous not only for its taste but also for its therapeutic properties. Particular grape varieties are distilled, aged in oak casks, and then transferred to glass containers. This *eau de vie* (literally, "water of life") dates back to the twelfth century.

The Romans introduced the grapevine to France, then the Arabians brought the alembic (a kind of pot still). Finally, the Celts (I think the author meant the French) developed the use of oak casks— "a divine union that could only have occurred in Gascony," according to the author. Because Armagnac is produced from a single distillation and at relatively low temperatures, it has more fruitiness and better balance than Cognac, its more famous and "refined"—and prolific—neighbor. (The rivalry between the two was quite apparent.) In addition, Armagnac is aged up to forty years in black oak casks, which apparently matures it more rapidly and gives it additional flavors. Only about 40% of Armagnac leaves Gascony and only one-fifth of the remainder leaves France.

We sat in the sun sniffing, smelling, and swirling samples of the fiery liquid. Not surprisingly, we learned that little sample bottles of 1982 Armagnac were for sale, and also not surprisingly, we bought at a price decreed by Annie.

I had been missing my son so I excused myself from the group and walked to the back of the garden to call Jesse on my cell phone. Standing alone in the back of the garden I felt overwhelmed with sadness and burst into tears. Maybe I was just tired of company and needed some time alone, even if only to cry. But there was no time or place to be alone except for a few moments in the back of someone's garden. Drying my eyes, I walked back to the group.

Sitting together in the garden, mellow from Armagnac, Gary and I agreed to walk with Irma and Wilhelm for the next four or five days, until we reached Condom. Condom was an arbitrary stopping place, but that was as far as Gary wanted to go.

Sometimes I thought, "I want to keep walking with Irma and Wilhelm all the way to Saint-Jean-Pied-de-Port! Let's *finish* this pilgrimage of gratitude!" But the next moment I would think, "I'm tired; I don't have much energy; I don't want to walk *anywhere.*"

It wasn't external circumstances that mattered but rather my reactions to them. It wasn't what happened to me but how I made meaning of it. After all, we were surrounded by fragrant flowers, drinking rare local brandy, eating delicious cherries, basking in the balmy sunlit afternoon, sharing animated conversations with interesting companions—and yet I depressed myself.

"Happiness isn't out there, it's within," I thought to myself. Only it wasn't within. And if it wasn't within, where was it?

Gary and I excused ourselves from the group and strolled down the country lane to see Annie's exotic fowl collection. At last I shared my feelings with Gary.

"I feel okay but then I get a wave of sadness. I think maybe it began after our conversation about what we'd do with our lives back in Boulder. You told me your plans but I didn't have any. Maybe I'm envious because you are a 'useful' human being while all I'm doing is recovering from cancer."

I started to weep and he held me close, stroking my hair. Calmly, he said, "I've seen you like this before. It's because you aren't writing."

I looked at him in surprise. He was right. Now I remembered. Whenever I started wondering about my purpose in life it was because I wasn't doing it: I wasn't writing. I used to think that when I got depressed, writing would bring me out of it, but Gary had observed during our ten years together that the reality was actually the reverse. I needed to be expressing myself creatively. Just remembering this helped my inner tension start to dissolve.

Gratitude, gratitude, for a partner who knew me better than I knew myself. Hand in hand, we strolled back to the garden.

Dinner was served at the big table in the main room. There were the four of us, Annie and husband, and five other guests and friends. Annie presented us with a mixed plate of pâté and a salad of dry, overcooked duck wing *confit*, local prunes, raisins, pine nuts, and tomatoes. Cheese was also served, but only after I complained in Spanish, "What, no cheese?"

In response, Annie went back into the kitchen and returned a short time later with a tray. "The cheese heard you call for it!" she said jokingly.

Despite the mediocre dinner, we had an enjoyable evening drinking and talking. The French sang songs and we joined in when we could. Gary and I sang a few songs in English, and Irma and Wilhelm sang a German walking song. As I listened to the joyful sounds I realized that in the US, informal a-capella group singing was a rare occurrence.

Eventually we excused ourselves and climbed into our very exposed bed at the top of the stairs. We tried to sleep but it was a difficult because of the revelry going on directly below us.

Sunday, May 18, 2003. Saint-Vincent-l'Espinasse to Miradoux. 28 kilometers (17 miles), but we walked only 24 (15 miles). We gave up in Flamarens and got a ride to Miradoux.

Breakfast was sparse: hot drinks and yesterday's bread with homemade jams. When Annie totaled up our bill, it came to more than the price of Irma and Wilhelm's room. How could that be, I protested! After all, we had practically slept in public and had not had a private bathroom. Then she suddenly realized she had added something twice (perhaps the charge for the sheets and towels, which we had thought were included with the bed) and deducted it. I felt taken advantage of but I didn't know how to say that in French or in Spanish.

Annie gave us directions to rejoin the GR 65 somewhat further down the road. Putting the financial unpleasantness behind us, we set off walking down the flat country road on a warm Sunday morning. Talking animatedly we marched along under the cloudless blue sky. Then Irma realized she had lost the damp t-shirt she had fastened on her daypack. Wilhelm volunteered to walk back to find it. He returned with Annie, who had given him a lift.

As Annie drove away, I confided to Irma, "I'm really unhappy about how much we were charged. We would have paid more than you did but I objected."

She commiserated.

"The calculations went by so fast," I continued, "that I couldn't keep track of what happened. I suppose I should have asked in advance about the charges, but Madame seemed so friendly."

"You have to be careful with French innkeepers. When I make reservations, sometimes the proprietor will tell me we will have a bathroom but it turns out it's not private. I have learned to be very precise, but sometimes I forget to write down the room number I have been promised and I am sure I get a different room."

Soon the day became quite hot and there wasn't much shade. Winded and sweating we struggled up a trail that zigzagged to the top of a hill and past a renovated *lavoir* (communal laundry washhouse with running water and stone basins) to the town of Auvillar, whose name comes from the Latin for "high house." At one time Auvillar was fortified and collected tolls for passage on the Garonne, but over the years it has faded in importance. Like so many towns in the region, it too suffered during the Cathar crusade, the Hundred Years' War, and the Wars of Religion.

But that day Auvillar bustled with activity. We had arrived during the "Day of Wood," a fair celebrating traditional crafts such as wood turning and sabot making. The event took place in and around the circular *halle†*, a medieval covered market that was rebuilt in the 1800s. The *halle* features Tuscan columns, a tile roof, and medieval grain measures, and is in the center of an arcaded square surrounded by red brick and half-timbered buildings. We wandered around admiring the folkloric revival—or perhaps it wasn't a revival; perhaps people had never stopped producing these crafts—and buying fruit at a market stand.

I took a photo of Wilhelm and Irma standing under a small statue of Saint Jacques on the side of a building. Two plastic grocery bags filled with purchases swung from the front straps of Wilhelm's daypack; Honey Bunny's legs dangled below the belt of Irma's fanny pack.

A brochure touted Auvillar as an active tourism center. It boasts a folk art museum; the Église de Saint-Pierre, originally a twelfth-century Benedictine monastery, later restored; a promenade on the site of the former viscount's castle; and a chapel dedicated to Saint Catherine, patron saint of sailors, apparently important because the Garonne River flows through the valley. Nearby sites of interest include Moissac with its summer jazz festival, various churches and castles, and the nuclear power plant of Golfech. Listing a nuclear power plant as a tourist attraction seemed a bit of a stretch.

We left town on the rue de l'Horloge, named after its seventeenth-century clock tower. When we reached the tiny village of Bardigues, it was in the midst of a flea market, but everyone wanted to sell and nobody wanted to buy. We wandered through town until we came to a sheltered picnic area behind the local school, where we spread out our lunch. A French family came in, saw us occupying the benches, and looked annoyed at our intrusion. The little boy came up to us, however, and said proudly, "This is my school." We thanked him for telling us.

After lunch we started back on the Chemin. What had begun as a balmy day had now become so hot I thought I'd faint. My thermometer indicated the high 90's F. We kept walking—what else could we do?—while I fought off heat exhaustion. During our 1997 pilgrimage I had nearly collapsed from the heat on the Spanish Meseta, and Gary had had to lure me step by step with juicy orange sections. This time we had no oranges and the alternative enticement, chocolate bars, had melted into a sticky mess.

At last we reached the village of Saint-Antoine, which took its name from the Catholic Order of Antonins. They had established a hospital in the twelfth century for people suffering from ergotism ("Saint Anthony's Fire"), so-named because it produced excruciating burning sensations in the extremities. Prevalent during the Middle Ages, people contracted it by consuming cereal grains contaminated by ergot fungus. Ergotism resulted in mental confusion, convulsions, hallucinations, and culminated in a dry gangrenous condition of hands and feet.

I was grateful I didn't have Saint Anthony's Fire but I was still in need of healing. We stumbled through town to the *gîte d'étape*, located in an old stone building, and I collapsed on a bench shaded by a large leafy tree. The woman in charge was a French version of a Spanish *hospitalera*, the well-trained host at a Spanish pilgrims' hostel. Marie told me to put cold water on my neck, hair, and face to lower my body temperature, and she gave me a towel to soak in the sink. I drenched myself and felt a little better. Although the Antonins were long gone, their tradition of healing lived on.

While we sat in the shade waiting for me to recover, several middle-aged men struggled into the *gîte*, loaded down with heavy backpacks. Soon one came back outside and washed his clothes in a bucket. I dowsed myself with water again.

While we waited for the day to cool down, we drank water and soft drinks and talked with an amiable dark-haired young woman from the south of Spain. For some reason, she started talking to me about the tau (the T-shaped cross) and gave me a brochure that included information about it and the local church.

I already knew something about the cross, having purchased one at a church outside of Castrojeríz, on the Spanish Camino. The tau is associated with the Antonins, Saint Francis of Assisi (who supposedly walked to Santiago), and the Templars. According to one story, Saint Francis told his followers that when they put on their monastic robes and stretched out their arms, they resembled a living, walking crucifix—thus they (and the tau, which resembled their pose) were a constant reminder of Christ's death and resurrection. In medieval times the tau was used as an amulet against the plague.

The brochure failed, however, to mention the tau's lengthy pre-Christian history. It was a symbol of the Roman god Mithras, the

Greek Attis, and their Sumerian forerunner Tammuz, solar god and consort of the goddess Ishtar. Tammuz' death and resurrection were celebrated every spring; marking one's forehead with a tau of ashes (as in Ash Wednesday rites) originated in Tammuz' rituals.

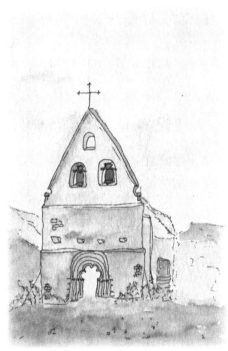

Saint-Antoine

Bored with just sitting, tired of talking, but not ready to face the uncertainties of the Chemin, we visited the small village church. It was cool and quiet. Its walls and domed ceiling were painted bright yellow and green, and rows of gold and colored medallions adorned the walls. We sat in comfortable stillness for a while, and then we introduced Wilhelm and Irma to our practice of singing "Ultreya" in churches.

Perhaps it was the soothing atmosphere inside the church or simply the hour or two we had rested, but I felt well enough to continue. Marie assured us that the remaining eight kilometers to Miradoux were shady and flat. She was wrong.

Even the occasional breeze failed to mitigate the blasting heat, now around 100° F. I poured more water on my head and back. Gary fed me sections of the orange we had bought at the *gite*. I called on willpower; I begged for Saint James's help as I staggered along on what seemed like an interminable journey.

Finally we reached Flamarens, a small village with a castle. We had walked twenty-four kilometers, much of it under the broiling sun. I could go no further. Gary used our cell phone to call the *chambres d'hôtes* in Miradoux and our hostess, Madame Lanusse-Cazalé, said she would fetch us.

Wilhelm and Irma were determined to continue walking. They wanted to walk all of the Chemin, every step of the way, and the heat didn't bother them as much as it did me. They would hitchhike if necessary but they didn't want to arrange in advance for a ride: that wasn't their idea of pilgrimage.

We said goodbye and they bravely trudged out of town. We followed very slowly, staying close to the walls of buildings to take advantage of a shrinking strip of shade.

A few minutes later a van drove up, lights flashing. Much to our surprise, Madame already had two passengers. She had mistakenly stopped for Wilhelm and Irma, thinking they were we, and they had not refused her offer. Apparently they considered her intercession divine, and perhaps it was. She drove three and one-half kilometers to Miradoux on a road that shimmered with the heat.

Madame was our angel of the day, as was the *hospitalera* at the *gîte*. I had been forgetting to acknowledge the day's angels, both known and unknown. Sinking into my disgruntled funk I had failed to hear the flapping of invisible wings.

Madame welcomed us into her tastefully restored *chambres d'hôtes*. Located across from the historic *halle* and next to the church, the elegant *chambres d'hôtes* had been featured in a glossy regional tourism magazine. We entered into a deliciously cool refuge. In a moment, we moved from agony to bliss.

Gilt-framed oil paintings hung throughout the house, furnished with antiques and Oriental rugs purchased at estate sales. After showing us the main floor, Madame led us up a large curving staircase to our accommodations. She gave each of us a two-room suite. Ours featured high ceilings, elegantly carved plaster over a marble fireplace, tile floors covered with Oriental rugs, and an onyx chandelier. The bed was dressed in high-count embroidered linens and piles of pillows. Our huge bathroom had marble counters, an electric towel heater attached to one wall, "Orient Express"-style faucets, and a large ceramic sink. I ran over to Wilhelm and Irma's suite to see it; it was equally attractive.

I asked Irma if she wanted me to take Honey Bunny back for the evening.

"No, I want Honey Bunny to stay with us."

"She sleeps in bed with us, you know," I said.

"I don't know about *that*, but she'll stay with us," she said, promptly putting Honey Bunny on a chair next to the bed.

Madame offered us cookies and tea in the garden terrace behind the house and explained that she had made dinner reservations for us at the Restaurant L'Etape, a few blocks away. The shady garden overflowed with roses, yellow bell-like flowers, white drooping flowers—I didn't know their names but they were lovely. Now I understood why the Arabic word for paradise is the same as the Arabic word for garden.

The garden view looked out over gently rolling hills and fields dotted with groves of trees, stretching into the distance. We could see where we would be walking for the next few days.

I washed, relaxed, and reveled in the opulence of our surroundings, rapidly recovering from my heat exhaustion. The night before Gary and I had slept on an uncomfortable sleeper-sofa on an open landing and shared Wilhelm and Irma's tiny toilet stall; tonight we would sleep in luxury.

We walked over to the Restaurant L'Etape, which reminded me of a typical Spanish bar, filled with cigarette smoke and loud conversations. The waitress was rather huffy at first. We learned, once she became friendlier, that L'Etape also rented rooms to travelers, so it viewed Madame as competition. The restaurant provided meals for their guests, which Madame didn't—but she expected L'Etape to do so. And she hadn't bothered to make the reservation until very late. Ah, the politics of tourism.

Paradoxically, the pungent cigarette smoke and strident voices made us feel nostalgic, so we started telling Wilhelm and Irma more about the Spanish Camino. They planned to walk it either that fall or the following spring and wanted to prepare for what lay ahead.

"How can we transport our luggage? Is there baggage transfer?" Irma asked.

I shook my head. "There wasn't in 1997, when we last walked the Camino."

"Surely there is a need?"

"Less than you might think," Gary replied. "The French Chemin follows the GR 65, and hikers often use baggage transfer services. The Spanish Camino is more religious or spiritual, and many pilgrims think that they should carry their own packs—perhaps because they feel it's more authentic or traditional, even though medieval pilgrims didn't carry backpacks. There are all kinds of metaphors that go along with it, like letting go of unnecessary stuff, carrying only what you need, learning how much you can do without."

I told Irma and Wilhelm that near the end of our 1997 pilgrimage, I had become ill and my doctor friend in Saint-Jean-Pied-de-Port told me I couldn't continue to walk and carry a pack. Since I was determined to finish the Camino, I arranged for a taxi driver to transport my backpack. The response I received from fellow pilgrims abruptly changed from friendly inclusiveness ("Buen Camino," they would say when I carried my backpack) to censorious glances and disapproving silence. Since I too had once thought that walkers without backpacks weren't "real" pilgrims, this gave me the opportunity to learn humility—and to learn not to be so judgmental.

Sitting in the restaurant in Miradoux with new pilgrim friends I was filled with gratitude. We had walked twenty-four kilometers in blazing heat with very little shade. I had survived relatively unscathed—demonstrating once again that, although there is an external reality of heat or pain or thirst, what really matters is the significance we give it, not the event itself.

Monday, May 19, 2003. Miradoux to Lectoure. 15 kilometers (9+ miles).

Madame provided an elegant breakfast in the terrace garden, complete with homemade cookies, breads, preserves, sugar-powdered beignets, yogurt, and fruit. Irma brought Honey Bunny down to breakfast.

"So tell me, did she sleep in your bed?" I teased.

"Oh no," Irma replied, looking a little scandalized. "She sat on the chair next to us."

Honey Bunny was no longer just "our" mascot; she was Irma and Wilhelm's as well.

We raved about the house to Madame and, encouraged by our response, she showed us a photo album of what the place had looked like ten years earlier. The previous owner, an eighty-year-old woman, had lived by herself for years, and the place had literally fallen down around her. There were holes in the ceiling and no heat or hot water, but Madame and her husband had seen the wonderful structural features buried beneath debris: the terracotta floor tiles, marble fireplaces, and carved plaster trim that had survived the gradual decay of the rest of the house. They had spent two years restoring it, doing the work themselves with the help of family and friends.

A bit sad to leave our comfortable accommodations, we said goodbye. On the way out of town we bought bread, *saucisson de canard* (dried duck sausage), and cheese. We walked through picture-postcard scenery of rolling hills, past a ruined château and scattered farmhouses with creamy stone walls and red tile roofs. Dark-green cypresses thrust into the sky. Fields of grain and garlic—the heads looking like little white turbans perched on top of green stems—and of leeks and green beans stretched out on either side of the Chemin. We picked some of the beans, so sweet and fresh that we ate them raw. Sunflowers were just beginning to come up. Soon they would fill the fields, turning their heads with the sun. No wonder they were called *girasol* in Spanish.

Irma asked whether I was Jewish. I had told her that I had gone to seminary to become a Unitarian-Universalist minister, and I'd told Wilhelm that my ancestors were Jewish. Obviously, Wilhelm and Irma shared our conversations just as Gary and I shared theirs.

Irma said, "My son had a Jewish girlfriend for a number of years. Max paid no attention to her religion. She was raised in Israel and then moved with her family to Germany. We were very sad when they broke up. But I don't understand your situation. Aren't you Jewish if your mother was?"

"Having a Jewish mother" was the deciding factor in Nazi Germany, an excuse for murdering secular Jews, Jews who had converted to Christianity, even people whose long-forgotten, distant relatives were Jews. This definition affected me directly, since my ancestors on both sides were Russian Jews. My father always considered himself Jewish, even though, after reading Marx and Freud in college, he no longer believed in any religion. Although my mother's relatives were Jewish, she vehemently denied that *she* was because she had been raised in the Chicago Ethical Cultural Society. I, in turn, was raised as a Unitarian-Universalist; all I knew about Judaism was that it could get you killed.

I told Irma, "It makes no sense to me that someone is Jewish just because their mother or their great-grandmother was. Judaism is a practice, maybe an ethnicity—but it's not a genetic code, even though intermarriage for centuries has limited the gene pool. Eastern European Jews share certain genetic similarities, and there are some specific genetic markers for the Cohen lineage—but many Jews share the same genetic stock as other Semites, including Arabs. And many have Chinese, Indian, Spanish, Ethiopian, indigenous or other ancestry as well, depending on where they fled in the Diaspora or who raped the women during persecutions."

Irma nodded thoughtfully.

Suddenly I had a new insight. Maybe "having a Jewish mother" really referred to the fact that children learned to be Jewish by observing what their mothers did at home: dietary observances, lighting candles, Friday night prayers and celebrating Shabbat. Practices continued the religion, not some putative bloodline. But my insight went counter to Israeli repatriation law, a New York Jewish religious court's decision—and the Nazis.

Was I Jewish? The answer depended on what one meant by "being Jewish": Genetics? Religious beliefs? Religious observances? Family upbringing? Ethnic patterns of food and interaction? All I knew was that I had been taught to honor all world religions, not to favor one. And the proof of it was that I was walking an ancient Christian pilgrimage route, singing "Ultreya," putting rocks on roadside crucifixes, and occasionally practicing Sufi meditations.

By early afternoon the hot, sunny day had clouded over and turned chilly. Just before a downpour hit, we struggled up a high ridge to Lectoure, one of the oldest towns in the Gers region, a *département†* in the heart of Gascony. D'Artagnan and Cyrano de Bergerac came from the Gers, as do Armagnac and *foie gras*.

Two Dutch pilgrims scurried for shelter. We waved at each other as we hurried off in different directions. Our accommodations were two apartments offered through Clés-Vacance (Key-Vacation), located in what appeared to be a medieval building complete with half-timbered construction.

Looking concerned, our landlord, a small, energetic dark-haired man, said, "I'm sorry to tell you that although Monsieur and Madame White's bags arrived, the Webers' bags aren't here!"

Irma was quite perturbed, but then Jules laughed and pulled their backpacks out of hiding. He was quite friendly, just a bit of a trickster. He showed us the neighboring apartment where he and his wife lived and offered to dry our laundry. We did several loads of laundry by hand and then brought them to him.

"Oh," he exclaimed, looking at our travel-worn clothes, "I'll take your fancy clothes and sell them at the market!"

This time, we all laughed.

Braving the wind and rain we ran over to the nearby church with its huge tower. The former Cathédrale des Saint-Gervais-et-Saint-Protais was built in 1325 on the site of a pagan sanctuary. The church was heavily rebuilt at some time and includes a bas relief of crossed crosiers, two on each side, with a bishop's miter at their intersection. Collette and Danielle would have known what that meant, but we didn't. The four of us sang "Ultreya" in the empty church, listening to the sound reverberate against the stone walls.

Lectoure's attractions include a mineral museum, an archeological museum—the Gers town was originally Gallo-Roman—and a thermal spa specializing in rheumatic afflictions, but the weather was too disagreeable to continue exploring. Instead, we dashed back to our spacious apartments and recuperated.

That evening we dined at La Rose du Chat, a tiny, six-table restaurant located at the end of a steep lane leading down to the city walls. We sat next to two ladies we had first met at Marcilhac-sur-Célé and greeted each other, enjoying being part of an extended pilgrim community.

We ordered the restaurant's premier assortment of *foie gras*: one dish arrived flamed in Armagnac; one was flavored with cardamom. The fragrant *foie gras* melted like butter in our mouths, tantalizing our taste buds with hints of apple and exotic spices. We tried the local aperitif, Floc de Gascogne ("flower" of Gascogne, a fortified rosé or white wine), and later, back in our apartment, we opened our little 1982 Armagnac bottles.

Made mellow by dinner and drink, we shared stories about how we had encountered our respective partners. Gary and I both attended the Unitarian Universalist Fellowship in Ames, Iowa, but we got to know each other at a weekly satsang ceremony for Mata Amritanandamayi, a Hindu saint known as the "hugging saint," who embodies unconditional love. Eventually we started doing Sufi practices together and were married in a Universal Worship Service, which honors all religious traditions on the same altar. Our religious eclecticism puzzled Irma and Wilhelm, but I was grateful for all that Gary and I shared.

Tuesday, May 20, 2003. Lectoure to La Romieu. 19 kilometers (12 miles). Gary walked but I hitched a ride with Factage.

I woke up with "the runs," feeling very weak. Too much *foie gras*? The reason didn't matter; I couldn't walk. We called Factage's emergency number, and the man who answered cheerfully agreed to pick me up with the baggage.

After a wistful goodbye to Irma, Wilhelm, and Gary, I waited in the dimly lit hallway for Factage. Eventually a slightly built man smelling of cigarettes came through the front door, swung our backpack on his shoulders, and motioned to me to follow. He slung the bag in the trunk of a slightly rusted Citroen and invited me to sit on the passenger's side.

As he drove we conversed in a mixture of fractured French and English. He explained—at least I think he did—that Factage was a group of five friends, each with his own car, who each worked approximately one day per week picking up bags and people on the Chemin. Unlike the more upscale Transbagage with its corporate vans, their operation was decidedly homegrown. Factage prided itself on personal service and planned to expand into Spain the following year. I made a mental note to tell Wilhelm and Irma about this development.

We drove over gently curving hills and through picturesque hamlets until we reached the Domaine de Pellecahus, our *chambres d'hôtes*, located a kilometer before La Romieu. The Domaine consisted of two separate guesthouses, the owners' small cottage, a cherry orchard, a large, tree-shaded pond, and several pet ducks. Trap horses were being put through their paces on the horse track next door.

Christine came out to greet me, surprised at my early arrival, and informed me that our room wasn't ready yet. When I explained I was sick, she led me to the attractive ground-level apartment that she and Brigitte were cleaning. I collapsed on the sofa in the living room, teary-eyed with gratitude.

Christine soon returned and took me to our *gîte,* a tastefully redone two-story building. The Webers would be staying next door. Downstairs was a multi-purpose room that included a dining table, sofa, kitchen, and washing machine. Upstairs were two bedrooms and a high-tech shower, complete with nozzles that sprayed your entire body. The room was warm; they had turned on the electric heat.

I was indeed held in God's hands—and taken care of by angels. I knew that Santiago was walking beside me, even if I couldn't see him and even if I wasn't walking. Lying down on the comfortable bed, I fell asleep.

When I awoke the weather had changed. It was cooler outside and raining occasionally. Christine brought me a picnic lunch of *bio* bread, ham, and cheese. Much to my surprise, I suddenly felt hungry.

My depression and irritation had lightened, but they were still there. Gary had told me I just needed to start writing again, but that was hard on the Chemin. I had wondered whether having private time would help. Now, because I was sick, I had been transported to a comfortable location where I would have an entire day by myself, even if I did spend part of it sleeping. My needs were being met. It was perfect. It always is, but sometimes it's harder to realize than other times.

I started to catch up on my journal.

> *Each day is so full that what happened two days ago seems like a month past; simultaneously, everything has begun to blur together.*
>
> *Irma brought a songbook with religious songs. Gary already knew many of the melodies; now he has the words. We've been lighting candles in churches and singing "Ultreya." The acoustics in the churches enhance the music. Yesterday after singing "Ultreya" in the cathedral in Lectoure, the space felt different. It felt vibrantly alive. Somehow our singing brought energy to the stones, the space, the building—energy that continued to reverberate after it was no longer audible.*

Suddenly exhausted, I fell back to sleep.

Gary and the Webers arrived mid-afternoon. They were wet and weary, and Irma felt a little sick to her stomach. But they immediately perked up when they saw the delightful accommodations.

Gary dried off, changed clothes, and rested for a while on the commodious sofa. Then we talked about our plans. Earlier he had been determined to stop at Condom. Now he was willing to continue with Irma and Wilhelm to Roncesvalles, the first stopping place on the Spanish side of the Pyrenees. I was delighted and gave him a warm hug and lots of kisses.

Crossing the Pyrenees had always been an enormous challenge for me, and one I had yet to overcome. When I made the pilgrimage in 1982, Michael and I left Saint-Jean-Pied-de-Port on the hottest day of the summer, unaware of how difficult the twenty-plus-kilometer climb would be. We got lost in the mountains en route to Roncesvalles, and I collapsed with heat exhaustion, intestinal flu, and low blood sugar.

Fortunately, Alan and Malou Anderson, an English-speaking Basque doctor and his wife, found us by the side of the road and drove us back to their home in Saint-Jean. They insisted that we stay with them until I recovered. Thanks to their ministrations I felt better within a few days. Then they drove us back up the mountain and walked with us part-way over the pass, carrying my backpack. Remembering that day, I realized that I had been held in God's hands even then.

Fifteen years later Alan and Malou offered to drive Gary and me up to the pass to start our pilgrimage. We accepted with gratitude, knowing how tough that day would have been, but I had always felt we had missed something by not walking over the Pyrenees. Now at last we would.

Now that we were going to continue over the Pyrenees, I felt our journey transform itself into a pilgrimage. We were not simply stopping at a randomly selected spot; instead, we would keep going to the finish. Of course, the only *real* end was Santiago—or perhaps Finisterre—but who knows? Maybe we would be inspired to continue on past Roncesvalles. At the very least, climbing through the Pyrenees would complete a part of the journey that I had never finished.

Gary and I suggested to the Webers that we spend another day at the Domaine. Although Wilhelm wanted to keep going, Irma really needed to recuperate. We pointed out that even medieval pilgrims occasionally rested a day or two in the same place. At last Wilhelm agreed.

Relieved, Gary and I went to ask Christine if we could stay another day. She checked the schedule and said, "You are lucky. I have room tomorrow but after that, no. A large group has reserved the *gîte*."

We were held in God's hands. I had to laugh at myself: I felt like I was reciting a mantra.

In the late afternoon Christine drove us a few kilometers to La Romieu. The town was on the medieval pilgrimage road to Compostela—the same route followed by modern pilgrims. La Romieu's name derived from the Gascon *roumiou*, a kind of pilgrim. It sounded similar to the Spanish *romero*, which originally referred to pilgrims going to Rome but later expanded to include other pilgrims.

I could see the large octagonal tower and the high walls of the church from nearly a kilometer away. The eight-sided tower resembles a gigantic gear with protruding teeth. In 1998 UNESCO classified the fourteenth-century gothic ensemble (cloister, tower, and church) as a world patrimony site.

Cardinal Arnaud d'Aux sponsored the original construction. A native of the area, he presided over the trial of the Knights Templar in 1307. He was also a friend and cousin of Clement V, the Gascon who moved the papacy from Rome to Avignon and began what the Italians referred to as the Babylonian Captivity of the papacy.

Although we seemed to be in the middle of nowhere, 700 years ago La Romieu was somewhere indeed.

Some churches we had visited felt empty and abandoned, but this one was well cared for—and very well preserved. We lit candles of gratitude for our journey, candles of healing for friends, candles of love for our children. Then we sang "Ultreya," our voices filling the chapel and soaring overhead.

Intriguing fourteenth-century frescoes cover the sacristy, located on the ground floor of the larger tower. Rows of faded medallions are painted on the walls and unusual esoteric paintings, including black angels with trumpets, decorate the octagonal dome. They reminded me of medieval frescoes in Spain and in Turkey. Since stonemasons and builders traveled widely at that time, presumably the artists did too.

Gary, Wilhelm, and Irma climbed up the east tower and sang "Ultreya" from high above the church. The sound echoed into the nave and I responded back.

We were not charged to enter the church, but there was a charge to visit the cloisters. Instead, we toured the village. Numerous cat sculptures and cat-themed plaques adorned the walls and buildings

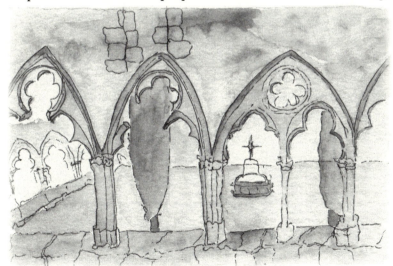

Cloisters, La Romieu

of the town. Some resembled an open book with a cat peeking out; others portrayed a woman's face with a distinctly feline nose and pointy cat ears.

The cat-woman was named Angeline. A medieval legend recounted the story of Angeline, a young woman born in La Romieu in 1338. The little girl was orphaned young and brought up by a neighbor. She had a great affection for cats, even allowing them to sleep with her. Then came several years of famine so great that there was nothing left to eat except cats.

Angeline's adopted parents kept a male and female cat hidden during the famine, and they managed to survive and multiply. More bountiful times returned; unfortunately, so did rats, which proliferated without natural predators. In response to the town's desperation Angeline released some of her numerous cats and the pesky rodents soon disappeared. Legend has it that over the years, Angeline's face began to resemble that of a cat.

Maurice Serreau, a sculptor from Orleans, heard someone's grandmother tell the story and decided to commemorate the tale. Cat sculptures, street plaques, postcards, and souvenirs now abound in La Romieu, forming an uneven mix of good intentions and kitsch.

We purchased dinner supplies in a small grocery store with an unexpectedly upscale stock. The shelves were laden with assorted goat cheeses, imported ham, canned *foie gras*, delicious *bio* bread, and *turrón*, a popular Spanish almond-nougat candy. I bought a box of *turrón* to give the Webers a taste of Spain. After careful consideration, they bought a bottle of good wine.

I also bought postcards, including one with a silly cartoon but with lovely words from the "Liturgy of Hours of the Feast of Saint Antoine":

> "Go pilgrim, pursue thy quest; go on thy way, may nothing stop thee! Take your share of the sun and your share of the dust, your heart aroused, forget the ephemeral! All is naught; there is no truth but love. Do not bind your heart to he who passes! Do not say: I have

succeeded, I have paid my penalty. Do not rest on your
works, they will come to judge you. Keep the Word in
your heart; this is your treasure."

*Wednesday, May 21, 2003. The Domaine du
Pellecahus. Not walking anywhere.*

Christine brought *bio* bread, homemade *confitures* and jams,
cheeses, and fresh cherries from the orchard for breakfast. Irma,
Wilhelm, and Honey Bunny soon joined us. I had given up retriev-
ing Honey Bunny from Irma. I could afford to be generous, after all,
since Honey Bunny would be going home with us.

It was a relief to spend another day in the same place—especially such a lovely place as this. It was tiring to always be moving on.
Medieval Irish monks made it their vocation to be peripatetic—they
referred to leaving Eire as the "Green Martyrdom"—but cloistered
monks stayed within the walled confines of their monasteries. Each
commitment required a different kind of devotion, a different sacrifice, and offered a different reward.

The day felt like a holiday, akin to an unexpected "snow day"
when school was cancelled. We could stroll to the village; we could
pick fruit from the organic cherry orchard; we could dawdle around
the large pond behind the buildings. There was time and space, lots
of space. I realized how confined we usually were in a cramped hotel
room—even though that was much more private than a communal
dormitory. Here we each had an apartment of our own and beautiful
grounds to explore. Gratitude, gratitude.

Christine spoke a little English so we were able to converse.
She and Brigitte had moved to the Domaine two years ago and had
spent a great deal of effort transforming assorted buildings in various states of disrepair into the current attractive accommodations. It
was hard to imagine that our *gîte* had once been a ruined barn.

Christine came from the 6th *arrondissement* in Paris, a chic, bo-
hemian, intellectual district, home to various high-end luxury design
houses. She had been in the garment business but had tired of it all.
A group of friends had decided to pool their money and fix up a
château. When that plan fell through, she and Brigitte bought the

Domaine. They had big plans for the property, including building an auditorium for music performances and theater.

"Why here?" I asked.

"The people in the Gers are happier than in the Dordogne. Tourist literature emphasizes the friendliness of the Gascogne people and it is true."

"Why on the Chemin?"

"The Chemin is magic. It brings people together from all over. Pilgrims share a cosmic connection, but mostly they share the search for inner meaning. They are different from tourists." With that, Christine excused herself and went back to work. Tending the Domaine was a full-time occupation.

Irma commented on how tedious it must be to keep telling your story repeatedly to new guests. To succeed in the hospitality business required a very special kind of person. On the one hand, you had to be polite to everyone and available even when you really wanted to be left alone. On the other hand, new guests came through with interesting stories.

I wrote in my journal:

> I am really happy we're going to walk to Roncesvalles. It feels important to close the Mobius strip of our pilgrimages. At last our journey has become a pilgrimage—which doesn't mean we can't take a taxi occasionally or catch a ride.

> I realize now that although I had strongly disagreed with Gary's decision to stop in Condom, I had not argued for what I wanted because I was grateful that he is willing make this pilgrimage, and I wanted to be accommodating. No wonder I had felt depressed and irritated. I still haven't learned to speak my truth—for one thing, it means I have to take responsibility for my feelings. Fortunately, the Chemin gives me many opportunities to practice.

It feels as if we have playmates staying in the gîte next door. We fight over who will get Honey Bunny. Irma wants her all the time, including at night. 'Well,' I joked, 'Honey Bunny is a bunny, and bunnies do sleep around.' Irma looked shocked.

I am intrigued by the way people make meaning out of Honey Bunny. Why is this soft, fuzzy bunny with floppy ears so alluring? Watching Wilhelm and Irma play, I am reminded of the innocence of children. Children live in the moment without worrying about the future; they accept whatever comes without judgment; they have no expectations. Children live effortlessly in the state of being that I am struggling to rediscover.

Gratitude for the incredible bounty of the Chemin.

Suddenly Gary started feeling chilled and dizzy. Irma, who was still very tired, blamed her fatigue on the low barometric pressure and the cloudy day. I thought she probably had a touch of whatever had made me so sick the day before, but we all try to make meaning of things in our own way.

Although Gary wasn't well, he still had an appetite. Christine recommended Le Cardinal restaurant and offered to give us a ride both ways. We accepted. When we got to town we saw pilgrims sitting at outside cafés and inside the restaurant. Its claim to fame was a buffet, the first I had seen in France, but it turned out to be the most mediocre food we had eaten in a country that prided itself on gastronomy.

While we picked at our food, we amused ourselves. I took photos of Irma and Wilhelm drinking espresso with Honey Bunny. Irma pretended to give Honey Bunny something to drink, and then Wilhelm wrapped a napkin around her like a bib. Unlike us, the Webers had no hesitancy about playing with a plush animal in public.

Irma explained that plush animals were quite popular in Germany among young people up to their early 30s. Her only hesitancy about playing with Honey Bunny was that people might think she was trying to act younger than she was. My concern was that people would think I was strange. I could almost hear Honey Bunny say, once again, "What do you care what people think of you, especially when you'll never see them again?" As usual, she had a point.

Thursday, May 22, 2003. La Romieu to Condom. 16 kilometers (10 miles).

Before leaving the Domaine we picked *bio* cherries from the orchard. We promised to keep in touch with Christine and exchanged cards. Several days of rest had helped me regain my strength, and Gary and Irma seemed to have recovered.

The weather looked promising: sunny, breezy, and not too hot. Six and one-half kilometers from La Romieu we reached the tiny twelfth-century Chapelle Sainte-Germaine, all that remained of a medieval monastery that once had accommodated pilgrims. A num-

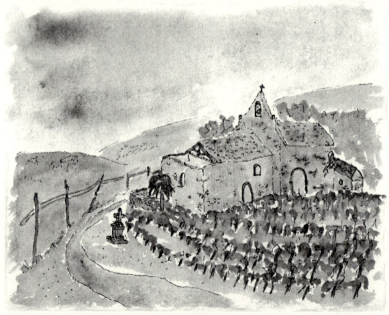

Chapelle Sainte-Germaine

ber of pilgrims rested in the shade of the ruins, including the couple from Lascabanes and the woman who had given me the tau booklet. Poppies sprouted alongside the old stone wall and vineyards thrived next to the church. Lichens and rock offerings covered an old stone wayside cross. Even this far along the Chemin, people still had burdens to leave behind.

After resting a while, we continued through a gently rolling landscape that reminded me of Spain. Vineyards and what appeared to be fields of rye were planted on either side of the path. The GR led us through a forest and around a lake. We perched on its bank, eating lunch. Irma tried to catch tadpoles while I tied a bronze scallop shell pendant on a string around Honey Bunny's neck so that she, too, would be recognized as a pilgrim.

I enjoyed watching Wilhelm and Irma interact. They would scold each other playfully, disagreeing vehemently in German. Wilhelm would shake his head and proclaim, "Oh Irma, Irma!" She would shake her head and do it—whatever "it" was—anyway. Sometimes they held hands while they walked. Sometimes they skipped together. He was tall and thin, she was short, but they hopped together briefly, legs moving in unison. They provided an example of how to make a relationship last a lifetime.

"This pilgrimage is just not like last time," Irma said wistfully, even though they had not hopscotched around and taken rides the way we had.

Somehow the Chemin from Le Puy to Conques had seemed more—something. Sacred. Traditional. Authentic. But as Gary kept pointing out to me, how could this pilgrimage be like last time? This was this time. We could never walk the Chemin the first time again, even if we were walking this part of the Chemin for the first time. Not only was this Chemin different because it traversed another part of France, with its own unique history, but we were different too.

We arrived in Condom at 2:00 p.m. Surprisingly, I still felt energetic, although we had walked sixteen kilometers. We entered town alongside a very high wall that separated us from the Convent of Carmel de Prouillan. Pausing at a crossroads, we wondered which way to go. Suddenly a sinewy workman jumped off the back of a truck, strode over, shook our hands, kissed mine, and gave us directions to the communal *gîte*. Ah, the Gascognes. Or more accurately, "les Gersois"!

Condom is a successful market town, the center of the Armagnac trade, with a population of 8000, not counting numerous tourists. It features a bustling plaza and wide streets lined with shops. One bar is called El Callejón (Spanish for "back street" or "alley") and advertises itself as a *bodega* (wine cellar) and tapas bar with Spanish (and Gascogne) specialties. Bullfighting posters and *espadrilles* (Basque slippers or shoes with a fabric upper and a flexible sole) dominate the shop windows, reminding me that although we were still in the Gers—the land of jocular good humor—we were moving closer to the French Basque country and Spain.

Condom, the self-styled "Pearl of Gascony," is situated on a spur between the rivers Gèle and the Baïse. The Baïse is the only navigable waterway in the *département* and connects with the Canal du Midi, thus giving Condom a major role in water tourism. That and local food products (ducks, geese, and chocolates) and the liquor trade (Armagnac and Floc) are central to the regional economy.

Rather than go directly to our hotel, located on the way out of town, we went sightseeing. Condom was buffeted between the French and the English during the Hundred Years' War and laid ruin during the Wars of Religion, but it was frequently rebuilt. During the eighteenth century, successful merchants erected luxurious mansions outside the medieval walls.

Rumor has it that the town's name referred to condoms. The wordplay is based on a homonym that is meaningful in English but not in French, since the French word for condoms is *préservatifs*. The name of the town probably derives from the Latin *condate* and *dum*, meaning confluence and hill respectively. Shrewdly taken advantage of a readymade marketing ploy, Condom built a Musée du Préservatifs. We skipped it and toured the Museum of Armagnac, which is filled with antique distillery equipment and farm machinery.

Next stop was the Cathédrale de Saint-Pierre, which was almost demolished in 1569 by the Huguenot army; the practical Condomois averted this disaster by paying a large ransom to the French Protestants. I lit candles in gratitude that Gary and I were going to continue walking instead of stopping in this town. I lit more candles for good companions, renewed endurance, and fine weather.

The sixteenth-century cathedral is in a style called late flamboyant Gothic, which means it is filled with filigree and baroque excesses. Usually I prefer more austere surroundings, but there was something energizing about the exuberance. Angels top a lacy stone choir, silhouetted against stained glass windows. There was no sign of Saint James, but I realized he hadn't been very visible on this part of the Chemin, at least not in material form.

Standing together in the spacious nave, the four of us sang "Ultreya," the sound resonating throughout the cathedral. A German couple came over to ask if we were singing "Taize"—an interdenominational chanting tradition developed at the Taize community in France. Irma and Wilhelm had never heard of it, but we had. We used to do Taize-style chanting at a Baptist church in Denver, as well as at a Methodist church in Boulder, where we would walk a labyrinth and sing sacred songs. We were so eclectic. The Divine was everywhere—even, as Michel had reminded us the year before, in a piece of bread.

After leaving the cathedral, Wilhelm remembered that a Dutch pilgrim had asked him to tell the innkeeper at our hotel that she would not be coming. He wondered if he should call immediately but then decided it would be all right to inform them when we arrived at the hotel. After all, what difference would it make?

We headed across the street to an upscale pub and sat on the second-floor balcony looking out at the church, drinking espresso and tea, eating cakes, and watching the people pass by. Then we strolled through the streets, visiting the tourist office and a variety of shops, many of which displayed Basque-style shoes and berets. A number of storefront Armagnac outlets offered *dégustation gratuite,* but we didn't feel like sampling, even if it was free.

We again encountered the star-crossed French couple from Lascabanes. The following day they would board trains in opposite directions and be separated for at least a month. Looking very sad, she asked about the *lapin* and smiled weakly when Irma pulled her out of the bag. Honey Bunny had acquired quite a following; she was no longer our and the Webers' mascot: she belonged to the Chemin.

Tired of sightseeing in the heat, we walked over to the Hôtel-Restaurant Relais de la Ténarèze. It was further than we thought because Condom was a long, dispersed town winding alongside the river. *Miam Miam Dodo* had awarded Ténarèze a welcoming flower, so we had high expectations.

When we crossed a bridge over the Baïse and saw our hotel, Irma and I shuddered. The sign dangling over the door was faded, the façade was peeling, and the hotel was at the edge of a busy street. However, we had no choice. We had made reservations and our bags were being delivered to the *relais.* Resigned, we entered and looked for the proprietor. Madame, a heavyset, overworked middle-aged woman, was cleaning up the dining room. She greeted us with a friendly but weary smile.

Irma told her a woman pilgrim had asked them to cancel her reservation. Madame was upset she hadn't been told sooner; now it was too late to fill the room. Grumbling, she pointed out the boot scrapers in the entrance hallway and led us up narrow worn steps to our rooms. I tried not to brush against the slightly crumbling stone walls. The room, like the building, was a bit decayed; fuzzy wallpaper covered up the cracked, probably mildewed walls. In spite of that, the room had a certain charm and, more importantly, a recently remodeled bathroom.

Soon I went back downstairs to inquire about a fax that our remodelers were supposed to have sent, but the fax machine was broken. So instead, I conversed with Madame, who told me that the hotel was 200 years old and that she and her husband had been running it for twenty-seven. Before that, three generations of another family had managed the establishment, going back to a time when horses were the mode of transportation—hence the name *relais*, which meant "post house," referring to the time when the mail, as well as people, was delivered via horseback.

While waiting for dinner, we treated ourselves to chilled white Floc de Gascogne and a *pousse rapière* (literally "rapier thrust," a layered cocktail of Armagnac, champagne, orange liqueur, and orange zest). The dining room was full of pilgrims and a few tourists; we took turns toasting each other. Madame took our orders, served us, cleared our plates, and did everything except cook. Her husband did that.

Dinner began with homemade soup with *fève* (broad) beans, followed by a traditional Gascogne appetizer assortment of shredded carrots, pickled beets, stuffed duck neck, pâté, and cooked new potatoes. Next came a marvelously fragrant sauerbraten beef roast with raisins, prunes, and Armagnac sauce, followed by spaghetti with vegetable sauce. Dessert was prunes soaked in Armagnac, served with vanilla ice cream topped with *chantilly* (whipped cream).

Honey Bunny was in evidence. Wilhelm had a spoon under her and used it as a lever to animate her. It was amusing to watch this retired business exec at play. It went contrary to my expectations—which started me thinking again about how expectations get in the way of appreciating what is.

Gary frequently reminded me that expectations bring disappointment and he was right. "Oh no," Irma and I had gasped when we saw the hotel because it was not what we expected. But our rooms were comfortable and dinner was delicious, also something we hadn't expected. I had the expectation that I should be strong, able to walk great distances, not have swollen ankles, and so on. Why on earth did I have such expectations? They certainly weren't based on reality, and they led me to criticize my performance instead of appreciating it. My goal was to live in a state of neutral curiosity instead of judgmental expectation.

Friday, May 23, 2003. Condom to Montreal to Eauze. 17 kilometers (10.6 miles) to Montreal-du-Gers, then 16 kilometers (10 miles) by taxi to Eauze.

We started at 6:30 a.m. to avoid the heat. The night before, Madame had asked what we wanted for breakfast and said she would leave it in the hallway near the front door. Apparently other guests thought it was for them—or maybe they just ate it anyway—so there was nothing left for us. Wilhelm and Irma were doubly upset that people had eaten our breakfasts and then left a mess. So much for the spirit of community and trust on the Camino.

Despite the inauspicious beginning, we were soon strolling alongside the river Baïse. We stopped at what our guidebook described as the Église de Saint-Jacques, our first sign of St. James in quite a while. The church was a boarded-up eighteenth- or nineteenth-century building and the statue over the doorway was Saint Joseph, not Saint James.

Our path took us along old railroad tracks with grass growing up between the rails, and then through oak forests. We followed the trail up and down gently rolling hills, past vineyards that would be transformed into Floc de Gascogne and Armagnac, alongside fields of sunflowers and wheat.

After an hour we met a middle-aged French couple resting by the side the road. The previous year they had walked from Le Puy to Condom; this morning they had begun their pilgrimage again. His pack weighed approximately forty pounds, hers about twenty. They carried a tent and planned to camp each day. She looked exhausted. I wished them well and she gave us a wan smile.

Five kilometers past Condom is the turn-off to the perfectly preserved medieval fortified village of Larressingle. Irma, Wilhelm, and Gary continued walking but I stopped, looking into the distance through a clearing in the trees. Clouds hung low on the horizon— but then I realized they weren't clouds, they were immense, snow-capped mountains.

"Gary! Irma! Wilhelm! Come look!" I shouted.

They turned, puzzled. I pointed. They looked but did not see.

"There! The Pyrenees!"

"Where?"

"There! On the horizon. They look like clouds."

"Oh my God," Gary gasped.

Irma and Wilhelm exclaimed something in German.

We continued in silence.

For a while that morning Irma and I walked together. She told me that she and Wilhelm had been talking about "choice points," those moments when you make a life-altering decision, whether you realize it at the time or not. Gary and I usually walked in silence, occasionally exchanging comments about the scenery.

The next time I was walking with Gary, I asked him about choice points.

He thought for only a moment before replying, "The biggest choice point was when I chose to teach music in Dolores, Colorado, instead of going to work for IBM." He had been offered a job with IBM the same day but a few hours after he had signed the teaching contract. He could have backed out, but he had given his word. "Another choice point was taking the teaching job at ISU instead of going to Michigan. Staying at ISU instead of going to Indiana. Early retirement and divorce. What about you?"

I realized that when I was young the major choice points were decisions I felt I had no choice about. For example, not going back to Stanford University in the middle of my sophomore year, and getting divorced from John. I had felt compelled by circumstances. In retrospect, however, I could see that I could have made other choices. Later, I made the important choice to study the Camino de Santiago for my Ph.D., despite pressure from my advisor to do something else. I never regretted my decision. I didn't choose to get cancer, but I chose how I would respond.

We crossed the Pont d'Artigues, originally a Roman bridge over the Osse River. Once there had been a pilgrims' hospital there, run by the Commandery of the Order of Santiago, but no sign of it remained. Encouraged by pleasant weather and easy terrain, we took a short detour to Routges, the oldest church in the region. According to Raju's guidebook, a small door on the side of the church was a *porte des Cagots*.

The Cagots were a group of outcasts who lived in the Basque country on either side of the Pyrenees. Mentioned as early as the eleventh century, they were subjected to stringent apartheid: they could not drink from public fountains; they had their own entrances and holy-water fonts in churches, as well as separate cemeteries; they could only marry within their own community; and they were usually employed as wood-gatherers and master carpenters. Although legends suggested that they originated as lepers, Moorish slaves, Cathar refugees, Visigoths, Saracens, or gypsies, modern research suggests they were probably all of the above—as well as renegade pilgrims who decided to settle in the Pyrenees.

They were forced to wear a goosefoot emblem or an actual goosefoot around their necks. Why a goosefoot? One long, convoluted explanation involves Mother Goose; Charlemagne's mother, the Good Queen Berthe the Goosefoot; and the goosefoot sign of the Companions, a secret guild that supposedly built the cathedrals along the Chemin as well as the Egyptian pyramids.

Eventually the Cagots began a massive civil rights battle against harassment, demanding equal rights as human beings. In 1789, with the French Declaration of the Rights of Man, the Cagots gained constitutional liberties and gradually ceased to exist as a marginalized minority—although nowadays some people proudly assert their Cagot ancestry.

We sat in the shade of the church resting our feet and legs, munching slices of stale almond cake I had purchased in Condom and puzzling over the Cagots and their affiliation with the goose. The goose had long been associated with a Celtic goddess and with Venus, so perhaps the Cagots really were the remnants of some ancient Pyrenean tribe. Or maybe not.

On the Spanish Camino we had occasionally seen a three-pronged symbol called the goosefoot carved on the side of churches. I had been told that this symbol represented the solsticial quadrilateral† measurement of the church, or indicated underground energy lines at that location, or stood for the mythic goose-messenger to the gods. Given that a stonemason had carved the goosefoot, perhaps the Cagots really had descended from the Companions who built the churches, and the goosefoot was a an obscure reminder.

We saw other pilgrims and talked with the French couple we'd met earlier in the day, who had caught up with us while we rested. The day had turned hot again. The temperature was 55° - 60° F in early morning, 70° F by mid-morning, and 95° F by noon, which was when we reached Montreal-du-Gers, a thirteenth-century bastide.

Gary's knee hurt, as did his right big toe. I could not tolerate the heat, especially when there was no shade. Although Irma and Wilhelm planned to walk the thirty-three kilometers to Eauze, we knew we couldn't. When we reached Montreal I located the tourist office, and a helpful young woman arranged for a taxi to take us to Eauze. It was a surprisingly easy transaction. I felt reassured: we could make it on our own. That should have been obvious by now, but I kept forgetting.

The local farmer's market was located across from the tourist office. Vendors were already packing up their goods but the four of us wandered through the stalls, admiring the variety of strawberries, cherries, cheese, farm chickens, and fish; we were grateful for the opportunity to buy supplies. Sharing our purchases, we ate lunch sitting on a shaded bench; then, with a farewell wave, the Webers headed off to Eauze. I wasn't sure if their resolve was based on a religious commitment or on Teutonic willpower.

While we waited for the taxi we had a conversation with a German man dressed entirely in black, with a watch on each arm. At one point he looked at his arm and said the barometric pressure was dropping and there'd be rain tomorrow and cooler weather. A video camera swung from his shoulder. Native American rings festooned his fingers, and he wore a silver and turquoise Native American wristband. Various pouches and objects dangled from his belt, which sported a US flag buckle. White roots showed beneath his bright red hair.

"Where are you from?" I asked.

He did a Heil Hitler salute, which he seemed to think was funny. Then he said, "I'm a journalist who wants to know why people are walking the Chemin."

I said enthusiastically, "I did my doctorate in anthropology on 'why.' That's a very good question!"

He ignored my pronouncement and repeated, "I want to know why they walk." Then he told us about meeting a German couple that didn't attend church anymore (Irma and Wilhelm, perhaps?), yet they were walking the Chemin.

I took a deep breath and was going to respond, but he turned away and had an unpleasant exchange with a woman he appeared to be traveling with. She left in a huff. We also left, deciding to explore the town in the brief time remaining.

Montreal-du-Gers was founded as a bastide in the thirteenth century. The town's attractions include restored half-timbered houses, an arcaded plaza, a thirteenth-century church, and nearby Séviac, a fourth-century Gallo-Roman village with amazingly well-preserved floor mosaics.

Wishing to avoid the heat and the self-proclaimed journalist, we sought refuge in the church. At 1:00 p.m. a car with a red cross on it pulled in front of the tourist office. After some confusion, we

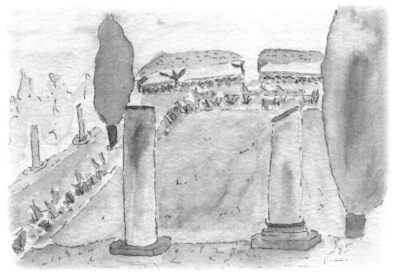

Séviac

realized this was our taxi. Genevieve explained that she delivered people to the doctor and the hospital, and occasionally she delivered pilgrims to the next stop on the road.

The road twisted and turned through countryside covered with trees; I hoped Wilhelm and Irma were walking in forest shade. After about twenty minutes, Genevieve dropped us off at our hotel in Eauze, the Hôtel de l'Armagnac. It was located on a noisy cross street and looked very shabby. I reminded myself that the previous night everything had turned out well despite my expectations.

One door, which was locked, appeared to lead into the hotel; the other, which was open, led into the adjoining restaurant. The restaurant was dingy, dark, and small, with two rows of tables, only three of which were filled. It was abnormally quiet. I felt as if I had walked into a still life.

We walked up to the bar and called "Hello!" to the corridor behind; then we also waited. Tattered bullfight posters were tacked on the wall, contributing to the forlorn decor. Eventually an annoyed woman with heavy makeup emerged from a back room, followed by her frowning husband. It seemed to be an imposition for them to give us our rooms, but we persevered.

I asked in French, "Do the rooms have *toilettes privéés?*"

"No!" Monsieur replied.

"We would like a room with a private toilet," I insisted.

"They're all alike! The bathroom is in the hall, " Monsieur retorted in French.

Well, there were worse things than sharing the bathroom. We took both room keys so we could check out the Webers' room as well as ours. Our room had one bed, which was what we had reserved. Furnishings included a red shag carpet used as a bedspread and a matching shag rug under the sink. A miniscule shower cubicle was wedged into one corner. Even though we didn't have a private bathroom, at least we had a shower and sink.

The Webers' room had one bed, not two, and faced the noisy street. Since we had arrived long before the Webers, we felt responsible for getting them the best room we could. We went back downstairs and requested a room with two beds.

"Two beds cost more," Monsieur snarled, "so why bother!"

Perhaps Monsieur wanted to keep his two-bed rooms for travelers who were not related to each other, but we insisted that the Webers must have two beds and the room should be quiet. We succeeded in achieving the first but not the second. We considered changing hotels but how would we tell Irma and Wilhelm? Besides, we had already checked in.

When we walked downstairs again, Monsieur and Madame were arguing—or maybe that was how they normally conversed. How awful to be linked by work and marriage. There would be no escape. We, on the other hand, could escape, and escape we did, heading uphill into town.

Construction work was in evidence all around us, but workmen were on their lunch break so it was relatively quiet. We went into a large, dimly lit bar across from the church and ordered two bottles of cold Schweppes tonic water.

The loquacious bartender spoke to me in Spanish and recommended we try the local specialty, *croustade d'Armagnac*, a puff pastry stuffed with vanilla sugar, a little Armagnac, and apples. He informed us that the *croustade* would not go well with Schweppes so we should order white wine.

I explained, in Spanish, "We're walking the Chemin and I can't drink alcohol and walk."

"How dreadful!" Jean replied, "That's as bad as having cancer!"

I responded—I don't know why, since it was not something I talked about in casual conversation—"I did have cancer last year. That's why we're walking."

Jean looked shocked and then embarrassed. Awkwardly, he turned away and disappeared into the kitchen. We went outside and sat down at a table, waiting for our Schweppes. Soon Jean returned with two glasses and two bottles, poured them for us, and left.

While we sipped the refreshing tonics, we admired the medieval half-timbered houses across the way, with their exposed wooden beams and red brick chevrons. Workmen were repointing the grey-white mortar.

Soon Jean returned with a warm *croustade*. I wondered if that were a special gesture or a common procedure. He tried to apologize.

"Don't worry about it," I reassured him.

When we paid him, he didn't have the correct change. Again I said, "Don't worry about it. Keep the difference."

"No," he insisted. "You will owe *me* fifty cents. Come back with it before 10:00 a.m. tomorrow or I will send the Mob after you!"

I feigned horror at the thought. Then we laughed and agreed.

We visited the thirteenth-century priory church of Saint-Luperc, downgraded from its previous status as the area's cathedral

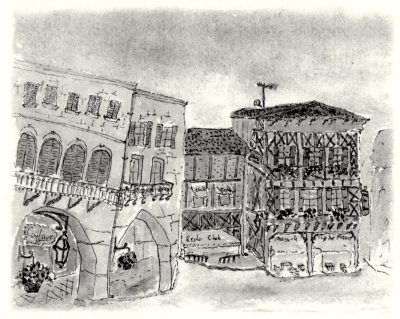

Eauze

because it no longer had a resident bishop. The church was being renovated. The interior plaster had been removed, leaving bare brick and stone.

I had once thought that the interior walls of medieval churches were originally bare stone and mortar, but this aesthetic austerity is a recent development. Many interiors—including that of Chartres Cathedral—were originally brightly painted. The walls of Chartres, for example, were covered with a thin plaster that was then painted to resemble stones and mortar—as if it was of great importance to visually acknowledge the no-longer-visible building blocks.

Frescoes depicting biblical scenes, daily life, the Heavenly Jerusalem, or decorative geometrical motifs often adorned church walls. In some churches, whitewash was later applied to cover the frescoes as a hygienic measure or because tastes had changed. When the whitewash was removed during later restoration, well-preserved frescoes were occasionally revealed—if the plaster hadn't "eaten" or "burned" the paint.

Next we visited the archeological museum. Eauze had once been the capital of the Celtic tribe called the Elusatti, hence its name. But its real claim to fame is the impressive Eauze Treasure of 28,000 Gallo-Roman coins and precious objects dating from the first to fourth century. Eauze had once been a Gallo-Roman metropolis; this is the only such intact treasure found in France.

After admiring the glittering hoard, we walked along the old ramparts. Trying to avoid returning to our hotel, we continued to stroll aimlessly through the town. We walked down a street lined with shops, many of which were run by individual Armagnac producers—not surprising, since Eauze (like Condom) claims to be the capital of Armagnac. This time Gary and I sampled the *dégustation gratuite* (free tastings) in one of the shops. The clerk was a young woman eager to practice her English, and we were eager to oblige. Besides, Julia kept plying us with Armagnac that was twenty and thirty years old.

I splurged on a pint bottled in 1942, as close to Gary's birthday (1937) as I could find. Julia's grandfather had bottled it during the war, before southern France was occupied. He had hand-written the label in ink, now faded. It seemed like the perfect present for Gary's upcoming birthday, since it was both lightweight and memorable.

On our way back to the hotel we stopped by the bar and gave Jean fifty cents plus two cents interest. He laughed heartily and shook our hands. Then we headed back to our dismal hotel to wait for the Webers.

They arrived around 5:30 p.m. and were quite disappointed with their room. We assured them we had done the best we could and that we had thought of trying to find another place, but how would we have gotten in touch with them if we had?

To make up for the disappointing accommodations we splurged at La Vie en Rose Restaurant. We had a wonderful meal, beginning with another *pousse rapière*, a delight for the eyes as well as the palate. Honey Bunny politely greeted the waitress and then, at the waitress's suggestion, settled into a place of honor next to a display of Armagnac bottles. She was underage but nobody cared.

During dinner, the waitress took Honey Bunny over to a nearby table. The guests had asked about the Chemin, so she showed them

Honey Bunny's scallop-shell symbol of the pilgrimage. They turned and smiled at us somewhat tentatively.

Saturday, May 24, 2003. Eauze to Nogaro. 20 kilometers (12.5 miles).

After an unpleasant night, we eagerly walked away from Eauze. The weather was cool and overcast, raining off and on, then sunny. The strange German journalist had been correct.

We walked through deep green forests, alongside fields of sunflowers, leeks, cereal grains, and occasional vineyards. While skirting a large fish farm we met a French pilgrim with a large elastic support on his knee. Claude explained that he had bent over while carrying his heavy backpack and, when he stood up, something gave out in his knee. Nonetheless, he was determined to keep on.

He and five friends had been walking the Chemin in weeklong stages for a number of years, but he had missed a few because he had been out of the country, so he was trying to catch up by walking thirty-four to thirty-eight kilometers a day. Claude had begun in Condom and would meet the group on Sunday or Monday night; then they would continue together to Saint-Jean-Pied-de-Port. I urged him to use Factage and lighten his load for a day or so, so as not to damage his knee further. He dismissed the idea.

We shared lunch at Chez Monique in Manciet, a long, narrow town just past the fish farms. The plat du jour was duck-leg *confit* with tomato-cheese sauce on pasta. The *confit* was so tough it was nearly inedible.

The waitress explained to a curious couple that we were walking the Chemin, sometimes covering as many as twenty-five kilometers a day. She hadn't asked us how far we walked, so she must have heard that number from others. Or maybe she just made it up. The couple was quite impressed and wished us a good journey.

There was a bit of confusion about our order and about the bill. Claude made some nasty comment about provincials who couldn't add. Later, when Irma and I were walking together, she confided that this sort of spiteful, critical exchange was common among their French friends, a sort of rude one-upmanship that they didn't appear to take personally. I was reminded of some of Collette's remarks to Danielle that I thought were rude but Danielle just ignored. Now I had a cultural rather than a personal context for them.

We stopped to admire an ancient stone cross, stubby and carved into a circular disk, pebbles piled on top of the square base. It resembled Basque tombstones, which often have a cross surrounded by a circle on one side and a six-petaled flower shape on the other. I wondered whether the symbol was a distant memory of a sun-worshipping cult.

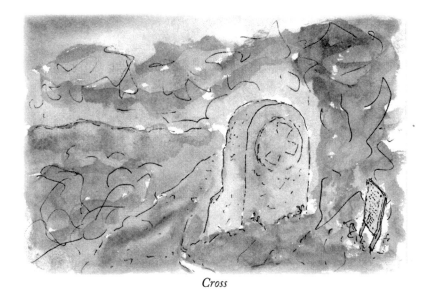

Cross

Unable to let go of expectations and comparisons, we all agreed that walking from Le Puy to Conques had felt more like a pilgrimage than our current journey. We discussed various reasons why this might be so. On last year's journey, Saint Jacques (or his usurper, Saint Roch) was visible in many of the churches, either by name or statue. The religious architecture was different: older, smaller, simpler, and still in use. In the area we were currently walking through, many of the cathedrals and large churches had been destroyed in the War with the English or the Wars of Religion; some of them had been rebuilt, others not, and many were closed.

In addition, the countryside from Le Puy to Conques was less developed, especially in the Aubrac. Cattle grazed in the fields but there was no large-scale agriculture with huge tractors and mobile irrigation systems, as there was in the Gers. Walking from Le Puy to Conques, we had had the feeling of traveling in a time centuries before industrialization. It was indeed *France profunde*.

When Gary and I had walked the Spanish Camino, it had never occurred to us to compare one part to another. The mountainous Pyrenees were simply different from the flat, dry Meseta, which was different from the green rolling hills of Galicia. The rural countryside was different from the cities, but each had their attractions.

When we walked from Le Puy to Conques, we hadn't compared one part of that Chemin to the other. So why were we doing it now? The current journey took us through a different terrain as well as through another part of French history. But that was no reason to feel that the first part was more of a pilgrimage than this one. I wondered if we were confusing our preference for medieval aesthetics and *France profunde* with our spiritual response to the Chemin.

Gary asserted, "This time we haven't seen anything like Le Puy, or Conques, or stunning Romanesque churches. We've being overcharged and dealt with unscrupulous innkeepers. We've had some terrible accommodations. And the weather has been very hot."

There we were again, caught up in judgment and expectations. Even Gary was doing it! How hard it was to break old patterns and simply enjoy what is. I tried, I really did, but I kept stumbling and forgetting and going back to an old, familiar lens through which I habitually viewed the world. A lens that compared and judged everything against what had gone before.

But there was more to it than that. We had had cold rainy weather during our first Chemin, yet we hadn't complained. We had simply accepted it and been grateful when we found shelter. Perhaps the excitement had worn off and we now realized how far we still had to go.

My feelings about the pilgrimage were like my recovery from cancer: elation followed by dismay. I now realized how long I had to go before I could feel safe from a recurrence—if I ever felt safe again.

I had a sudden insight. "What's a pilgrimage without challenges and tribulations? After all, that's part of the process. We heard the call of the Chemin. We started out on a quest—for healing, or understanding, or deeper faith. We are encountering tests and trials along the way. Ultimately—perhaps at the end, or maybe even before—we will receive a reward for our efforts. Perhaps we'll achieve some kind of inner transformation, gain some new clarity. Why are we surprised to encounter difficulties? After all, we are *pilgrims*, not hikers!"

I was greeted with thoughtful silence.

Irma changed the topic. "Wilhelm and I are trying to decide how to do the Spanish Camino 'right.' Do we have to make reservations to have a place to stay?"

"Not if you're staying in *refugios*," I replied. "They don't accept reservations."

Gary added, "Remember, there is no 'right' way to walk the Chemin. There are just different ways, each with its own rewards and risks."

That didn't seem to satisfy them. They continued the discussion in German.

Pilgrims and pilgrims-to-be spend a great deal of time discussing how to make a real pilgrimage. I used the word "make" intentionally, since it emphasizes the creative, decision-filled nature of the journey: one doesn't simply "do" it, one constructs it.

In my dissertation I explored the culturally constructed meaning of being a "real" pilgrim. One set of definitions focuses on one's means of transport: traditional (on foot, carrying one's own backpack) vs. modern (by bicycle or car). Another set of definitions focuses on something less tangible, something related to "traditional" reasons for the journey, which often places a high value on suffering. Using this definition, walking and carrying your own pack is more authentic than having someone else carry your pack. Never mind that medieval pilgrims didn't carry backpacks, and many traveled by horse and/or carriage if they could.

Some pilgrims think the only authentic Camino is to begin from home (difficult for Americans) and to only stay in *refugios*. Judgments and distinctions abound, even among presumably spiritually motivated pilgrims. After all, why should they be any different?

It was simpler in medieval times. Pilgrims went through a blessings ceremony before leaving home and donned special travel attire, including the iconic staff with water gourd, a cape to keep off the rain, and a wallet (flat bag with a strap) for papers and money. They joined other pilgrims for safety and followed established routes to important shrines. Only modern pilgrims worry about authenticity. Ironically, not all medieval pilgrims were authentic pilgrims—some were thieves or vagabonds taking advantage of the hospitality of the Camino; some were people who were paid to go for others; and some were criminals sentenced to walk a particular pilgrimage road.

Gary and I had had lengthy debates in 1997 about how to make a real pilgrimage. I wanted to put myself in God's hands and just walk, trusting there would be a place to stay at the end of the day, the way I had in 1982. But Gary's comfort level required hotel reservations.

I understood Irma and Wilhelm's agonizing over how to do the Camino right, but there is no single right way. After all, I had gotten sick in 1997 on the Camino and needed a taxi to carry my backpack. Did that mean I wasn't making a real pilgrimage? One could argue that my determination to continue despite serious health concerns made it more real, even if it didn't look that way to casual observers.

If discomfort was any measure, we were definitely making a real pilgrimage. Chilled and shivering from a sudden shower, we arrived at our two-star hotel, Hôtel-Restaurant Le Commerce, in Nogaro. Claude, the Frenchman with the bad knee, was staying at Les Arènes, a few blocks away, so we said goodbye for the time being, confident that we would meet again.

The hotel looked well maintained. Attractive brickwork around a large entry arch framed the front door; fresh white plaster brightened the walls. Irma and I sighed with relief and went inside.

Madame seemed friendly and helped carry our luggage upstairs. When we got upstairs we realized that the hotel was being completely renovated—the hallway floors were bare concrete; the walls had been stripped of wallpaper; uncovered light bulbs dangled from the ceiling; and signs proclaimed "wet paint" on various doors. Madame gave us a newly repainted room that smelled badly of cigarette smoke. Gary opened the balcony doors and the wind blew in.

Irma went with me to ask Madame for a no smoking room. Madame looked annoyed, came back to our room, saw the open door, and rudely demanded that we close it immediately—the newly redone paint would get wet. Gary was furious and thought of leaving immediately.

She gave us another room but complained loudly as she did so. Then she left.

I looked around and realized that there was only one pillow on the bed. While Gary fumed I went downstairs to ask for a second pillow.

Madame looked me in the eyes and said in French, "No, there is only one pillow for the bed."

I responded in my best French, "Two people, one pillow?"

She nodded yes.

I repeated in disbelief, "Only one pillow?"

She nodded again.

I knew she was lying but I thanked her politely and left, reporting my unsuccessful venture to Gary. He became even more furious.

A few minutes later there was a knock on the door. I opened it and Madame tossed me a second pillow.

Madame seemed uncomfortable interacting with foreigners, or perhaps she was awkward with social interaction in general. However, she was the proprietress and being polite should have been part of her job description. Instead of being angry, I tried to be compassionate. How difficult it must be for her, I thought, to deal with all these demanding guests.

Since we were all dissatisfied with Mme's behavior, we went into town to find somewhere else to eat dinner. The other restaurants, however, like most of the shops, were closed.

Our hotel's restaurant billed itself as a gastronomical location so we hoped it was. A table of twelve people, part of an organized tour group, was already being served. Madame took our orders, brought the food, bussed the tables, and calculated the bills while her husband cooked. We had an excellent meal.

That night I couldn't sleep. My feet felt hot and burning, as if they were on fire. They looked red and irritated. Maybe the thin cotton socks I had bought in Figeac were letting my feet slide around too much. I was also afraid I was developing tiny blisters on the striking edge of my heels, so I decided to switch back to thicker socks the next day.

Sunday, May 25, 2003. Nogaro to Aire-sur-l'Adour. 28 kilometers (17.4 miles). We did it!

In the morning Madame wasn't much friendlier. Her affable husband served us hot chocolate, bread, and jam.

At Arblade-le-Haut, about one and one-half kilometers down the road, we passed an attractive *chambres d'hôtes* called the L'Arbladoise. We soon passed some pilgrims who had spent the night there. L'Arbladois, they assured us, provided a warm welcome, lovely rooms, and excellent food. Next time we would stay there, we told each other, even though there was no reason to think that we would ever be in Nogaro again.

We walk up and down gentle hills in the cool morning rain, through forests, across fields. Often the route was flat but hard to walk because of uneven footpaths. Signs advertised *accueil* or *étape* specifically for pilgrims—a welcome sight that reminded me of the Spanish Camino. We were indeed on a pilgrimage road, not just a long-distance hiking trail.

Irma and Wilhelm walked ahead of us part of the morning. She had apologized in advance and explained that her head hurt from speaking English and French. She had found it tiring to discuss economic development topics with Claude in English and was quite frustrated because her English wasn't at the level she would like. I assured her that her English was fine. Besides, we didn't have to talk. Silence was good.

I began to wonder if we had traveled together too long. Without us, Irma and Wilhelm would walk faster. Perhaps Irma was disappointed because she had wanted to improve her French, absorbing colloquial expressions into her heart not only into her brain, but instead she was spending her days speaking English.

Then I realized Irma and Wilhelm could travel alone if they wanted to. I was taking unnecessary responsibility, an old pattern I struggled to overcome. The Chemin was offering me another opportunity to change.

Later on, Irma and I walked together again, and she told me that German history was a heavy burden.

"Do you think the French react badly to you because of it?" I asked.

"Sometimes," she said.

"Sometimes that happens to us, too, because of the Iraq war."

"Yes, but what Germany did was different: premeditated state-sponsored genocide of its own citizens. That is *quite* different from what happens in a war setting."

Then she recounted an incident that had occurred a number of years before, when she and Wilhelm were living in Paris. She had chatted with a little girl in a grocery store queue; the girl's grandfather was genial until he realized she was German. It had ended up all right, but she had never forgotten how she felt. The sins of the fathers....

We ate lunch in a small village churchyard next to a recreation building, with tennis courts below. Wilhelm photographed Honey Bunny sitting on the stone steps smelling the flowers. My heel felt sore. The thicker socks I was wearing were apparently not helping. Hoping to avert a catastrophe, I lubricated my feet and tied my boots tighter.

It rained off and on, chilling us, but then it got hot again. I didn't know which was worse or better. During a rest break I took the advice of seasoned walkers: air out your feet every hour or so. Unfortunately, my socks were a little damp when I put them back on. Damp feet or damp socks are almost guaranteed to cause blisters.

Although our road was relatively flat, the day had turned very hot. Much to our relief we encountered a rest stop near Barcelonne-du-Gers sponsored by the Berdoulet family. "Ultreia," proclaimed a sign posted on the trunk of a tree that shaded a bench, a chair, a table, and a cooler filled with bottled water.

What an unexpected gift of hospitality for weary pilgrims: a place to sit in the shade, fresh water to drink. The *livre d'Or* was filled with appreciative comments. We saw the sponsor working in the farm across the railroad tracks and called out our thanks. She waved.

Gratitude, gratitude. It had been a while since I felt gratitude. I certainly hadn't felt it for the accommodations in Nogaro, nor had I felt it for the sun that warmed the fields and helped the plants to grow. I had been too uncomfortable to do anything but complain.

After about twenty kilometers Gary's knee began to hurt again, so we decided to hitchhike. Irma and Wilhelm went on without us. Since we were on a flat road with lots of traffic, we thought it would be easy, but no one stopped. After five or ten minutes we gave up and began walking again. Irma and Wilhelm saw us and waited.

Rain splattered down as we crossed the bridge over the l'Adour. Fortunately, we were only a few kilometers from Aire-sur-l'Adour, our stopping place for the night. As we walked along the side of the country road, the rain-driven wind whipped Irma and Wilhelm's ponchos. Irma and I walked together, talking, while Gary and Wilhelm strode on ahead.

Two stone memorial plaques with fresh cut flowers stood by the side of the road. One was engraved, "To the members of the Resistance killed and 'carbonized' by the Germans in June 1944." Irma stopped next to the plaque to look at tadpoles in the stream; I stepped in front so she wouldn't notice the memorial.

(Gary informed me later that Wilhelm noticed both monuments and was distressed. He told Gary that it wasn't until the 1970s that Germans started examining the atrocities committed by their armed forces. People didn't want to know. According to Wilhelm, the shadow of the war didn't extend to his son's generation, and Irma had indicated that neither did anti-Semitism.)

Irma and I started walking again. Suddenly I realized I had a row of tiny blisters along the striking edge of both heels. They hurt with every step I took. In addition, my right ankle felt a bit wonky, and if I took a longer step than usual, a sharp pain ran up my left calf. Fortunately, we reached Aire-sur-l'Adour just as the rain let up. Gary and I had walked twenty-eight kilometers, more than we had ever walked in one day. I had a fleeting sense of accomplishment.

On the way to the hotel we stopped to visit the Cathédral Saint-Jean-Baptiste, originally built in the twelfth century but severely damaged in the fourteenth century during the wars between the French and English. Later it was partially reconstructed, only to be destroyed again during the sixteenth-century Wars of Religion, and finally rebuilt in the nineteenth century.

We stopped in a chocolate specialty store to ask directions to our hotel, so I took the opportunity to purchase some sweets to share. Aire-sur-l'Adour, population 6200, is a lively commercial town just over the border from the Gers, in the Landes region. It has a circular, nineteenth-century *halle*, several sporting goods shops, bookstores, clothing shops, chocolate and pastry specialty stores, and much more to delight tourists and foot-sore pilgrims. It also has several churches, including the Église de Sainte-Quitterie, the patron saint of Gascony, complete with healing fountain and a crypt that had originally been a Roman temple to Mars.

We were staying at the Hôtel Chez L'Ahumat, so-named because the grandmother of the owners had sold smoked sausages in the market in front of what was now the hotel. From such humble beginnings she had started the hotel and restaurant. The hotel was a hodgepodge collection of interconnected buildings. Although L'Ahumat wasn't fancy, uniformed staff carried our luggage up an impressive central staircase. On our way to our rooms we greeted a number of familiar pilgrims.

Our room contained a shower, a sink, and a bidet screened off from the rest of the room by a plastic, pink polka-dot shower curtain. The toilet room was down the hall. Furnishings included an impressive but somewhat threadbare velvet-upholstered armchair with fringe trim. Nothing, of course, could compare aesthetically with the red shag bedspread and matching rug in the sleazy hotel in Eauze. At least I thought it was Eauze. My memories of the towns, churches, and hotels on the Chemin were beginning to run together like butter melting in the sun.

I wrote in my journal:

> *So many days on the Chemin. Something triggers a memory and I have a momentary vision of a place; but like sunlight piercing through fog, the vision soon blurs and then disappears. All we do each day is walk a few kilometers (or perhaps as many as twenty-eight), but as we walk hour after hour, day after day, I experience sensory overload. Traveling by car, the scenery whizzes by so fast*

I don't realize how much there is to see. I don't experience the minute-to-minute changes in the weather, in the path under my feet, in the scent of the air.

I try to recall images from the day: the lovely scallop shell and the sign on the stone wall saying, "water ahead." A shaded bench under a tree with a cooler filled with water bottles, a livre d'Or to write a message. The rest has already faded from memory.

That evening Gary and I arranged for Factage to transport us along with our baggage. Gary's knee needed a rest and I hoped my blisters would heal if I gave them a day off.

Monday, May 26, 2003. Aire-sur-l'Adour to Arzacq-Arraziguet. 34 kilometers (21 miles) by Factage.

We ate breakfast with Irma and Wilhelm, then wished them "Buen Camino" as they set off down the road. Factage didn't arrive until noon. Less than thirty minutes later, we were in Arzacq-Arraziguet.

The day was cool and overcast—a fine day for walking, if one was able.

We checked into our hotel, La Vielle Auberge, located at one edge of the vast central plaza. As the name suggested, La Vielle Auberge was an old inn. It was also decrepit. Wallpaper peeled off the walls and cobwebs festooned the ceiling of our room. The toilet cubicle was down the hall, tucked into a diminutive space under the stairs, too small to stand up in. Our room had two beds, one of which collapsed when Gary sat on it. A few pegs hammered into the wall substituted for a closet. Irma and Wilhelm's room was equally dirty and unkempt, and lacked even the clothing pegs.

In 1982 on the Camino I had felt gratitude for refuge of any kind. Sometimes my companion and I had slept in the rain because there was no shelter. I had been grateful for a toilet that flushed, for hot water in the shower at the end of the hall, grateful for much that I had previously taken for granted—and which apparently I took for granted once again.

"Gratitude, gratitude for all that life brings," I repeated as a silent mantra, but I wryly added, "as long as it's clean, pleasant, and meets my expectations!"

Lunch in the Vielle Auberge was surprisingly innovative. It began with the chef's invention, an egg poached in cream and local Cantal cheese, followed by roasted *pintade* (guinea hen) with Brussels sprouts. For dessert we had a choice of numerous misshapen cakes or cheese with cherry jam.

My ankles swelled badly after lunch. I started to worry again about my health, something I preferred not to think about. I told myself perhaps they had swelled because I had walked so far the day before. Or because I hadn't walked today. Or because of something I ate....

Having nothing else to do, we decided that a stroll around town would do us no harm. Besides, walking had become a habit, despite my blisters and Gary's aching knee.

Arzacq-Arraziguet was a bastide, founded sometime in the thirteenth or fourteenth century. It looked, however, as if much of it had been torn down for urban renewal. Its central plaza resembled an immense empty parking lot.

We found the church and took numerous photos in case Irma and Wilhelm didn't arrive in time to visit it. A life-size statue of the Madonna drew our attention. She sits on a throne, holding a squirming baby Jesus, who reaches toward a bowl of fruit held by an angel. Two stained-glass windows feature Saint James—the first sign of him in some time. Near the entrance to the church, a laminated world map was propped on a table; a note requested pilgrims to indicate their homeland. All the pushpins were in use, so Gary and I debated the ethics of removing one and placing it in Colorado.

Then we hobbled to a large pharmacy on the edge of town that advertised itself as an herbal and homeopathic center. Gary needed to buy a different knee brace, since the one he had bought in Moissac was so tight, itchy, hot, and irritating that he refused to wear it. I searched for blister remedies. I had a lengthy exchange with a white-jacketed clerk who asserted that she spoke English. If she did,

I didn't. In desperation, I purchased several products, but I wasn't very hopeful. I'd had blisters before. Nothing much helped except time.

Around 5:30 p.m., Irma and Wilhelm staggered into the hotel along with Claude, whom they had met on the road. Exhausted, they told us they barely managed the last two kilometers. Wilhelm had tied his boots too tight and had some swelling and pain in his shins, so Gary offered to massage his legs.

Not surprisingly, their squalid room was a great disappointment. They, and we, had been promised a private toilet but none of us had one. Claude, however, who had only made his reservation that afternoon at their suggestion, was given a private bathroom. Perhaps it was because his was a single room or because he spoke Parisian French. Later that afternoon the plumbing sprung a leak. What seemed like a better room actually wasn't.

Despite the marginal accommodations, the dining room provided palatable food. It was the day before Gary's birthday, but since we were all together, we decided to celebrate early. Our celebration included birthday cards as well as duck and noodles.

Jean Georges, the cook and proprietor, joined us at the end of the dinner and began comparing Armagnac to Cognac. "Armagnac is not as refined, so it still has the *heart* in it. That's why my fellow Landesmen and Gascognes like it more."

In response, Gary fetched his birthday bottle of 1942 Armagnac. Not to be outdone, Jean Georges brought out a nearly empty bottle of 1952 Armagnac and poured it for us. Although the rooms were a disappointment, the conviviality was all one could ask for.

Tuesday, May 27, 2003. Gary's Birthday. Arzacq-Arraziguet to Pomps. 20 kilometers (12.5 miles), plus 3 kilometers by car to Morlanne.

While skirting a large artificial lake in the early morning, we watched a heron take off and land. Then it was back to walking rocky trails up hillsides and down, through forests and around fields, and past numerous tiny settlements. We took photos of unusual folk art: scallop shells strung diagonally on a tree trunk with half-filled water bottles dangling from branches. Honey Bunny spent much of the morning peering out of Wilhelm's daypack; the rest of the time she was sandwiched between Irma's waist and the belt of her fanny pack.

My blisters hurt at the start, but after walking for a while I quit feeling the pain. The nerve endings must have become exhausted from firing so much. So far so good, I thought.

We stopped in several small churches along the way, lit candles, and sang "Ultreya." When we reached Larreule we took a lunch break, sitting across the street from a school with a sign on it urging solidarity for the ongoing teachers' strike. We took off our socks during our lunch break to cool off our feet. Although I didn't realize it, I had damp feet when I put my socks and boots back on.

A van was parked by the side of the road; soon two familiar couples joined the driver. When our paths crossed, we struck up a conversation, and they explained that they took turns driving the van with their luggage and providing lunch for each other.

"Why are you walking the Chemin?" I asked.

The person who spoke the best English replied, "We wanted to do something together, and we got the idea of walking the Chemin in stages. Le Puy to Lectoure, Lectoure to Saint-Jean-Pied-de-Port. We scout the route and make our reservations at least six months in advance." They planned to continue into Spain and wondered how to make reservations. We gave them some advice before continuing down the road.

In Uzan a scallop-shell-decorated sign on a gate offered hospitality: "Pilgrims going to Compostelle, if you want coffee or tea, come in and serve yourselves." Eager for a break we walked around the house to the garage, which had been converted into a pilgrims' rest stop. There were chairs, a table, and an assortment of drinks, including tea, coffee, and water. Gratitude for the generosity of the Chemin.

A poem was taped on top of a tin box with a cake inside:

"Sur le Chemin, il y a du monde devant, et il y a toujours du monde derriere." (On the 'Road of Life' there are some people ahead of us—and always some behind.)

We rested in the welcome shade, drinking water and eating a piece of cake. Honey Bunny had a chair to herself and Irma posed her as if she were eating cake too. We took a photo. There was a "kitty" for a free-will offering. After leaving a donation, we started walking again.

Centuries ago, Arzacq-Arraziguet was at the boundary between Bearn and old France; as we walked deeper into the Bearn I fancied that this historic separation was still visible. Rural architecture and Chemin waymarkings varied from what we had seen before. The new signposts gave the estimated time to walk to the next village (based on fifteen minutes per kilometer) and clear directions. In addition, meter-high stone posts engraved with a scallop shell appeared periodically; their presence affirmed that we were on the pilgrimage road to Saint-Jacques de Compostelle. Once again, I could almost feel Saint James walking beside me.

The attractive houses we walked past were often constructed of rows of rounded stones set in grey mortar, with an occasional row of flat bricks or larger stones, creating a stacked sandwich appearance. They reminded me of Anasazi ruins in Chaco Canyon in New Mexico; those indigenous people had also used flat stones to stabilize rows of small round ones. Dormer windows adorned the steeply sloping red-tile roofs. The houses were tidy and well kept, with fragrant flower gardens.

That day our route included rocky trails, hilly country lanes, and relatively flat country roads. Sometimes the Chemin was lined with blossom-filled hedges. Gorgeous butterflies—some iridescent blue, some red and black, one with two "eyes" on each wing, yellow ones, white ones—fluttered alongside. One kind of butterfly and then another predominated, as if each species had its own territory.

The day had gotten warm and we were tired, but at last we reached Pomps, where we were to call our hosts in Morlanne, a few kilometers off the Chemin. As we walked into town to find a phone booth, we passed a small château with an octagonal tower. A young couple strolling up the walk met us at the gate. They were from Chicago, staying with their friends who owned the château. They offered to show us around outside and we eagerly accepted.

What to us was a picturesque castle was in fact a family burden. The château has been in their friend's family for 400 years but it had been abandoned for most of the last four decades. It would cost a fortune to restore, they explained, which the current owners (a young couple with two small children) did not have. There was no heat so it was uninhabitable in winter. In summer it was chilly. But their friends couldn't bring themselves to sell the place. They were wondering if opening a *table d'hôtes* would be a successful way to bring in money. We all thought it would work. After all, who wouldn't be interested in eating in a château, if the price was reasonable?

Waving goodbye, we walked into town and called our hosts in Morlanne. We waited at the seventeenth-century Église de Saint-Jacques, admiring the statue of the saint, until Madame Geyre came and drove us to our Clés-Vacance *chambres d'hôtes*. There was a highly recommended *chambres d'hôtes* across the street, but its three rooms had been reserved long before—perhaps by the walkers with the van.

Our *chambres d'hôtes* was a renovated stone building that included the owners' own apartment. It was modern and sparkling clean, with a kitchen, dining room, and two bedrooms, each with private bathroom and shower (the British called this *en suite*, for some reason using French, not English, to describe hygienic arrangements). After the previous night's decrepit lodging this was luxurious.

Madame offered to do our laundry so we sorted through our clothes and I brought the dirty ones to her. I asked her if she could make something special for Gary's birthday dinner. With such late notice, she was doubtful.

That day was Gary's sixty-sixth birthday. The weather had been beautiful, and we had walked twenty kilometers across rural France without his knee causing him pain. He had developed a red oozing rash on his calves, however, that resembled a heat rash. But even that didn't bother him. He had never expected to be so happy and healthy.

Sitting around in our shared living room we discussed again how easy it was to have expectations and judgments.

"In 1982," I mused, "we made no reservations and were grateful for shelter, no matter what it looked like. The pilgrimage was a process of letting go. Of doing without."

Gary said, "But in 1997 when we walked the Camino we made reservations in advance. I felt more comfortable that way."

I added, "And we've had to do that on the French Chemin as well. What I've noticed is that we make reservations, we have a place to stay—and then we have expectations about what it should look like, how clean it should be, what amenities we expect to have."

Irma commented, "Maybe the solution is not to make reservations."

"That might solve one issue but it creates another, so it's a trade-off," I replied. "It's harder to walk carrying a heavy pack, and we need reservations so Factage knows where to take our bags."

Irma was adamant. "In Spain I want to walk with my backpack and not make reservations. That feels like the right way to do it."

This dispute wasn't going to be resolved. Actually, it wasn't a dispute, it was a difference in perspective. What really mattered was that we gave meaning to the pain, the discomfort, the effort we expended each day.

We decided to stroll around the village, beginning with a visit to the fortified church across the street from our lodgings. There were narrow slits high up on in the four towers, presumably for military defense. It seemed strange to mix warfare and religion, but in the Middle Ages (as well as now), those two often went together.

Most of the shops were closed, their windows covered. Madame had informed us that there was no *supermarché* in town, so we would not be able to purchase supplies for the next day.

That evening we gathered in the dining room for Gary's birthday dinner, the second in two days. It began with a Basque *pipérade*, an omelet filled with sweet red and green peppers, tomatoes, and onions, followed by a delicious *daube* (slow-braised beef stew with carrots, onions, and dark gravy). We hadn't known if the omelet was the entire meal, so we were quite full by the time the *daube* appeared, but we managed to eat all of it. Then came a course of luscious Camembert and ripe goat cheeses presented on a platter. In honor of Gary's birthday Madame surprised us with ice cream and cake.

Wednesday, May 28, 2003. From near Pomps to Maslacq. 18.5 kilometers (11.5 miles).

Monsieur Geyre drove us back from Morlanne to Pomps, where we could buy lunch supplies. He dropped us off at a house with a large open garage; inside, a vendor sold fruit, cheese, sausage, and toothpaste from a well-stocked van. Unfortunately, the vendor had no bread. He told us the nearest place to buy it was nine kilometers away in Arthez-de-Béarn, a town on our route.

The trail became hilly again. Bushes lined the path and trees covered the neighboring hills. The snow-capped Pyrenees spread out like low-lying clouds on the horizon. They didn't look much closer than they had a few days before, but in about a week we would be climbing through them from the foot of the pass at Saint-Jean-Pied-de-Port.

A mixture of fear, awe, and gratitude flowed through me. I imagined myself a medieval pilgrim seeing the Pyrenees for the first time after months of walking. I thought again about continuing to Santiago. What would it feel like to walk through the Pyrenees with Santiago instead of Roncesvalles as our goal? How the journey beckoned!

Gary pointed out that the Camino in June would be too hot and too crowded. In truth, I didn't *really* want to continue on to Santiago, I just wanted to savor the idea. For a moment, just a moment, I had had the wonderful taste in my mouth of being a pilgrim who continued on, always on—Ultreya, ultreya—to the far-distant goal of Compostela.

Some two kilometers before Arthez-de-Béarn we passed the Chapelle Caubin, but since we were on a mission to find bread, we didn't stop. Arthez-de-Béarn was a sinuous town that stretched out nearly two kilometers along a ridge. As we neared the commercial center, we shared greetings and information with familiar pilgrims: Where was the nearest pharmacy? Where were a *boulangerie* and a good restaurant?

We chose a café and sat outside to avoid the acrid cigarette fumes inside at the bar. The *menu* choices were typically Spanish:

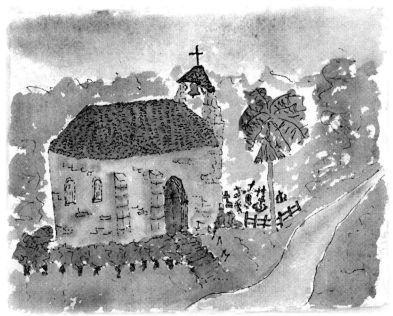

Chapelle Caubin

an appetizer of air-dried *Serrano* ham, followed by fried steak and French fries. This was a good introduction for Irma and Wilhelm to the food they would find on the Camino. Even the architecture reminded me of the Spanish Basque country: massive buildings with stone trim around the windows and doors.

While we waited for lunch to be served, Irma made reservations for the next four nights, which would get us to Saint-Jean-Pied-de-Port. We had different ideas of how we wanted to spend our time there. Gary and I wanted to visit our friends Alan and Malou, my saviors from 1982, who had driven Gary and me to the top of the pass in 1997.

Wilhelm and Irma wanted to spend the evening with fellow pilgrims. They wanted to see them disembark at the train station, then walk in the streets in the evening and share the enthusiasm of soon-to-be pilgrims. A friend had told them this was a not-to-be-missed experience, but it was one Gary and I looked forward to missing. Unlike Wilhelm and Irma, we were nearing the end of our pilgrimage. Instead of excitement I felt a nagging disappointment.

I called Alan and Malou; Alan sounded pleased to hear my voice after so many years. I explained we would be in Saint-Jean on Sunday and invited them for dinner. He said they would look forward to seeing us.

Lunch arrived. While we ate, we discussed how to cross the Pyrenees together. I suggested that we stay in a combined *chambres d'hôtes* and *gîte* located partway up the mountain pass. That would make the stiff ascent—twenty-plus kilometers up a 3000-foot gradient—more manageable. Irma telephoned, but the *chambres d'hôtes* was full. We would either have to stay in the *gîte*, problematic since we lacked sleeping bags, or we would have to make the journey from Saint-Jean to Roncesvalles in one day. Pilgrims did it all the time, but it was a feat of endurance. Gary and I wouldn't make it. Irma and Wilhelm thought they could.

Our heavy lunch had time to digest while we made our phone calls, so we started walking again. My blisters were now soft and tender, filled with fluid that created intense pressure on my heels with every step. When I walked the Camino in 1982 I had had blisters inside of blisters and the pain had been excruciating. This time the pain wasn't so bad. At least not yet.

Rather than following the GR 65 we took a purported shortcut, the Cami Salíe—the prehistoric (and medieval) salt route through the valley. The country lane was flat and shadeless, though trees beckoned in nearby fields. There was a refinery in the distance, which several pilgrims had told us belched foul smells. We didn't notice. All we felt was heat.

It was 100° F under the blistering sun. We stumbled down the road in a daze. The asphalt began to melt. I poured water on my back to cool off, remembering the advice of the *hospitalera* in Saint-Antoine. We staggered on in silence, putting one foot after the other. At last we reached the Hôtel-Restaurant Maugouber in Maslacq.

As soon as we walked inside the cool reception area I began to feel better. The thick stone walls insulated against the heat. Our attractive and pleasantly cool room on the second floor had a small balcony that faced a lovely garden and a large swimming pool. Our room had a bidet, a shower, two beds, and a TV. Out of curiosity—or old habits unexpectedly surfacing—I turned it on. For a few minutes I watched a CNN program in which Amnesty International condemned the US "War on Terror" for making the world less safe and causing the loss of civil liberties around the world. With a shudder, I turned off the TV.

Walking our pilgrimage road through deepest France, we had paid scant attention to the world outside. Occasionally we had conversed about the war in Iraq and President Bush with fellow pilgrims or innkeepers. We simply said he was insane and shook our heads in bewilderment. We were pilgrims walking the Chemin, praying for peace. That seemed the most effective way to combat such destructive policies.

It was time to tend to my feet. I took off my boots. I was afraid to look. The rows of tiny red dots had merged into huge, throbbing, fluid-filled blisters on both heels. Since both heels were equally afflicted, I hadn't favored one foot over the other, which was a blessing. Altering my gait would have led to other problems.

Using a sterilized needle and thread I punctured the blisters, but they immediately reappeared. I cleaned them carefully, left a tail of thread on either side of each blister to help it drain, and covered them with loose gauze and tape. Advice differs on how to deal with blisters. Some authorities warn against leaving a thread dangling because it can become a source of infection; others claim it is the best way to keep a blister open and draining, which will hasten healing. All agree that the best advice is to avoid getting any.

Later, we sat near the pool, enjoying the colorful roses that bloomed in the garden. The landscaping included pines and palms, cedar and cypress, bamboo and cacti, and fruit trees of all sorts. Other guests were also enjoying the garden. The melodious sound of French flowed over me, peppered with bits of German, larded with Dutch. Languages blended harmoniously into a soup of sound, lulling me to sleep until Irma and Wilhelm sat down beside us.

While we rested in the cool shaded garden, we again discussed our plans for climbing out of Saint-Jean-Pied-de-Port. A few days earlier I had been thrilled with the idea of climbing through the Pyrenees, but now I wondered whether the whole conversation was moot. Would I be able to walk the Chemin the next day, let alone climb the Pyrenees?

In 1997 I had had similar blisters and had stopped walking for five days so they would heal and I could recover from heat exhaustion. This time we didn't have five days to wait, not if we wanted to walk with the Webers. Not if we wanted to have time to visit Danielle and Collette, the Loire Valley, and Paris.

I realized that unlike the previous year—and unlike our other pilgrimages—we were trying to fit our pilgrimage into other priorities, rather than making it the central event. Instead of reflecting on this insight, however, I struck up a conversation with some of the pilgrims sitting at the table next to us.

One of the women was German, married to a Frenchman for forty years. When she saw my bandaged heels, she commiserated in English. Her companion, who had very bad bunions, explained that she wrapped a self-sticking bandage around her feet to keep from getting blisters. Everybody had a theory about how to avoid blisters, including Irma, who swore by a certain kind of sock. But even Irma and Wilhelm had blisters.

Another woman suggested Compeed. When I said that I had tried it already but it hadn't helped, she informed me that I should have used it as soon as I noticed the blisters forming. She thought it would have helped the blisters dry out at that early stage, something I'd never heard. Putting Compeed on after I already had blisters, someone else asserted, would result in major loss of skin when it peeled off. There was much advice, but all of it retrospective. What to do now was my question, and the consensus was that "now" was too late.

In 1997 we had met a Spanish pilgrim in his mid-seventies. His feet were so badly damaged that a doctor had wrapped them in bandages and insisted that he quit walking. We saw him the next day hobbling up the pass to O Cebreiro. "Santiago will take care of me," he had said with a faith-filled smile. Maybe so.

Time had passed quickly while we rested in the shade and chatted with fellow pilgrims. Dinner was being served. I ate too much—as if I were afraid I would run out of energy on the Chemin. I joked that I had a very efficient metabolism since even with all the exercise I was still gaining weight.

I brought Honey Bunny down from our room, curled up in Gary's hat.

The waitress saw her and asked, "Is he your 'fetish'?" She thought Honey Bunny was a boy.

I smiled enigmatically.

"Does he sleep with you?" she wanted to know.

"Oh yes," I said.

"Oh, the three of you—oolala!" she exclaimed.

She went on to say that Honey Bunny was the best of all of us. She wanted to take him home for the weekend. Her mother-in-law and husband were both gone, she explained, so she would sleep with Honey Bunny. We laughed. Irma looked miffed, however, and grabbed Honey Bunny to take up to her room for the night.

Back in our room I asked Gary if he wanted to continue walking even if I couldn't. He said that would be all right, unless I needed him to stay with me. I had to rephrase the question several times to find out if he *wanted* to keep walking even if I didn't, which was a different response than "that would be all right." Sometimes it was hard for him to express his own desires, although at other times he could be adamant.

When we finally understood each other, I was delighted to learn that he wanted to continue on the Chemin even if I couldn't. Walking the Chemin was not just something he was doing with or for me; it was also something he was doing for himself.

"How's your knee holding out?"

He rubbed it. "It's doing okay. It's good for about twenty kilometers, and we walked a little less today."

My ankles were swelling again and my neck started to go into spasm. Gary massaged it. I sighed. "I'm worried you'll leave me for someone without all these malfunctioning body parts. But be warned. If you do, you'll never find anyone else to take you on such excruciating adventures!"

He laughed and gave me a big hug.

Thursday, May 29, 2003. Maslacq to Navarrenx. 20 kilometers (12.5 miles). Gary walked; I took Factage.

Gary and I discussed whether I should try walking to Navarrenx. I had finally managed to get my blisters drained, more or less, but my left heel was very tender. I had put Compeed over the blisters to protect them but that didn't stop the pain. If it became excruciating while I walked to Navarrenx, then what? I wouldn't be able to walk the final part of our pilgrimage of gratitude.

We considered options. If I didn't walk the next four days my blisters would heal enough for me to climb through the Pyrenees. That seemed like a reasonable plan but I still wanted to walk. Gary left the decision up to me, of course, but he reminded me that I often tried to do more than was advisable. The Chemin was giving me the opportunity to do things differently.

Still undecided, I put on my boots and walked around the hotel, feeling some discomfort. But striding around the hotel for a few minutes was quite different from walking twenty kilometers.

On previous pilgrimages I had walked with the pain, but this time I wasn't interested in putting myself through so much trauma. It didn't seem healthy. Call me a wimp or call me wise, but I wasn't interested in self-mortification. I wanted to *heal* my body, not hurt it. Saint Jacques didn't require me to walk every kilometer—nor did I.

I decided not to walk. While Gary and our friends walked the Camino, I would go to mass. The desk clerk had told me that today was the Day of the Ascension of Jesus, so there would be a special mass in the parish church. And then I would catch a ride on Factage, the modern equivalent of a passing oxcart. Gratitude, gratitude.

When Gary, Wilhelm, and Irma left early in the morning, it was already hot. The hôtel-restaurant was closed for the day, although they let me stay while I waited for my early afternoon lift from Factage. For a while I sat in back in the beautiful garden listening to chirping birds. The pool sparkled. The roses were a little past their prime but still lovely. I wrote in my journal:

> *I've learned to look French people in the eyes and listen intently when they speak. Then I understand them much better. Something really is communicated through the glance.*

> *Last night my ankles swelled badly. I don't know why, so I am worried that the swelling could be related to the*

possibility of a recurrence of cancer. Note the cautious "could be" and "possibility." But I don't know what to do.

Maybe it's just like getting blisters. I tried to avoid them but I got them anyway. Maybe that was another lesson of the Chemin: things happen. You do what you can to avoid blisters or cancer, you try to be vigilant—but ultimately, all you can do is have faith and find meaning in whatever happens.

Bless all that we receive, including not walking. Gratitude for time by myself. Gratitude for whatever life brings.

I put away my journal and went out, mailed postcards, and bought lunch supplies at the only open grocery store. Because it was a holiday, all the other shops and restaurants were closed. Cars kept pulling up to the grocery and people hurried in to buy supplies before it shut its doors at noon.

Then I went to mass, sitting near the doorway so I could leave if I felt the urge. Two swallows flew in and landed on the flower-covered crucifix. The music director sang and led the congregation, her graceful hands demonstrating the tempo and pitch. I sat in silence, then left after half an hour.

I learned later from the hotel staff that this "visitation of the birds" had never happened before. The event quickly turned into a modern miracle: the birds had come to celebrate the Ascension of Jesus. "All acts and blessings are sanctified by You O my Lord," according to one of the prayers I had recited during the mass—which was just another way of making meaning out of seemingly random events.

The day was breathtakingly hot, given that this was not the Sahara: it was late May in southwestern France, near the Pyrenees. According to my thermometer it was 113° F in the sun on the patio in front of the hotel, 93° F or so in the shade. Inside the hotel, because of the thick stone walls, it was a temperate 79° F. I had made the right decision to stay behind. I learned that hundreds, perhaps thousands, of people were dying all over France because of the unprecedented heat wave.

The next day was supposed to be even hotter. Although just that morning I had hoped I could walk the final day through the Pyrenees, now I began to wonder if maybe we should give up and return later in fall or next spring.

I sat at a table outside in the shade in front of the hotel, writing in my journal and giving directions to exhausted pilgrims who straggled by, looking for the *gîte d'étape communal.* One couple asked where they could find water. There was no municipal fountain, so I directed them to the grocery store. A group of pilgrims walked by, apparently in the wrong direction; they returned a little later and headed the other way down the road. The extreme heat dazed everyone.

By 2:00 p.m. Factage had not yet arrived. I hoped Gary and the Webers had reached Navarrenx before it had gotten so unbearably hot. I moved inside and waited in the relatively cool room with the baggage.

At last Factage arrived. The driver was hot and tired; his car lacked air conditioning. About half an hour later he dropped me off at the *gîte d'étape* Charbel in Navarrenx. Gary, Irma, and Wilhelm were already there, relaxing at a picnic table outside the main building, drinking something cool under a large shade umbrella. Gary jumped up when he saw me and gave me a hug. Irma and Wilhelm raised their drinks in a silent toast.

"We wondered when you would get here!" Gary exclaimed.

"How was the Chemin?" I asked.

"Terrible," Gary replied, shaking his head. "The asphalt was bubbling on the road and there was no shade. You wouldn't have made it. I hardly made it. Near the end I was in an altered state. I didn't know if I was alone or with Wilhelm and Irma—I didn't even know where I was. I thought I would pass out by the side of the road." Then he smiled. "But after resting for a few hours in this wonderful *gîte* I feel revived."

We went into the main building, where several pilgrims were relaxing in the refreshingly cool living room. After greeting the people we knew we continued to our room. The proprietor had given Gary the "Bridal Room," perhaps because it had a large bed and a private bath. I sat down on the comfortable bed and listened to frogs croaking outside.

Gary showed me photos he had taken of terraced fields with the imposing Pyrenees in the background and of the Église de Saint-Jacques at La Sauvelade. The church is all that is left of a monastery founded in 1128, sacked by the Huguenots in 1569, restored around 1630, and sold during the French Revolution. It is a marvel that anything remains, but inside is a gilded statue of Saint James. A real scallop shell hangs from a cord around his neck. In his right hand he holds a bent hiking staff.

We walked outside and Gary showed me around the *gîte,* named after Charbel, a nineteenth-century Lebanese Maronite† saint. A wall surrounds the *gîte,* whose extensive grounds include a stream, two spring-fed ponds filled with reeds and frogs, and a bridge that leads over one of the ponds to a diminutive stone circle. The *gîte* consists of a new two-story building with private rooms and a dormitory, and an older building where the owners prepare meals and from which they run the business.

We walked through an arch and over the bridge to a circle of twelve small standing stones with a tree in the middle. Farther on was a dolmen (stone table), with a menhir (large upright stone) behind that.

"Manée, the owner, is from Brittany. That's why they erected the stones," Gary explained. Brittany is a region in northwest France famous for its variety of megaliths, including the miles-long alignments at Carnac.

While circumambulating the standing stones, we decided not to continue the pilgrimage. How quickly our plans had changed. Just a few days before I had fantasized about walking all the way to Santiago—and now we had abruptly stopped at Navarrenx.

Next time. There would be a next time, I consoled myself, and my mood immediately lightened. Our pilgrimage of gratitude wasn't over yet; once again, it was just on pause. We would complete the pilgrimage the following April or May. I would be able to look forward to it for the entire year and to practice the many lessons I had learned.

We went to tell the Webers, who were sorry but not surprised. Since this was our last evening together we again talked at length about the Spanish Camino. I explained how to make hotel reservations if they chose to do so. They might want to learn some Spanish but if not, they could get along with French, German, and English.

After examining a map showing the intimidating elevation gain to the pass above Saint-Jean-Pied-de-Port, Irma and Wilhelm decided to call the *gîte* on the mountainside again. This time they made reservations to stay in the dormitory even though they didn't have sleeping sacks or sheets. It would all work out. Everything worked out just the way it was supposed to, whether we knew it or not.

Gary and I decided to rent a car, go back to Rodez to pick up the bag we left behind at the hotel, visit the Aubrac to see the wildflowers and then spend time with Danielle and Collette in the Loire while we waited for our house remodel to be completed.

Everything fell easily into place. We made a phone call to AutoEurope in the States and half an hour later we received a fax confirmation that a rental car would be waiting for us in Pau the next morning.

By chance—or synchronicity—we discovered a *Miam Miam Dodo* for the Spanish Camino for sale at the *gîte*. We bought a copy and showed the Webers how to interpret it. Since I spoke Spanish, I made reservations for the Webers in Roncesvalles for Tuesday night. I was glad to be able to help them as they had helped us.

Some twenty pilgrims gathered for dinner. While we ate, someone's cell phone rang, playing the "Toréador Song" from Bizet's *Car-
men*. We all burst spontaneously into song. Honey Bunny joined us
for this last supper, but suddenly she disappeared. A balding Frenchman at the far end of the table had kidnapped her and was pretending to feed her. Ah, the child-like innocence of pilgrims on the
Chemin. Everyone laughed except Irma.

Irma and Wilhelm were both sad that we were leaving. So were
we, but my disappointment was tempered with excitement. We
would return the following year!

Friday, May 30, 2003. Navarrenx to Pau
by taxi, and then on by rented car.

After an early breakfast we wished "Buen Camino" to our dear
friends. Honey Bunny waved goodbye; Irma wiped away a tear. I
whispered to Wilhelm we would try to find another flop-eared plush
bunny for Irma.

Our taxi arrived at 9:00 a.m.; a half-hour later we were in Pau.
We rented the car and reached Aire-sur-l'Adour at noon, just in time
to go to a sporting goods store where I bought a pair of sports sandals that wouldn't rub against the edge of my heels. We also bought
cheese, bread, and fruit for lunch, just before all the shops closed.
Everything was perfect, "as good as it gets," even if it was nothing
like what I had expected it to be.

We picnicked on the bank of l'Adour, then drove over to the Église de Sainte-Quitterie, which we hadn't seen during our overnight
stay in Aire-sur-l'Adour four days earlier. Four days ago. It seemed
like much longer. That was another feature of the Chemin: so much
happened in so little time and space.

Sainte Quitterie is the patron saint of Gascony. Medieval pilgrims traveling to Compostela visited her shrine and carried tales
of her miracles up and down the Camino. We were continuing our
pilgrimage by stopping there, even though we were going home instead of to Santiago.

Sainte Quitterie was a fourth-century Christian princess who
refused to marry a local Visigoth lord; instead, she ran away and

began performing miracles. The jilted lord found her and cut off her head. Her body then picked up its head and, head in hand, she walked over to the site where she wanted to be buried. A miraculous fountain immediately sprang forth. Her legend of martyrdom is similar to the legend of Sainte Foy, who is also associated with a healing spring. I wondered how many ancient goddesses had been renamed and baptized, how many ancient holy wells had been Christianized over the millennia.

The exterior of the medieval church was badly abused by wars and weather. We paid a fee to visit the eleventh-century crypt, originally a shrine to the Roman god Mars. Roman paving stones, some decorated with laurel leaves, cover the floor. The dark, dank crypt contains a chapel to Saint Desiré, its eleventh-century frescoes still more or less intact, and others to Saint Roch and Saint Philibert. Across from them is Sainte Quitterie's remarkable fourth-century sarcophagus of polished white marble, exquisitely carved with scenes from the Hebrew Bible and the New Testament.

What is now called Sainte Quitterie's sacred spring, originally dedicated to naiads, can still be seen outside the church. I was intrigued that the healing qualities of the spring continued, despite the management turnover.

By 5:00 p.m. we were back in Rodez. It had taken less than a day, including shopping and sightseeing, to drive a distance that had taken us three weeks to walk. At the Hôtel de la Tour Maje, we again checked into Room 301. Purely by chance, Christine assured us.

We went shopping and I replaced my hiking attire with a summery outfit, transforming myself from pilgrim to tourist. It was an effortless transition in some ways but wrenching in others. This was not how I had expected to end our pilgrimage.

I promised myself that while we waited for our final journey on the Chemin I would continue to let go of expectations and judgments. I would embrace with wide-open arms whatever life sent my way. After all, I was held in God's hands.

September 2004 Pilgrimage

Early September 2004. Back to France via England.

In early September we returned to France to finish the final stage of our pilgrimage of gratitude. We had hoped to go in spring but Gary's son, Greg, and his wife, Kristin, were expecting their second child in late April or early May. We wanted to be on the same continent for that event. Summer would be too hot for me to walk, so we scheduled our return for early fall. This gave us extra time to get in shape for the journey—but once again we had other priorities. Besides, we told ourselves, "How hard can a week-long walk be?"

I had spent the past year "on pause," always aware of the unfinished Chemin. That awareness was a mixed blessing. I was tired of thinking about the pilgrimage, tired of thinking about cancer. I was eager to get on with the rest of my life—so eager, in fact, that I decided not to take a travel journal on this final stage of our pilgrimage. I told myself I wanted to be "in the moment," but I really wanted to be in the future: cancer definitely in the past, pilgrimage of gratitude complete.

This time we traveled not only with Honey Bunny but also with her new companion, Brown Bear. We had found him during our search the previous summer for a flop-eared bunny for Irma. Unable to locate one (Honey Bunny smugly assured us they had "broken the mold" after making her), we instead had purchased two small teddy bears that matched Honey Bunny in size (about 13" tall) and style. We mailed one to Irma and kept the other for ourselves.

When we got home and took Honey Bunny's sweater out of storage, we discovered that she and Brown Bear had matching sweaters with the same logo at the bottom, "Lola et Basil." They were, indeed, meant to be together. I took this as a sign that we were still in the flow of life, that synchronicities were still occurring. The events in our lives had meaning—or at any rate, I chose to make meaning out of seeming coincidences. I comforted myself with this perspective, just as I comforted myself by snuggling with Honey Bunny and Brown Bear.

Honey Bunny was a reminder of a meaningful intervention in my life (even if I hadn't understood its import immediately). She and Brown Bear were also opportunities for me to break out of a restricting view of what was acceptable behavior, to take risks, to not care so much what other people thought. They were opportunities for play and playfulness. They reminded me of the interconnected web of existence and that *everything* is alive—something children haven't yet forgotten—including plush animals who became enlivened through ongoing interaction. They reminded me that we choose how we look at the world. As they found their voices (Gary and I spoke for them but, in fact, they spoke for us) they leavened our habitual seriousness.

We made our plans and flew not to France but to England, where we had arranged to study with Sig Lonegren, an expert on geomancy (earth energies) and dowsing. We spent five days with him in Glastonbury and surrounding areas, visiting stone circles, Avebury, and Bath cathedral. Under his guidance, we learned how to dowse for underground energy lines and use a pendulum. On our own in Glastonbury, we explored the abbey ruins and the Chalice Well Gardens, sites rich with intriguing Grail and Arthurian associations.

As Companions of The Chalice Well, we were able to sleep in Little Saint Michael's Guesthouse and wander through the gardens at night. Our stay coincided with the one night of the month, however, when the flow of rusty-red spring water was diverted so that the garden's fountains could be cleaned. Nonetheless, it was a blessing to walk quietly through the grounds after the hordes of visitors had left.

Our next stop was St. Ives, on the northern coast of Cornwall. It was to be our base camp for walking the twelve-and-one-half-mile Saint Michael's Way. I had a small booklet that described the footpath, which extends from nearby Lelant to Saint Michael's Mount on the southern coast. Medieval Irish and Welsh pilgrims on their way to Santiago supposedly had favored Saint Michael's Way because the day-long journey on foot enabled them to avoid sailing the rough seas at Land's End. We hoped the trail, waymarked with the European Union's stylized scallop shell, would be a gentle yet authentic prelude to the long hike ahead of us.

Although we expected St. Ives to be a quiet little seaside town, we quickly discovered that it is one of the most popular tourist destinations in England. It wouldn't be the only thing that wasn't what we expected.

The next morning, following the directions in the Saint Michael's Way brochure, we went by taxi a few miles south to the church of St. Uny in Lelant, located on an estuary to the southeast of St. Ives. Once there we were supposed to head back north along the coast, then turn west and climb assorted hills to Knill's Steeple. It seemed counterintuitive that pilgrims would have walked in a direction that led them away from their goal to the south, but that's what the directions indicated. Despite my misgivings, we started back up the sandy trail.

I felt surprisingly nostalgic when I saw the scallop shell waymarkers again. Soon they would be leading us to the end of our pilgrimage in France.

The weather was chilly and blustery.

"At least it's not horribly hot," I said, trying to make the best of it.

"You're right, there," Gary replied, as he braced himself against the wind.

Daunted but not discouraged, we made our way up the trail to Knill's Steeple, a singularly unattractive granite pyramid built as a mausoleum by John Knill in the mid-eighteenth century and overlooking Carbis Bay. Knill had been mayor of St. Ives in 1767 as well as an audacious smuggler. Who would have thought you could be both? In honor of himself, he established a trust to pay for a ceremony at his steeple every five years on Saint James's Day, July 25. This celebration involved "ten young girls, two widows and a fiddler processing to the Steeple" to perform a dance and sing the 100th Psalm. It was hard to imagine such a festive event at this dreary site. I wondered if it still was celebrated or whether the funds had long run out.

When we tried to leave the mausoleum, we became almost hopelessly confused. The scallop-shell waymarkers were nowhere to be found, and we lost all sense of direction as we pushed our way through shoulder-high brush. At last we freed ourselves from the entrapping vegetation and struggled on to the Iron Age hill fort at Trencrom Hill—or rather, we saw the archeological site in the distance.

At that point we decided not to continue following the way-marked path. No self-respecting pilgrim would have followed such a route, nor were some of the touted sights present in the Middle Ages. Saint Michael's Way might be a fine day-hike designed to offer scenic views and interesting monuments, but it was not a tra-ditional pilgrims' route, of that I was sure, even if it was waymarked with the scallop shell of Saint James.

Worn out from fighting the biting wind and backtracking sev-eral times to find the trail, we stumbled onto a road. A few hun-dred feet away was a large restaurant, its parking lot full of cars. We hurried over to find food and shelter. Huge sizzling haunches of roasted meat were piled high on the carvery table, and the dining hall overflowed with noisy, solid English citizens tucking into heap-ing plates of food. While we tried to warm up by drinking hot tea, the bartender called a cab to take us back to St. Ives. This did not bode well for our pilgrimage, I thought, but after all, this was Saint Michael's Way, not Saint James'.

Tuesday – Wednesday, September 14 – 15, 2004. St. Ives to Bordeaux to Aire-sur-l'Adour. Too many kilometers to count.

Eager to get on with our pilgrimage of gratitude, we took a train to Bristol and the following day flew to Bordeaux. The next day we traveled by train and bus to Aire-sur-l'Adour. We had decided to begin at Aire-sur-l'Adour rather than at Navarrenx so that we could get into condition before climbing the Pyrenees. Besides, I wanted to walk the parts of the Camino I had missed the year before because of heat, blisters, and exhaustion.

Thursday - Saturday, September 16 - 18, 2004. Aire-sur-l'Adour to Maslacq. 70 kilometers (43.5 miles).

After three difficult, exhausting days we reached Maslacq, where I had a nagging sense of déjà vu. I had an excruciating blister on the striking edge of my left heel. How this could have happened—and happen so quickly—I did not understand, since after last year's debacle I had taken extensive preventive action. I had bought a slightly larger pair of hiking shoes and had worn them on several hikes to break them in. I had also bought the high-tech German socks that Irma and Wilhelm recommended. Boots and socks had seemed to fit just fine. In addition, I had regularly slathered my feet with salve each day on the Chemin to make them more slippery. Nevertheless, I had suddenly developed a huge, squishy blister. To make matters worse, I had some kind of vague malaise that was sapping my energy.

I was dumbfounded. My precautions had been for naught. I wondered why this was happening at Maslacq, the town where I had quit walking the year before. Was it serendipity or synchronicity? And if the latter, what did it mean?

Sunday, September 19, 2004. Maslacq to Navarrenx. 20 kilometers (12.5 miles)—but only a few on foot.

When we started out the next day, I was in agonizing pain and feeling quite weak—but I was determined to finish this pilgrimage of gratitude. As I limped down the Chemin, however, I realized that I just couldn't do it. It was one thing to be determined, quite another to acknowledge one's limitations. Gary and I agreed we would call a taxi as soon as we found a phone booth, even though it was only mid-morning and we had only walked a few kilometers.

Our route led down a country road lined with massive stone houses on either side. As we passed one, a man working in a well-kept garden called out, "Bonjour!"

We replied, "Bonjour! Hello!"

Wiping his hands on his trousers he came over to greet us. Speaking perfect English, he inquired about our pilgrimage. Then he introduced us to his son, who was working in the garden with him, and invited us into his home. Rarely do French people invite strangers into their homes and offer them hospitality. The generous offer couldn't have been more appreciated, given my pain and fatigue.

Soon his wife was bustling around offering us refreshments while he showed us photos of the French Caribbean, where he had lived. Before we knew what had happened he had called his parents, who lived nearby, to come over and meet us. He seemed genuinely delighted to be interacting with us. Did our pilgrimage status made us special or was he just eager to speak English? I didn't ask.

Did we need anything? Could his wife do our laundry? I hesitantly explained that I was not feeling well so we needed to call a taxi to take us to Navarrenx. Immediately our host offered to drive us there. After spending an appropriate amount of time visiting with his family, we said goodbye and piled into his car. Fifteen minutes later we were there.

As we got out of the car in front of our hotel, I asked our host his name. "Jacques," he replied, with a mysterious smile. Then he drove off.

Gary and I checked into the Hôtel-Restaurant du Commerce and I passed out on the bed. When I woke up, we discussed Plan B (not walking for a while), since Plan A (walking the Chemin in a week) was clearly not going to work. If I didn't irritate the blister on my heel, I thought it would heal in about five days.

Last year on the Chemin we hadn't had five days to wait—or at least we didn't think we had, since we wanted to visit Collette and Danielle and go sightseeing. This year, our only commitment was to complete our pilgrimage of gratitude. To conclude it as soon as possible would have been preferable, but we would have to be patient.

Perhaps this time the Chemin was teaching us patience, a lesson that would help me as I waited three more years before I could be declared cancer-free. Or maybe it was teaching me, once again, to let go of expectations.

Monday, September 20, 2004. Navarrenx.

We spent another day in Navarrenx, where I bought a pair of walking sandals that didn't rub against my heel. Déjà vu. Bored and restless, we explored the town. We visited a church with a Cagot entrance, similar to that at Routges; intrigued, I went on a quest to learn more about this ostracized minority. The local bookstore offered several books devoted to the subject. I was not the only one who found this mysterious people fascinating.

Since neither my blister nor my general malaise had improved, we activated Plan B: rent a car for a week and drive into Spain. Just as we had the year before, we arranged to take a taxi to Pau to pick up a rental car the following day.

Tuesday - Friday, September 21 - 24, 2004. Navarrenx to Haro. Too many kilometers to count and all by car.

We planned to stay on the Camino de Santiago or its variants, traveling by car to Spanish pilgrimage sites we wouldn't have visited on foot, including Jaca, San Juan de Siresa (located in the nearby Valley of Hecho on one of the ancient, original Caminos across the Pyrenees), San Juan de la Peña, San Millán, and the Monasterio de Leyre. We told ourselves we would still be on pilgrimage even though we weren't walking. We propped Honey Bunny and Brown Bear on the dashboard and took off across the Pyrenees into Spain.

After exploring architectural gems on the Camino, we headed off to Haro, a town famous for its wineries and Beethoven's Restaurant. I had eaten there in 1981 and hoped it was still there. Although I didn't think Haro was on the Camino, we had decided to make an exception for nostalgia's sake. After settling into our hotel, a monastery that had been transformed into elegant tourist lodging, we went for a stroll around the town.

While looking at a window display I noticed a book entitled *El Camino de Santiago en su paso por La Rioja*. I went inside the store and paged through the book: Haro is on the Camino! The Camino is always with us.

We ate lunch at Beethoven II, a spin-off from the original; the garlic-scented roast lamb was just as good as I remembered. We spent the rest of the day relaxing in our hotel room, a former monastic cell with thick stone walls and the faint resonance of prayers.

At dinner in the hotel's restaurant, eight Americans on a bicycle tour regaled us with their adventures. They were biking part of the Camino, staying in upscale hotels and drinking lots of the local Rioja wine. When I inquired about the Camino as a pilgrimage, they looked puzzled. Pilgrimage? For them the Camino was simply an interesting route replete with excellent accommodations and fine dining.

Five days had passed since we had quit walking the Chemin. My blisters still had not healed, nor had my energy-sapping malaise disappeared. I wanted this pilgrimage of gratitude to be over so I could get on with my life, but events had conspired so that I couldn't.

I reminded myself that this *is* my life, the whole messy catastrophe—and it was pointless to wait for something to be over so I could get on with living. I tried to tell myself that everything was perfect, if I would just realize it—but everything wasn't perfect at all. It was a disaster. All our plans, all our intentions were coming to nothing. I urged myself to let go of expectations and then I berated myself because I couldn't.

At last I took responsibility for my feelings. I remembered that I was the one making meaning out of events—and I was choosing to view our situation as frustrating and unsatisfactory, rather than as an opportunity to enjoy Spanish Camino sites that I had long wanted to visit.

A Hawaiian kahuna once pointed out, "The truth isn't that 'it's a beautiful day'; the truth is that 'it's a day.'" Lovely or disastrous, irritating or delightful, we are the ones who choose how we experience the day.

The Spanish poet Antonio Machado said much the same thing in a poem that pilgrims often quote:

> Caminante, son tus huellas
> el camino y nada más;
> caminante, no hay camino,
> se hace camino al andar.
> (Walker, your footprints are the path
> and nothing more;
> Walker, there is no path,
> It is made by walking.)

With a grateful sigh, I realized I was being given the opportunity to learn more lessons on the Camino, lessons that would serve me well during my ongoing pilgrimage through cancer. I was the one making meaning of the events in my life.

Saturday, September 25, 2004. Haro.

At 3:00 a.m. an epiphany woke me up from a sound sleep. Of *course* I couldn't finish my pilgrimage of gratitude. You can never finish a pilgrimage of gratitude! What had I been thinking? That we'd reach the Pyrenees and I could wipe my brow, take off my hiking boots, and say, "Whew, glad that's over. Now, on with my life"? Suddenly I understood. A pilgrimage of gratitude is a life-long journey, not a destination. It is a way of living, not a one-time hike.

I hadn't understood that, the previous year when I had been forced to stop walking at Navarrenx. And I hadn't understood it this year either, even though I had had to stop walking at the same place. I could almost hear Santiago chuckling as he said, "I tried to help you out, but you're a slow learner, aren't you?"

I rolled over in bed and shook Gary until he woke up. He looked at me blearily.

"What's wrong?"

"Nothing's wrong! I finally understand what's been going on! I've learned the lesson. You can never finish a pilgrimage of gratitude. There's no end to it. It will continue for the rest of my life."

With a big smile, Gary nodded. He understood. He hugged me, and we laughed and wept in each other's arms.

As I lay in bed snuggling with Gary, I looked to the future with open-hearted curiosity. The pilgrimage we had already made had been filled with unforeseen difficulties and unexpected delights, with pain and pleasure, with challenges and opportunities. Just like life. Just like having cancer. I couldn't control what happened to me, but I could decide how I would respond: with hope, enthusiasm, and gratitude.

EPILOGUE

When we returned from France I put away my travel journals and the manuscript I had begun in 2002. I didn't want to keep thinking about cancer. That didn't mean that my pilgrimage of gratitude was forgotten; how could it be? I felt grateful every day, and I tried to remember the lessons I had learned on the Chemin. Breaking old patterns takes time and vigilance—and practice—but I knew the pilgrimage had changed me forever.

According to my surgeon, five years without metastasis would mean that I had passed the "magic milestone" and was no longer at any higher risk for cancer than the rest of the population. When that date arrived in June 2007, I told Gary that I should be in a *less*-at-risk population group since I'd already had cancer. But statistics don't work that way. I am thankful to be alive and to be cancer-free—at least for now, as far as I know.

Honey Bunny and Brown Bear have become more enlivened as the years pass. Not only are they ongoing reminders of the importance of synchronicity and playfulness in our lives, but their conversations have also taken on greater depth.

At one point, Honey Bunny was horrified to discover she wasn't alive. We were able to reassure her that she is real, though not alive, a situation that has many advantages: she doesn't need to eat or find a bathroom; she doesn't get sick; and she will never die. Brown Bear has discovered that when Honey Bunny gets too wound up, he can lean over and whisper, "Now Princess...." in her ear and she will calm down immediately. After extensive nagging, they convinced us to give them their own blog.

Are they our alter egos? Not exactly. I am not, nor do I aspire to be, the flighty material girl that Honey Bunny personifies; nor is Gary the stoic, contemplative being that Brown Bear embodies. Besides, they have frequently surprised us with their wise observations—much wiser than anything we could come up with.

They have acquired extensive wardrobes, for the most part given to them by our friends who have become their friends—though sometimes their friends have become ours. They have hand-knit scarves and sweaters, hand-embroidered vests (Honey Bunny's has a tiny cell phone attached), crocheted ponchos, and assorted jewelry, including a gold Saint Christopher's medal (the saint of travelers) given to Brown Bear by Foxy, our dental technician. She knew that the "fuzzy kids" travel with us on our journeys and she wanted us to have a little extra protection.

Several of our friends have disclosed that they, too, have "fuzzy kids"—some with names, some without. They seemed almost relieved to discover that they are not alone in this eccentricity. Sometimes we have fantasized about a coming-out party where all the "fuzzy kids" could meet—but that would require bringing them together from all over Europe and the US. In the meantime, Honey Bunny and Brown Bear's blog will have to do.

It had been six years since I heard the call of the Chemin. I went on pilgrimage, following a sacred way. I experienced both successes and tribulations—normal parts of any pilgrimage. And I persevered. Then I returned home, forever changed by the experience. It was time to give something back, to share what I had learned.

I took out my notes and re-read what I had written. I decided the manuscript was worth completing because I hoped my experience walking through cancer could be helpful to others. I had learned that cancer wasn't the enemy—it was an opportunity, however unexpected, however unwelcome. What matters is not what we experience in life but rather the meaning and significance we give to it.

A few months after I began reworking the manuscript, Gary and I went to a dinner party. Our hostess suggested that I tell the other guests about my writing project. She added that the woman sitting next to me had also had cancer and walked the Camino.

After I talked briefly, the woman turned to me and asked, "What kind of cancer did you have?"

I replied, "Uterine cancer."

Dismissively, she said, "Oh, that's the *easy* kind!"

I was taken aback. Easy? I hadn't thought so. After all, it could have been fatal. Then I realized that she was partially correct: although the cancer diagnosis and subsequent uncertainty were not easy, the treatment was. And for that I am grateful.

Regardless of what kind of cancer I had, or what kind of treatment I underwent, I will always stand on the other side of an unbridgeable divide, the abyss between those who have had cancer and those who have not. There is no going back. But there is going forward in gratitude for the rest of my life, however long or short that may turn out to be. And that is as good as it gets.

Resources

I. Pilgrimage Resources

Websites

Numerous websites are devoted to the Caminos in Spain (the Camino del Norte, Camino Francés, Vía de de Plata, etc.) and the Chemins in France. The American Pilgrims on the Camino (**http://www.americanpilgrims.com/**) holds annual gatherings in the US and provides support and training for pilgrims and volunteer *hospitaleros*. The website contains excellent resources and links. The Confraternity of Saint James (**http://www.csj.org.uk/**) is a British association with an extensive website and online bookstore; CSJ also organizes walks and conferences. The Société Française des Amis de Saint-Jacques de Compostelle, founded in 1950, conducts extensive research on the Chemin, promotes the pilgrimage, and provides assistance for pilgrims: **http://compostelle.asso.fr/**.

The following website provides specific information on the Chemin de Saint-Jacques: **http://www.chemindecompostelle.com/**

In addition, numerous list-serves provide ongoing interactive support for pilgrims. Several popular list-serves include Santiagobis on Yahoo and GoCamino. Also check out **http://www.pilgrimage-to-santiago.com/**. An excellent blog by a pilgrim and *hospitalera* is Rebekah Scott's **http://moratinoslife.blogspot.com**. Another worthwhile blog is **http://honeybunnyandbrownbear.blogspot.com**.

Books on the Camino/Chemin mentioned in the text (NB: There is a plethora of books on the pilgrimage roads; additional resources can also be found by googling the Way of Saint James, Chemin de Saint Jacques, and Camino de Santiago):

Elyn Aviva. *Following the Milky Way: A Pilgrimage on the Camino de Santiago*, 2nd edition. Pilgrims' Process, Inc., 2001. The first contemporary account by an American walking the Camino de Santiago, first published in 1989 by ISU Press. The second edition includes a new introduction describing the Camino twenty years later.

Jacques and Lauriane Clouteau. *Miam Miam Dodo: GR65, la Voie du Puy 2009*. Editions du Vieux Crayon, 2009. Available from the Confraternity of St. James bookstore: http://www.csj.org.uk/.

Paulo Coelho. *The Pilgrimage*. Harper Perennial, 1998.

Hannah Green. *The Little Saint*. Random House, 2000.

Alison Raju. *Way of Saint James: Le Puy to the Pyrenees - A Walkers' Guide*. Cicerone Press, 2003.

Sentier de Saint-Jacques-de-Compostelle - Le Chemin du Puy - GR 65. A three-volume set in French with informative text and IGN maps on facing pages. Part of the FFRP's *Topo-Guides des Sentiers de Grande-Randonée* series. Note: be sure to obtain the latest edition. Available from the Confraternity of St. James bookstore.

Annie Shaver-Crandell and Paula Gerson. *The Pilgrim's Guide to Santiago de Compostela - A Gazetteer with 580 Illustrations*. Harvey Miller Publishers, 1995.

Miscellaneous books drawn on for this text:

William Anderson. *Green Man: The Archetype of our Oneness with the Earth*. HarperCollins, 1990.

Philip Ball. *Universe of Stone - A Biography of Chartres Cathedral*. HarperCollins Publishers, 2008.

Ean Begg. *The Cult of the Black Virgin*. Chiron Publications, 2006. (Includes extensive gazetteer)

Jean Shinoda Bolen. *Crossing to Avalon: A Woman's Midlife Quest for the Sacred Feminine*. HarperOne, 1995.

Jon Burke and Kaj Halberg. *Seed of Knowledge, Stone of Plenty: Understanding the Lost Technology of the Ancient Megalith-Builders*. Council Oaks Books, 2005.

Simon Coleman & John Elsner. *Pilgrimage Past and Present in World Religions*. Harvard University Press, 1995.

Paul Cousineau: *The Art of Pilgrimage: The Seeker's Guide to Making Travel Sacred*. Conari Press, 2000.

Paul Devereux. *Places of Power: Measuring the Secret Energy of Ancient Sites.* 2nd edition. Blandford, 1999.

——————. *The Sacred Place: The Ancient Origin of Holy and Mystical Sites.* Cassell, 2001.

Barbara Freitag. *Sheela-na-gigs: Unravelling an Enigma.* Routledge, 2004.

China Galland. *Longing for Darkness: Tara and the Black Madonna.* Viking, 1990.

Robert Hodum. *Reflections on Spain's Saint James and His Way.* Seaburn Books, 2005.

Roger Housden. *Sacred Journeys in a Modern World.* Simon & Schuster Editions, 1998.

Georgiana Goddard King, *The Way of Saint James, Volumes I – III.* Pilgrims Process, Inc., 2008. (Completed in 1917, this three-volume masterpiece is a wide-ranging exploration of the history, literature, legends, and architecture of the Camino de Santiago.)

Robert Lawlor. *Sacred Geometry: Philosophy and Practice.* Thames & Hudson, 1989.

Sig Lonegren. *Labyrinths: Ancient Myths & Modern Uses.* Revised edition. Sterling, 2001.

Miranda Lundy. *Sacred Geometry.* Walker & Company, 2001.

John Matthews. *The Green Man: Spirit of Nature.* Red Wheel/ Weiser; Book and Access Edition, 2002.

Joanne McMahon (Author) and Jack Roberts. *Sheela-na-Gigs of Ireland and Britain: The Divine Hag of the Christian Celts - An Illustrated Guide.* Mercier Press, 2001.

Blanche Merz. *Points of Cosmic Energy.* Essex: C. W. Daniel Company Ltd, 1995. Distributed by www.beekman.net.

John Michell. *The New View over Atlantis.* Thames & Hudson, 2001.

Nigel Pennick. *Sacred Geometry: Symbolism and Purpose in Religious Structures*. Capall Bann Publ., 2001.

Mark Pogacnik. *Sacred Geography: Geomancy: Co-Creating the Earth Cosmos*. Lindisfarne Books, 2007.

Michael S. Schneider. *A Beginner's Guide to Constructing the Universe: Mathematical Archetypes of Nature, Art, and Science*. HarperPerennial, 1995.

Gordon Strachan. *Chartres: Sacred Geometry, Sacred Space*. Floris Books, 2003.

Henri Vincenot, *The Prophet of Compostela*. Vermont: Inner Traditions International, 1996.

Tim Wallace-Murphy. *Cracking the Symbol Code*. London: Watkins Publishing, 2005.

Tim Wallace-Murphy and Marilyn Hopkins. *Rosslyn: Guardian of the Secrets of the Holy Grail*. Element Books, 1999. (An unusual take on the Camino that claims it starts in Santiago and goes backwards through France to Scotland.)

Marina Warner. *Alone of All Her Sex: The Myth and the Cult of the Virgin Mary*. Vintage, 1983.

II. Cancer Resources:

Websites:

American Cancer Society: **http://www.cancer.org/**

Caring4Cancer: **www.caring4cancer.com**

Center for Disease Control Cancer Prevention and Control: **www.cdc.gov/cancer**

National Cancer Institute Cancer Information Service: **http://cis.nci.nih.gov**

Alternative Medicine: **www.alternativemedicine.com**

The Cancer Project: **www.cancerproject.org**

Healthweb: Alternative Medicine: **www.healthweb.org/alternative**

M. D. Anderson Cancer Center Complementary/Integrative Medicine Education Resources: **www.mdanderson.org/departments/CIMER**

WholeHealthMD: **www.wholehealthmd.com**

Books:

Jeremy Geffen, MD. *The Journey Through Cancer: Healing and Transforming the Whole Person.* Three Rivers Press, 2006. Extensive appendices filled with resources, including books, numerous websites, music, and much more.

Jimmie Holland and Sheldon Lewis. *The Human Side of Cancer: Living with Hope, Coping with Uncertainty.* Harper, 2001.

Julie K. Silver, MD. *After Cancer Treatment: Heal Faster, Better, Stronger.* The Johns Hopkins University Press, 2006.

Puja, A. J. Thomson. *AFTER SHOCK: From Cancer Diagnosis to Healing - A step-by-step guide to help you navigate your way.* ROOTS & WINGS, 2006.

GLOSSARY

(A somewhat idiosyncratic selection of words and phrases, marked with a † in the text)

albergue A Spanish hostel; some are specifically for pilgrims. Not to be confused with the French *auberge,* which is a restaurant, inn, or lodge, sometimes quite luxurious.

Año Santo or *Año Santo Compostelan*a A Compostelan Holy Year is declared whenever Saint James's feast day, July 25, falls on a Sunday (every 6-11-6-5 years). The next two are 2010 and 2021. Catholic pilgrims can earn a plenary indulgence† if they go to Santiago de Compostela during the Holy Year and perform certain rites. Millions of pilgrims travel to Santiago during an *Año Santo.*

AOC (Appellation d'Origine Contrôlée) Government certification that a product comes from a particular region and conforms to certain standards.

archivolt Curved carving on the arch over a doorway. A church's main portal may have a series of archivolts, each one framing the next.

aromatherapy Use of fragrances (e.g., essential oils) for therapeutic purposes. Lavender is relaxing; frankincense relieves depression and anxiety. There is recreational aromatherapy as well as medical aromatherapy.

basilica Originally a "hall of kings"—a stately hall with a particular quadrilateral shape. More generally, public buildings of ancient Rome with a central nave with an apse at one or both ends and two side aisles, used as an assembly hall. A Christian church of similar design.

bastide Carefully planned towns built in France by the French and English during the Hundred Years' War (1337 – 1453). Based on a grid with a central market square and fortified perimeters. Some have survived and form a modern bastide tourism circuit.

boulangerie Bakery, specializing in bread and rolls.

buron Stone house that shelters shepherds and their flocks in summer.

cabécou A small, soft, raw-goat's-milk cheese from the Midi-Pyrénées region of southern France. Means "Little Goat" in Occitane. Said to have originated with the Moors who brought goats to the region in the eighth century. Received AOC† in 1996.

Camino de Santiago The Way of Saint James across Spain. 1000-year-old, 500-mile-long pilgrimage route from the Pyrenees to Santiago de Compostela in northwestern Spain. Also known as the Camino Francés because of its popularity with French pilgrims. The four French routes join together and become the Camino in Spain. In 1987 it became the first European Cultural Itinerary.

canon Christian priest who lives with others in a clergy house near a church and follows rules and regulations of a particular church chapter; priest who is a member of a certain body of the Christian clergy and subject to an ecclesiastical rule.

capital In architecture, the crowning member of a pillar, column, or pier. From Latin *capitellum*, diminutive of Latin *caput*, head. Has a spreading contour fitting its function as the weight-bearing member beneath the lintel or arch supported by its shaft. Often elaborately carved.

cathedral A church with a bishop. "Cathedra" means chair and refers to where the bishop sits. Cathedrals are often large, impressive, and beautiful.

causse(s) Ancient eroding limestone plateau(s), found in the Massif Central†. The *causses* average 700 – 1200 meters (2300 – 4000 feet) high.

CE Common Era (the preferred, contemporary substitute for AD).

cépes Latin name, *boletus edulis,* means "superior mushroom"; most common name for this meaty mushroom is porcini.

chambres d'hôtes French equivalent to a guesthouse or B&B (bed and breakfast) establishment, often located in rural villages, with a garden or scenic surroundings. The owner is personally responsible for guests. Select *chambres d'hôtes* are members of the Gîtes de France organization and ranked from one to four *épis* or wheat heads.

chambres et table d'hôtes French B&B with dinner available by reservation for guests.

charcuterie Sausages, ham, pâtés, and other cooked or processed meat foods; a delicatessen specializing in such foods.

Chemins de Saint-Jacques de Compostelle The four French pilgrimage routes to Saint-Jacques de Compostelle (Santiago de Compostela) that become the Camino de Santiago† in Spain. (Not to be confused with the Camino Francés, which is another name for the Camino de Santiago—the most popular of numerous Spanish routes that lead to Santiago de Compostela.) The four routes begin in Paris, Vezelay, Le Puy, and Arles. The first three join at Ostabat, near Saint-Jean-Pied-de-Port, and then cross over the Pyrenees. The fourth route, from Arles, crosses the Pyrenees at Somport Pass and joins the Camino de Santiago at Puente la Reina in Spain.

cloisters An interior, quadrilateral, covered walkway with open colonnades on one side and a wall on the other. Faces a quadrangle, often with a garden in the center. Found in many medieval monasteries or extending out from one side of a cathedral or church.

confit (1) meat, such as duck or goose, that has been salted, cooked, and preserved in its own fat (also known as "potted" meat); (2) a condiment made by cooking seasoned fruit or vegetables, usually to a jamlike consistency. Not to be confused with *confiture.*

confiture Jams and preserves.

conversos Medieval (or later) Spanish Jews who converted to Christianity, either willingly or under duress. Often regarded with distrust because of fear that their conversion was inauthentic and that they continued to practice Judaism in secret—even when that was not the case.

demi-pension "Half-board." Lodging-and-meal rate that includes room, breakfast, and dinner (as opposed to *pension complete*, which also includes lunch). The *menu†* is selected by the innkeeper and is usually more limited than the regular menu.

département Administrative division roughly analogous to a United States county. France has 100 *départments*, grouped into 22 metropolitan and four overseas regions, further subdivided into 342 *arrondissements*.

dolmens Approximately 5,000 – 6,000-year-old megalithic ("large stone") monuments constructed with two or more upright stones supporting a horizontal stone slab or capstone. Often thought to have been tombs, it is likely that they served other purposes as well or instead. Originally covered with earth, what remains millennia later is a bare, table-like stone structure. They occur from the Baltic and North Sea coasts south to Spain and Portugal.

épicerie Small French grocery that carries dairy products and cold meats.

European Union (EU) An economic and political union of at least 27 member states, located primarily in Europe.

FFRP Fédération Française de la Randonnée Pédestre (literally, French Federation of Pedestrian Excursion Trails). In charge of the GR's†; publishes guidebooks and maps.

fleur-de-lys or **fleur-de-lis** Device consisting of a stylized three-petaled iris or lily, used as the heraldic armorial emblem of the kings of France and in artistic designs. Old French for "flower of the lily."

fromage Cheese. Charles de Gaulle, one-time president of France, once commented: "How can anyone rule a country that has 246 varieties of cheese?" In 2008 France produced more than 1,000 varieties of cheese and was the world's largest cheese exporter.

furta sacra "Sacred theft." Refers to the medieval belief that relics of saints could be stolen and taken to another religious setting only if the saint (whose relics they were) agreed to the move. A novel excuse that justified stealing Sainte Foy's relics from Agen and bringing them to Conques.

Gaia Pre-Olympian Greek earth goddess, worshipped as Mother of All. Although not the first to propose it, James E. Lovelock popularized the modern Gaia hypothesis of the earth as a living organism. His books propose a dynamic interaction between life and environment, with earth regulating life, and life regulating earth, virtually a single self-regulating entity.

gite In the most general sense, a simple, inexpensive, rural vacation retreat in France. Those that are part of the Association des Gîtes de France are ranked with from one to four *épis* (wheat heads).

gîte à la ferme Hikers' hostel in a farm; may rent sheets and towels.

gîte d'étape Provides lodging for hikers (in preference to motorists), often has large or small dormitories; may have private rooms. May provide cooking and laundry facilities; may rent sheets and towels. May provide breakfast.

gîte d'étape privé Privately run hikers' hostel.

Grande Randonnée 65 (GR 65) Well-marked long-distance hiking trail (*grande randonnée*) from Le Puy-en-Velay to the Pyrenees. Closely follows the Chemin de St-Jacques. The number indicates the particular trail (e.g., GR 10 runs along the Pyrenees). Part of the network established by the FFRP†.

GR 651 Northern variant of the GR 65; goes along the Célé river valley.

Green Man Popular vegetal image in medieval and Renaissance European art, often portrayed as a face with tendrils and leaves coming out of its mouth. Occasionally takes the form of a Green Woman. Carved in stone capitals of churches; also carved in wood on church choir seats. Thought to represent the vital life-force of green and growing things; perhaps a carry-over from pagan imagery. Popular today as garden décor and furniture decoration.

halle Covered market.

Hundred Years' War Sporadic conflict (1337 - 1453) between the English and the eventually successful French. French House of Valois was pitted against the English House of Plantagenet, which claimed both France and England.

infusion Herbal tea; hot water is infused with herbs.

liminality Comes from *limen* or threshold. Refers to the special qualities of sacred space and time—a time "in-between," outside of normal daily life. A fluid time filled with possibilities for transformation (e.g., a bride steps over the threshold to enter married life; Mardi Gras occurs at the beginning of Lent and is a time of role reversal, masquerade, and license). Pilgrims, especially if their pilgrimage takes a long time, have the opportunity of leaving behind their usual status and roles for an extended period, thus opening themselves to significant personal change.

livre d'Or Visitors' book or guestbook. Found along the Chemin and sometimes in guesthouses.

Maronite Lebanese Syriac Eastern Orthodox church that dates back to
the fifth century. Maronites share the same doctrine as other
Catholics but retain their own liturgy, theology, spirituality, discipline, and hierarchy. Saint Charbel (born Youssef
Antoun Makhlouf in 1828 in north Lebanon) became a
Maronite priest and took the name of Charbel, a second-
century Antiochan church martyr. After Charbel's death in
1898, many healing miracles were attributed to his relics. He
is buried at Saint Maron's Monastery in Annaya.

Massif Central Mountainous plateau of south-central France that includes
the Cévennes and Auvergne mountains; covers one-sixth
of France. Average height, 300 meters (1000 feet); highest
point, 1886 meters (6188 feet).

menu See *table d'hôte menu†*.

nave Central part of a church, extending from the entrance to the transept†
or the area around the altar. Traditionally runs east to west.

patisserie A bakery specializing in fancy French pastries.

pilgrimage credential Official document provided by the Pilgrims' Office of the Cathedral of Santiago de Compostela; different
pilgrims' associations issue approved variants. It is not an
international passport. By getting this small, folded document stamped at least daily along the way, pilgrims may gain
access to inexpensive pilgrimage *refugios†* and *albergues†* in
Spain. If they have walked the entire last 100 kilometers to
Santiago, as demonstrated by the stamps on their credentials, they can receive a *Compostelana* (sometimes called a
Compostela, just to make things confusing) pilgrimage certif-
icate in Santiago de Compostela at the Oficina de Acogida
de Peregrinos (Pilgrims' Office, Rúa do Vilar 1). The *Compostelana* is modeled after medieval pilgrimage certificates.
The credential makes a great memento.

plenary indulgence In Roman Catholic usage, remission before God of all one's temporal punishment for one's sins committed up to the time one receives the plenary indulgence. Confession obtains forgiveness, but punishment is still due (either in this life or in purgatory) unless remission is received. Available to pilgrims who go to Santiago de Compostela during an *Año Santo†* and perform certain rites. It is retroactive but not anticipatory. Also available at select other pilgrimage shrines (e.g., Rome, Le Puy) at specific times. If you want a more detailed explanation, ask a priest.

priory A house of men or women under religious vows, headed by a prior or prioress. Priories may be houses of mendicant friars or religious sisters (e.g., Dominicans or Augustinians), or monasteries of monks or nuns (e.g., Carthusians). Originally Catholic institutions; however, the Taizé Community in southwestern France is an ecumenical priory.

randonnée French term for excursion, hike, or walk.

refugios Inexpensive Spanish pilgrimage hostels, privately run or run by pilgrimage support groups. Often have large dormitories with bunk beds; may have smaller rooms, kitchens, and laundry facilities. Usually request a small donation.

relais Originally a post-house where horses were exchanged and mail collected; now, another name for an inn or restaurant. Range from simple to luxurious accommodations (as in the exclusive Relais & Chateaux association).

rillettes Minced, well-seasoned meat spread, similar to pâté. Originally pork, may also be made from goose, duck, chicken, game birds, rabbit, and sometimes from fish such as anchovies, tuna or salmon.

Saint James the Greater First martyred apostle; patron of Spain. Known as Santiago† in Spain.

sandre Perch-like fish.

Santiago (1) Saint James the Greater, the first martyred apostle, the religious patron of Spain; (2) Informal way to refer to Santiago de Compostela, the location in northwestern Spain where Santiago is supposedly buried.

Sheela-na-Gig From the Irish *Sile na gcíoch,* "Julia of the breasts." Figurative carving of a naked woman (often emaciated in appearance) squatting with knees apart, one or both hands holding open her large vulva. Sheelas are found carved on Irish, British, and continental European churches built before the sixteenth century; some still remain (especially in Ireland), though most have been destroyed. The Sheela's true origin is unknown and her meaning controversial. Some scholars think she is an ancient good-luck or apotropaic (ward-off-evil) symbol; others suggest she represents fertility; others propose that her off-putting appearance was the Church's effort to discourage lust.

solsticial quadrilateral Rectangle or square whose dimensions are based on measurements of the solstices and equinoxes at a particular latitude.

table d'hôte menu or *menu* (similar to Spanish *menú*) Not to be confused with the American "menu," which is similar to *à la carte.* In France, an all-inclusive, multi-course meal usually offered at several different prices, each with preset choices selected by the chef. The least expensive includes three courses (soup or salad, meat or fish, dessert, and wine); the more expensive menu includes an extra course, more elaborate preparations, and perhaps more choices. The *menu* contrasts with *à la carte,* in which one selects whatever one wants to eat. The Spanish *menú del día* (like the French *plat du jour)* is usually a relatively inexpensive, three-course meal that provides better value than selecting *à la carte.* Restaurants on the Camino de Santiago frequently offer a low-priced *menú del peregrino* (pilgrim's menu) for verified pilgrims (see pilgrimage credential†).

topo-guide FFRP guidebook with topographic maps of the Chemin.

traiteur Caterer.

transept Architectural term. In a cross-shaped (cruciform) Romanesque or Gothic church, the transept is set crosswise to the nave† (the long, central corridor that usually runs east-west) and separates it from the sanctuary.

transhumance Annual seasonal migration of livestock and their caretakers from one part of the region to another (from mountain to valley and back). The Aubrac transhumance festival is in late May.

trumeau A central pier between double entry doors or sections of a door; helps support the tympanum† of a wide doorway.

tympanum Located in the area above the lintel over main entrance(s) to a church, the tympanum is framed by an arch above it. Often filled with elaborate carvings that present important religious themes.

Via Lactea "The Milky Way"—another way of referring to the Way of Saint James and the Camino de Santiago†. "There were as many pilgrims on the Camino as stars in the Milky Way," according to one medieval source.

Via Podiensis The Way of Le Puy: the Chemin de Saint-Jacques de Compostelle† that starts in Le Puy-en-Velay and stretches 460 miles in a southwesterly direction toward Saint-Jean-Pied-de-Port, at the foot of the Pyrenees. It joins the routes from Tours and Vezelay at Ostabat, just north of Saint-Jean-Pied-de-Port.

Wars of Religion Long, bloody struggle (1562 – 1598) between French Catholics and Protestants (Huguenots). A struggle between the House of Bourbon and the House of Guise (Lorraine) allied with the Catholic League; at the same time, a war by proxy between King Philip II of Spain and Queen Elizabeth I of England. Ended with the Edict of Nantes issued by Henry IV of France, which granted a degree of religious toleration to Protestants.

Index

Printed in the United States
212284BV00001B/3/P

9 780979 090981